PERENNIAL
PSYCHOLOGY
OF THE
BHAGAVAD GITA

PERENNIAL
PSYCHOLOGY
OF THE
BHAGAVAD GITA

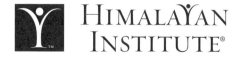
HIMALAYAN
INSTITUTE®

HONESDALE, PENNSYLVANIA USA

Himalayan Institute, Honesdale, PA 18431
HimalayanInstitute.org

Printed in the United States of America

23 22 21 20 19 18 17 16 15   9 10 11 12 13

ISBN-13: 978-0-89389-090-2

The paper used in this publication meets the minimum requirements of American National Standard for Information Sciences—Permanence of Paper for Printed Library Materials, ANSI Z39.48-1984.

Library of Congress Cataloging-in-Publication Data:

Rama, Swami, 1925-1996
        Perennial Psychology of the Bhagavad Gita.
            1. Bhagavadgita—Commentaries. 2. Bhagavadgita—
            Psychology.
            1. Bhagavadgita. English. 1984.
            II. Titles
            BL1138.66.R36 1984   294.5'924 84-25137

∞ This paper meets the requirements of ANSI/NISO Z39-48-1992
                    (Permanence of Paper).

Contents

Acknowledgments

The completion of this work would not have been possible without the generous and untiring assistance of Carol Kingsbury, who spent long hours typing; Aparna Bharati and Dr. Arpita, who assisted with the editing; and Anne Morrow, who managed our household in India while we worked on the commentary. Pandit Usharbudh Arya provided the translation of the Sanskrit text. The cover photograph was taken by Carol Kingsbury.

Swami Ajaya, a practicing clinical psychologist, acted as consultant throughout the writing of the book, and his input served to enhance the final product.

Introduction

The Bhagavad Gita is the fountainhead of Eastern psychology, and this commentary is designed to draw out its psychological concepts and make them accessible to all students. These profound psychological insights are intertwined in the Bhagavad Gita with philosophical concepts, so the task undertaken here is to separate the psychological principles and to explain their practical application.

Self-realization is the goal of human life. The purpose of Eastern religion, philosophy, and psychology is to fulfill that goal. Philosophy as it is understood in the East is neither a mere speculative exercise nor an intellectual adventure. The word "philosophy" is a compound of two words: *philo* and *sophia,* which mean "love for knowledge." But this term is not applicable in the East, for those who consider the prime questions of life such as: Who am I? From where have I come? Why have I come? and Where will I go? are not interested in only the intellectual answers to these questions. The subject matter of Eastern philosophy leads the student through a systematic way of directly experiencing the truths of existence and the height of Self-realization. After realizing one's real Self, one knows that this Self is the Self of all.

In the Vedantic tradition the term *Brahma Vidya**is used instead of the term philosophy. It has a different connotation and a deeper meaning than the word philosophy conveys, and it is unique in its approach to knowledge. Brahma Vidya means the knowledge that leads one to realize *Brahman,* the Self of all. The Bhagavad Gita conveys that wisdom in its entirety and teaches the practical methods for the study and transformation of one's inner being. Philosophy and psychology are thus intermingled. Without the help of psychology—knowing, analyzing,

*Sanskrit terms that are defined in the Glossary are italicized upon first mention in the text.

and learning to use our inner potentials—we cannot fulfill the goal of human life: Self-realization.

In contrast. Western philosophy is intellectual and deals with man's relationship with the universe. With the knowledge he gains, he tries to understand his status in the universe. In Brahma Vidya, however, one comes to know all the levels of his being and finally to realize his true Self. According to the Eastern system, knowing the real Self is the first and foremost purpose of life. After Self-realization all the mysteries of the universe and one's relationship with the universe are revealed. Because of their contrasting approaches, there is a wide gulf between philosophy and Brahma Vidya. One is only theoretical, but the other is practical as well.

Though the Bhagavad Gita is composed of only seven hundred verses, it contains all the principles of the philosophy and psychology of the East. There are eighteen lessons in the Bhagavad Gita, each describing a different aspect of the process of self-transformation. This commentary emphasizes the psychological principles found in each chapter of the Bhagavad Gita. The *sadhana* (spiritual practice) described in each section is explained so that aspirants can help themselves progress in the inward journey and attain the highest state of bliss. The aim of the Bhagavad Gita is to teach the aspirant how to establish equanimity both in his internal life and in his activities in the external world; to help him develop tranquility within, and to explain the art and science of doing actions skillfully and selflessly.

The teachings of the Bhagavad Gita help one to understand the distinction between the real Self and the mere self. The mere self is subject to change and destruction; the real Self is not. The aspirant should understand both and should finally establish himself in his essential nature: Atman. Then he can live in the world without being affected by it. In the domain between the real Self and the mere self lies our *antahkarana* (internal instrument), which plays a most important part in both our internal and external life. If not understood, both goals of life—living in the world and Self-realization—are defeated. Our psychological life needs profound and deep study if we are to free ourselves from the quagmire of emotionality, egotistical preoccupations, and self-delusion and if we are to realize our fullest potentials for the unfoldment of consciousness. The perennial psychology of the Bhagavad Gita deals with analyzing and training the internal processes of the human being so that one becomes creative in the external world and attains a state of tranquility at the same time. That which needs detailed analysis, understanding, and unfoldment is the mental life, which is vast in its characteristics. The outside world can be mastered only when the inner potentials are systematically explored and organized. Without understanding one's inner potentials, it is not possible to function effectively and harmoniously in the external world, for all things happen within before they are expressed externally.

The wise man knows the distinction between the real Self and the mere self, but he still does sadhana so that barriers are not created for either. Sadhana is for the inner level that creates delusion or mirage; it is not Atman or the external world that creates confusion but one's mental life. The internal and the external are two inseparable aspects of one single life. Practice or sadhana should be modeled in such a way that it does not lead the aspirant from one extreme to another. Some aspirants think that retiring from the world will help them attain the purpose of life. Others believe that doing actions and performing their duties in the world will fulfill the purpose of life. It is the moderate path, however, that creates a bridge between these two extremes and that is the most useful for the general public. This commentary is neither written specifically for the renunciate nor for those who are scratching the surface of the mundane world for the sake of their self-existence, without understanding that if the world is meant for them, they are also meant for the world. If one is to live life happily, he needs to be aware that others are also striving to attain happiness. Consideration for others is a primary requisite for finding happiness and building a good society.

One may wonder why the Bhagavad Gita came into existence when we already had such scriptures as the *Vedas* and *Upanishads*. The great Vedantic sage *Shankara* explained, "The Vedic *dharma* was practiced over a long time. But eventually discrimination and wisdom declined. Unrighteousness became more predominant than righteousness." * The

*From Shankara's introduction to the Bhagavad Gita.

Vedas are the source of all streams of Indian philosophy and psychology, and the Upanishads are the later parts of the Vedas. With the decline of discrimination and wisdom, it became difficult for those who were not scholars to understand the teachings of the Vedas and Upanishads. So it was necessary to restate these teachings in a way that could be appreciated and assimilated by all.

The Bhagavad Gita contains in condensed form all the philosophical and psychological wisdom of the Upanishads. It is said that the Upanishads are like a cow that Sri Krishna milks to bestow its nurturing wisdom to his dear friend and disciple, Arjuna. Sri Krishna imparts all the wisdom of the Vedic and Upanishadic literature through the teachings of the Bhagavad Gita. Rather than imparting a new trend of thought or expounding a new philosophy, Sri Krishna modified and simplified the Vedic and Upanishadic knowledge. He speaks to humanity through his dialogue with Arjuna. The word *Arjuna* means "one who makes sincere efforts," and the word *Krishna* means "the center of consciousness." One who makes sincere efforts inevitably obtains the knowledge that directly flows from the center of consciousness.

The unique dialogue between Sri Krishna and Arjuna deals with all aspects of life. It is useful for modern therapists, psychologists, and philosophers to study the Bhagavad Gita in order to understand the way Sri Krishna counsels Arjuna. Arjuna, like many patients who seek therapy, is in a state of despair and feels unable to cope with the situation before him, so he seeks Sri Krishna's advice and guidance. But there are major differences in the way Sri Krishna treats Arjuna and the approaches used by psychotherapists today. Modern psychotherapists attempt to help the client modify his conscious attitudes and unconscious processes and behaviors, but their analysis lacks the depth and profundity found in the Bhagavad Gita. Most modern therapists do not explore the purpose and meaning of life. They are loath to discuss and give advice on basic philosophical issues such as activism verses pacifism, one's duty in life, and the nature of life and death. They limit the depth and range of counseling and focus primarily on bringing out the patient's complex. Most modern psychologists do not go to the root of the problem but analyze it without understanding the fundamental cause. They deal with specific problems and symptoms, and the untouched cause then expresses its agony in different ways. They work in this way because of lack of time and fear of becoming involved with the unknown.

By contrast, Sri Krishna presents a philosophical foundation for understanding the purpose of life and the way to live harmoniously, and he offers Arjuna practical advice on living and on coping with the world. In Eastern psychology the teacher helps the student plan a self-training program and observes all the possible hindrances that may rise to the surface. In Eastern psychology the whole being is treated—the focus is not merely on the obvious problem. The Eastern method leads one to become a therapist for himself. The path of sadhana is perfect and profound.

Modern psychology is still in an evolving state; it is not a finished product as yet. Counselors and therapists play an important role in society, but many of them lack the depth and insight to adequately analyze and advise their patients. They lack self-confidence and are insecure. Because of that, the counselor is unable to guide the client effectively toward the resolution of his problems. Counseling is a very noble profession, but it is taken too lightly. It is often practiced by erratic and egotistical people who are not interested in developing themselves but who are only interested in teaching. The same problem exists with those modern gurus who can theoretically explain but do not ever practice. Therapists and gurus can be more dangerous than anyone else when they exploit the innocence of others. We must find a way to keep this noble heritage and this wonderful profession from degeneration. It is through sadhana (spiritual practice) alone that one can come in touch with his inner Self. Without that, trying to help others is like building a castle in the sand: it will crumble in the first rain shower.

In the Bhagavad Gita, the protagonist Arjuna is a most brilliant *sadhaka* (one who follows the spiritual path) and warrior. He had been trained to skillfully fight the battles of life, yet even he becomes confused like any other person. According to the Bhagavad Gita, confusion can lead to serious conflict, and if the conflict seems unresolvable, one can lose all incentive and become desolate. The purpose of his life will then remain unfulfilled. Like many clients in psychotherapy, Arjuna is not at first receptive to the guidance of his preceptor, Sri Krishna. In the second chapter, after his initial arguments with Sri Krishna, Arjuna finally begins to listen to the teachings imparted to him. It is important to stress here that modern therapists and teachers need to establish rapport with their clients and students, who will be more receptive to advice when a sincere and friendly atmosphere is created.

According to the Bhagavad Gita, Atman (the real Self or center of consciousness) is never-changing, everlasting, eternal, and infinite, whereas the body is constantly changing and prone to decay. Between the body and Atman is the mental life, which needs to be understood in its totality. The antahkarana should be understood, analyzed, and trained to allow the light of Atman to be expressed and to enable one to live in the world while remaining undisturbed by worldly fetters. After explaining both the immortal and mortal aspects of existence, the Bhagavad Gita describes all aspects of yoga psychology.

Atman cannot be known in the same way we usually know something, that is, as an object to be perceived, understood, or acquired. For Atman already exists and is the source of all of one's knowledge. It is the basis of knowing rather than an object to be known. That which is the subject matter to be known is our mental life and the way we should function in the world. All the systematic efforts and practices described in the Bhagavad Gita are means to organize the internal life so that human beings can attain a state of tranquility and thus become useful to themselves and others. The psychology of the Bhagavad Gita leads the student first to awareness of the center of consciousness, then to training that focuses on the understanding and mastery of one's internal states, and lastly to the skillful and selfless performance of actions in the external world. Comprehension and knowledge of Atman are essential to fully understand the internal state of mental life. And without an understanding of the various aspects of one's mental life, coordination between mind, senses, breath, and body is impossible. So knowledge of Atman in itself is not enough: application of this knowledge is paramount.

It is Atman alone that gives light to the prime faculty of our internal being called *buddhi* (intellect). Buddhi has three main functions: discrimination, judgment, and decision. In Western psychology these three qualities of buddhi are considered to be aspects of the ego. In other words, they are intimately connected with one's limited, subjective sense of I; it is "I" who discriminates, judges, and decides. Eastern psychology, however, shows that these three functions of the intellect are distinct from the ego. That is, they are not necessarily connected with one's limited, subjective sense of I. In this view the powers of discrimination, judgment, and decision need not be expressed within the more circumscribed perspective of one's ego.

No action can be performed without the help of the mind: all the actions and speech of a human being are governed by the mind. Therefore, that which needs the most attention in developing a practical way of living is our mental life. Training the mind means making the mind free from all complexes, and in sadhana all the faculties of mind are trained in a unified way. This is important because one-sided progress is exactly like knowing half a truth, which is not a truth at all.

Commentaries on the Bhagavad Gita

There are many ancient and revered commentaries on the Bhagavad Gita, each of which has a unique emphasis. The most prominent are those of Shankara, Ramanuja, and Madhva. The most ancient commentary on the Bhagavad Gita known to the modern world is that of Shankara (A.D. 788-820). He refers to still earlier commentaries, but they are not available. According to Shankara the Bhagavad Gita leads one beyond action and beyond all the distinctions of the phenomenal world to the realization of the Absolute. Shankara views the Bhagavad Gita as an expression of Advaita philosophy, and he uses the Bhagavad Gita to support his assertion that there is only one Reality without a second. His commentary emphasizes the identity of the Self with Brahman as the only Reality. In his view the phenomenal world is illusory, and taking it to be real creates bondage and suffering. Only direct knowledge of the ultimate Reality can bring freedom. Though selfless actions help to purify the mind, ultimately one goes beyond action and renounces all involvements in the mundane world.

Ramanuja's commentary (eleventh century A.D.) emphasizes the devotional aspect of the Bhagavad Gita. Ramanuja interpreted the Bhagavad Gita in accordance with his dualistic philosophy, rejecting the view that the Self and Brahman are identical. His commentary argues against the renunciation of action and asserts that the phenomenal world is real rather than illusory, although it is totally dependent on God. In Ramanuja's view God is not beyond form (*nirguna*) but is a personal being with form *(saguna)*. God is immanent within every human being, but the human being always remains distinct from God. According to Ramanuja the Bhagavad Gita teaches that devotion to *Vishnu* is the highest path. Madhva's commentary (thirteenth century A.D.) also interprets the Bhagavad Gita from a dualistic framework and criticizes the monistic view that there is only one Consciousness. He asserts that devotion is the only means for attaining liberation, and he attempts to show that the Bhagavad Gita supports his view.

Of the many twentieth century commentaries on the Bhagavad Gita, a small number are widely read and respected. Each of these has a unique emphasis. In the first half of this century, a number of those who led India to independence from alien rule wrote commentaries that focus on karma yoga. Tilak, a prominent leader in India's quest for independence, asserts in his Gita Rahasya that the Bhagavad Gita emphasizes *karma yoga*. Tilak stresses the importance of undertaking action, not for personal reward but based on selflessness. Mahatma Gandhi also wrote a commentary on the Bhagavad Gita that stresses action based on truth, non-violence, and selflessness. The commentary by his follower Vinobha emphasizes "actionless action," that action which combines action with renunciation.

Sri Aurobindo wrote a collection of essays which assert that the Bhagavad Gita offers a synthesis or integration of the various paths of yoga, notably *jnana yoga*, karma yoga, and *bhakti yoga*—the yogas of knowledge, action, and devotion, respectively. Aurobindo attempted to reconcile the dualistic and non-dualistic interpretations of the Bhagavad

Gita. Krishna Prem, an Englishman who lived in the Himalayas as a *yogi* during the later part of his life, contributed a commentary that has given insight into the symbolic significance of the Bhagavad Gita. He emphasizes that the battle is taking place within between the negative forces of greed, selfishness, and desire and the noble qualities of the human being that can lead to Self-realization.

One of the most thorough and meticulous commentaries is the four-volume work of Satwalekar. His commentary makes many comparisons between the Bhagavad Gita and the Upanishads and other scriptures. He refers to previous commentaries and presents detailed discussions of the fine points of many verses. Since he was a practicing yogi as well as a great scholar, he was able to bring out many subtleties in his translation and commentary that are missed by other translators and commentators.

Dr. S. Radhakrishnan has written a well-known commentary that is primarily philosophical in nature. He often refers to previous commentaries, particularly that of Shankara, and to relevant passages in the Upanishads. However, he does not give much insight into the practical application of the teachings of the Bhagavad Gita. The present commentary is unique in emphasizing the practical application of the many facets of the Bhagavad Gita's teachings. It does not exclusively emphasize action, devotion, or renunciation but delves into the way in which each of the paths and practices described in the Bhagavad Gita may be utilized to attain the Absolute.

Historical Background of the Bhagavad Gita

The Bhagavad Gita is unique among philosophical and psychological teachings, for it begins as two great armies confront one another at the start of a battle, and the teachings continue for eighteen days in the midst of the battlefield. Most Western readers who read this scripture for the first time become confused by the first chapter, which describes the battlefield, for there is no introduction to inform the reader of the cause of the war and who the protagonists are. Many readers are not aware that they are reading a scripture from the longest epic poem in the world, eight times longer than the *Iliad* and *Odyssey* combined. The Bhagavad Gita is a mere seven hundred verses out of the one hundred thousand verses of the *Mahabharata*. If the reader were familiar with the Mahabharata, the events of the first chapter would be easily understood rather than being enigmatic. But without knowing what came before, the reader will be confused and will not fully appreciate Sri Krishna's counsel.

The Mahabharata records all the events leading up to the battle, explains the battle itself, and tells what came after. These events are said to have taken place some five thousand years ago, but for our purposes the epic's historical authenticity is not important, for we are concerned with the profound psychological insights conveyed in the Bhagavad Gita. The Mahabharata is a source of great wisdom about how to conduct one's life skillfully and harmoniously, and it should be studied as a work of profound insight into psychological functioning. A brief sketch of it is provided here in order to clarify the context of the Bhagavad Gita.

Dhritarashtra is the eldest son in a royal family. Ordinarily he would have become king, but since he had been born blind, his younger brother *Pandu* assumed the throne. In time Pandu had five sons, of whom Arjuna, the protagonist in the Bhagavad Gita, is the second. Dhritarashtra had one hundred sons, the eldest of whom was *Duryodhana*. The war is between the sons of Pandu, the *Pandavas,* and their cousins, the sons of Dhritarashtra, who are called the *Kauravas*. Duryodhana is the leader of the Kauravas, and Arjuna leads the army of the Pandavas.

Pandu died at an early age, so his five sons grew up under the care of their uncle Dhritarashtra, who usurped the throne. All the cousins were brought up together in the same household and had the same teachers, the most notable of whom were *Bhishma* and *Drona*. Dhritarashtra favored his sons over his nephews, and he tolerated their wicked acts. But the sons of Pandu had many outstanding qualities: they were virtuous, superior in archery, and favored by the elders. Thus Duryodhana became envious of them.

Yudhishthira, the firstborn of the Pandavas, is the rightful heir to the throne, but Duryodhana conceived several plots to kill his cousins and to send them into exile so that he could become the king instead.

For example, he built a palace made of wax for his cousins. This was extremely flammable, and when he thought they were asleep it was set afire. But as a result of divine intervention, Arjuna and his brothers escaped. Duryodhana also tried to poison and drown the Pandavas but failed. Twice appealing to Yudhishthira's sense of honor, Duryodhana goaded him into a crooked game of dice. The first time Yudhishthira lost the entire kingdom, but it was soon restored to the Pandavas. On the second occasion Yudhishthira was again cheated, and lost. As a result the five brothers were not allowed to enter the kingdom for twelve years, during which time they went to the forest where they led an austere and spiritual life. After twelve years of exile, they were permitted to return to the kingdom, but it was required that they live unknown and in disguise for one year. If their identity were discovered, they would be exiled again.

As with all of the Mahabharata, these events are symbolic, for the Mahabharata is not merely a story concerning a historical event. It is symbolic of the inner process of self-transformation and Self-realization. The entire epic explains through symbols the sequential stages in that process and the experiences that one must undergo in the heroic journey of self-discovery. For instance, a period of exile in which one lives in the wilderness and purifies oneself in preparation for spiritual awakening is a common theme that occurs in history, myths, and initiation ceremonies throughout the world. For example, consider Jesus' forty days in the wilderness before returning to Jerusalem, Moses' retreat to the mountain for forty days before receiving the Ten Commandments, and Buddha's prolonged period of meditation under the bodhi tree before he was enlightened.

Once the Pandavas successfully completed their trial, they sought to have their kingdom restored, but Duryodhana would not give them their legal and moral rights. The Pandavas would have been content with a small village for each brother, but Duryodhana told them that he would not even allow them as much land as could be placed on the point of a needle. The Pandavas tried every means to avoid fighting to regain their rights, but the battle was forced on them. The war was not fought merely to regain mundane wealth and power but was in fact a war between the just and unjust, between good and evil.

Symbolically the armies represent the positive and negative forces functioning within the human heart and mind. The battle is waged to decide whether the positive or the negative forces govern the city of life within the human being. There is a constant battle going on within each person to regain the lost kingdom of peace, happiness, and bliss. Duryodhana and his ninety-nine brothers represent the evil desires that exist within each human being, whereas the five Pandavas represent the virtuous and noble qualities. When one's reason is blinded by evil designs, it is impossible for him to live peacefully in the world. The Pandavas tried their best to solve the serious problem that arose as a result of the unjust and unrighteous ways of Duryodhana. Finally there was no choice left for the Pandavas but to decide to fight with full will and determination.

As the two sides began gathering their armies, both went to Sri Krishna and sought his support, for he possessed the strongest army, as well as being revered as the wisest teacher and the greatest yogi on the earth. Both Duryodhana and Arjuna requested Sri Krishna to support them in fighting the war. Sri Krishna, the center and source of all consciousness, wisdom, and knowledge, offered to give his vast armies to one of them and to become the chariot driver and counselor for the other. Duryodhana chose Sri Krishna's vast army, for he was greedy and materially oriented. Arjuna preferred to have Sri Krishna as his counselor and guide. Before the battle, *Sanjaya,* considered to be a wise counselor, was sent to the Pandavas' camp in order to confuse them and weaken their resolve. He tried to dissuade them from fighting, but disappointed that they did not agree to call off the war, he returned to Dhritarashtra, the blind father of Duryodhana.

At the start of the Bhagavad Gita, the two armies are facing one another on the field of *Kurukshetra,* and the battle is about to begin. Dhritarashtra is standing on a hill with Sanjaya overlooking the battleground, and he requests Sanjaya to narrate all that is taking place on the battlefield. The first chapter of the Bhagavad Gita offers a glimpse into those who are taking part in the battle and sets the stage for the dialogue between Arjuna and his preceptor, Sri Krishna.

Chapter One
Arjuna's Despondency

धृतराष्ट्र उवाच
धर्मक्षेत्रे कुरुक्षेत्रे समवेता युयुत्सवः।
मामकाः पाण्डवाश्चैव किमकुर्वत संजय।। १

Dhritarashtra asked
1. *What did my sons and the sons of Pandu do, O Sanjaya, gathered together on the battlefield of righteousness, Kurukshetra, with the intent to fight?*

The first chapter is prefatory. Dhritarashtra, the blind king, is standing on a hill overlooking the battlefield. In his anxiety, the unrighteous and unjust Dhritarashtra wants to know what is happening. So he asks his counselor and charioteer, Sanjaya, to describe the scene to him. Sanjaya, the narrator of the Bhagavad Gita, is a man of special attainments. He has inner vision and is able to describe exactly what is taking place even though he is far away. Sanjaya thus gives Dhritarashtra a complete account of what is happening on the battlefield.

Ignorant and unjust people are spiritually blind. Because of their selfish way of life, they do not accept reality. Dhritarashtra usurped the kingdom of the innocent and righteous, refusing to hand over the lawful rights of his nephews. In every family, society, or organization the elders must give the younger members their proper rights. When that is not done, frustration develops and creates a reaction in the minds of those whose rights have been snatched unjustly.

People forget that their span of life in this transitory world is brief and should be utilized to perform those actions that are helpful on the path to enlightenment rather than to perform actions that will create further bondage. Self-realization is the ultimate goal of life. Not realizing that fact, the ignorant waste the precious moments of life that could be utilized for spiritual progress and for the benefit of others. Selfishness contracts the personality rather than allowing it to expand to universal awareness. Ignorant people like Dhritarashtra live only for themselves and do not show consideration for others.

Arjuna was aware that without profound knowledge of the Eternal, external and mundane power and wealth are not at all helpful in fulfilling the purpose of life. The central theme of life is to awake, arise, and gain knowledge. If that is not constantly remembered, one becomes lost in the jungle of the external world. One should always be aware of the purpose of life, for it is only awareness of the Eternal that prevents one from being dissipated and distracted by the charms and temptations of the world. When a student like Arjuna constantly remains in contact with his teacher, and a competent teacher like Sri Krishna is teaching him, liberation becomes easy and is attained here and now.

संजय उवाच

दृष्ट्वा तु पाण्डवानीकं व्यूढं दुर्योधनस्तदा।
आचार्यमुपसंगम्य राजा वचनमब्रवीत्।। २

पश्यैतां पाण्डुपुत्राणामाचार्य महतीं चमूम्।
व्यूढां द्रुपदपुत्रेण तव शिष्येण धीमता।। ३

अत्र शूरा महेष्वासा भीमार्जुनसमा युधि।
युयुधानो विराटश्च द्रुपदश्च महारथः।। ४

धृष्टकेतुश्चेकितानः काशिराजश्च वीर्यवान्।
पुरुजित् कुन्तिभोजश्च शैब्यश्च नरपुङ्गवः।। ५

युधामन्युश्च विक्रान्त उत्तमौजाश्च वीर्यवान्।
सौभद्रो द्रौपदेयाश्च सर्व एव महारथाः।। ६

Sanjaya replied

2. *King Duryodhana, seeing the force of the Pandavas deployed in battle formation, approached his preceptor, Drona, and addressed him in these words:*

3. *O Preceptor, see this great army of the sons of Pandu deployed in battle formation by your intelligent disciple, the son of Drupada.*

4. *Here are brave men like Bhima and Arjuna, with their great bows, intent upon war; Yuyudhana, Virata, and Drupada, each commanding eleven thousand chariots.*

5. *Dhrishtaketu; Chekitana; the virile King of Kashi; Purujit Kuntibhoja; and Shaibya, the bull among men.*

6. *Here are the strident Yudhamanyu; the virile Uttamaujas; Abhimanyu, the son of Subhadra; and the five sons of Draupadi, all of them great commanders.*

Duryodhana sees the army of the Pandavas ready to fight and takes note of its great leaders. He describes their qualities to Drona, his general and teacher in the art of military affairs. Bhima and Arjuna are the foremost leaders of the Pandava army; along with their brothers, they represent the virtuous aspects of life. Yudhishthira, the eldest of the brothers, represents righteousness; Bhima is a symbol of strength undisturbed in all conditions. Arjuna is the greatest of all warriors; he has both inner wisdom and external strength. Nakula is able to attain inner peace. Without such peace and tranquility, one cannot have presence of mind. Sahadeva has wisdom that comes from faithfulness, sincerity, and one-pointedness. The five brothers create a unique team, for their qualities are complementary.

In this righteous battle of life, Duryodhana, the eldest of the one hundred sons of Dhritarashtra, leads the negative forces. He is an evil, destructive, and unjust leader. On the other side the five Pandava brothers collectively represent the positive qualities that already live as a treasure within each person. Both the positive and negative forces remain dormant within every human heart, and their characteristics are totally adverse to one another. The negative forces are numerous, shallow, seemingly powerful, misleading, and distracting. Though individually each is very powerful, they conflict with one another and so lack collective power and a sense of unification. Because the Pandavas are well organized, methodical, balanced, and aware of the truth, they will finally become victorious though they are few in number.

A human being need not waste his time and energy gathering great means to fulfill the purpose of life. He can live with few means if he knows how to utilize those few means correctly and at the right time. That skill is developed as one learns to coordinate his different faculties and modifications of mind. It results from sincere efforts made by the aspirant to develop full clarity of mind, which is the very basis of actions performed successfully in the external world. Mind and action are virtually one and the same: one is a seed and the other a plant that bears flowers and fruit.

It is important for one to be aware of both his strengths and his weaknesses, for without such awareness, success in life remains a mere dream. An aspirant should first learn to strengthen the faculty of discrimination and judgment. That faculty enables him to recognize both sets of qualities as they exist within himself: those that inspire him to attain his goal and those that create barriers for him and dissipate his will power. Every sadhaka should first learn to examine and be aware of those two factors.

The strength of the Kauravas lies in material might. Their army is much larger, and they have the best weapons and a great treasury to supply their needs. Bhishma and Drona are great military leaders and have never been defeated in battle. In terms of material strength, the Pandavas are inferior in every way, but the Kauravas have a great weakness: their side is in the wrong and is spiritually and morally corrupt. The Pandavas, by contrast, are far superior in spiritual and moral strength. Bhishma and Drona believe that their duty is to fight on the side of the Kauravas, who hold the throne, but they are aware that their side is unjust. Though they are sure to fight with honor, their hearts and sense of justice lie with the Pandavas.

A strong army that lacks moral courage is not capable of successfully fighting a war, for inner courage is the very center of that strength which motivates one toward concentrated effort. A king or hero who possesses the strongest army but does not have moral courage will finally be defeated. But the army that is fighting for a just cause and has moral courage and inner strength to support it will be victorious.

One whose mind is imbalanced due to a lack of moral courage can use brute force to support his ideas, but he can never remain in peace and happiness. What good is life when one is torn by anxiety, which weakens his inner strength? Such a person experiences defeat in fighting the battle of life, although he has many external means to support him.

Parents play a significant role in shaping the lives of their children, and thus the sons of Dhritarashtra follow in the footsteps of their unjust father. When parents are greedy, egotistical, conniving, and unjust, their children consciously and unconsciously develop the same characteristics. Human society suffers as a result of self-created misery because the elders do not realize that children trained in an unjust atmosphere will also become unjust. As one rotten fish pollutes the whole pool, so one man can mislead an entire society. Therefore, a king or leader should be righteous and just and should stand as an example for others to follow. Dhritarashtra is the antithesis of such an example.

Many great civilizations have been destroyed by foolish, selfish, and greedy leaders. For instance, Nero was delighted to see his kingdom burning, and in the second world war Hitler was obsessed by war hysteria and became imbalanced, thinking of nothing but killing and destroying other nations. Many examples of such atrocities committed by kings and leaders in the past and present could be cited. Why do we forget that this world is a field of action and that if we learn to perform our actions skillfully and righteously, our journey will become a perennial song?

अस्माकं तु विशिष्टा ये तान्निबोध द्विजोत्तम।
नायका मम सैन्यस्य संज्ञार्थं तान् ब्रवीमि ते।।७
भवान् भीष्मश्च कर्णश्च कृपश्च समितिंजयः।
अश्वत्थामा विकर्णश्च सौमदत्तिस्तथैव च।। ८
अन्ये च बहवः शूरा मदर्थे त्यक्तजीविताः।
नानाशस्त्रप्रहरणाः सर्वे युद्धविशारदाः।। ९

7. *Now, O Drona, the best of the twice-born, learn of those who are distinguished among us, the leaders of my army. I tell you of them so that you may recognize them.*
8. *Yourself, Bhishma, Karna, and Kripa, conquerors and victorious ones; Ashvatthama, Vikarna, the son of Somadatta, and Jayadratha.*
9. *And many other brave men ready to sacrifice their lives for my sake, they who attack with many weapons, and all of them experts at the art and science of combat.*

Chapters 164 through 171 of the Mahabharata give a detailed description of the warriors who are participating in the battle. The foremost commanders of Duryodhana's army are Drona and Bhishma, who are revered as generals of unparalleled skill; Karna is also a great warrior on Duryodhana's side. Duryodhana calls them "conquerors and victorious ones," and others are also mentioned who are ready to die for him. Duryodhana is confident that he has highly skilled and powerful generals in his army. Although these generals are very old, they are strong and skilled in the art and science of combat, knowing all the strategies of battle. Bhishma is one hundred and seventy years old, and Drona is ninety years old, but despite their ages these veterans fight fiercely.

The modern mind might take these ages as an exaggeration in the same way that everyone used to laugh at scientists when they began preparing to go to the moon. There is nothing that is impossible, however, for one who practices *samyama* (self-discipline) on all levels. It amazes the modern mind that the ancients knew the methods of prolonging the span of life and led a healthy life of more than one hundred and twenty years. The way in which they used to think, eat, and practice discipline kept them both healthy and wise, but we do not find such examples in our modern world. Today there are people who live ninety to one hundred years and occasionally up to one hundred and fifteen years, but they remain bedridden invalids and are usually senile. This clearly shows that our lives are not correctly organized; we have forgotten the secrets by which we can arrest the aging process. Bhishma and Drona were great yogis who knew the secrets of perpetual youth as well as the technique of dying. They could drop their bodies willfully, according to their desire. As a result of technological attainments, modern man has been able to acquire the means for living comfortably, but external comfort without inner strength is not enough for one to lead a healthy and useful life.

If we read the conclusion of the Mahabharata, we will find that Drona and Bhishma, the greatest of all warriors, lose the war because in their heart of hearts, they know that they are fighting for an unjust cause. One who does not do his duty wholeheartedly and with full attention is not successful. Drona and Bhishma fight for Duryodhana because of their loyalty to the King, but their hearts are with the Pandavas. In such a serious division of loyalties within and without, it is not possible to win a battle, whether that battle is taking place within oneself or in the external world. When one acts in a manner contradictory to what he feels and thinks, he becomes disoriented. In such instances, neither success in the external world nor peace within is possible.

The first task for a seeker of truth is to understand the words "coordinated effort." This means that one should always follow the dictates of his conscience; he should not do anything that does not agree with his conscience. When a normal human being considers doing something, his conscience helps him to choose what he will do by placing the consequences of his actions—good and bad, helpful and damaging, right and wrong—in front of him. And if he has a firm will, he will be able to carry out the action he chooses. *Samkalpa shakti* (will power) is a powerful force in the human being. If it is not utilized, there will always be failure, regardless of the external efforts made and the means applied. True sadhakas are taught to be vigilant, to not allow the light of samkalpa shakti to be diminished or extinguished. If the knowledge of that light is protected and allowed to grow, the aspirant becomes self-reliant, and self-reliance is an essential virtue. Self-reliance, courage, a one-pointed mind, and determination all unite to build the force of samkalpa shakti, without which the aspirant cannot fearlessly tread the path of life.

अपर्याप्तं तदस्माकं बलं भीष्माभिरक्षितम्।
पर्याप्तं त्विदमेतेषां बलं भीमाभिरक्षितम्।। १०

10. *This force of ours supervised by Bhishma, is large but inadequate; however, the force of these (Pandavas) supervised by Bhima, is small but adequate.*

Although Duryodhana has superior strength, he has an inferiority complex that shows itself in his jealous feelings toward the Pandavas. He knows he is fighting a war for unjust and unrighteous motives. When enveloped in selfishness, even the mightiest cannot be victorious, for inner strength alone motivates one to successfully fight in the battlefield of life and to skillfully perform his actions and duties. By contrast, selfish motivation weakens the will and inner strength. One who is selfishly motivated cannot persuade the conscience, which judges one's intentions before he decides to act, to take his side. Such a human being continually creates a division within himself by ignoring his conscience and continuing to follow the path of unrighteousness. He knows what truth is, but his actions are motivated by selfishness, greed, and possessiveness. Duryodhana's situation is exactly like that: his inner strength is weakened by the division he has created within himself. Although Duryodhana has the stronger army and skilled generals, he is unsure of his victory.

When a king suffers from an inferiority complex, he may act as though he is superior, but such a person actually feels inadequate underneath his false show of bravado. There is no such thing as a superiority complex: there is only one complex, and that is inferiority. When one is aware of his weaknesses but does not know how to rid himself of them, he creates a shield for his protection; when one does not want to accept and confront his weaknesses, he puts on a false front and acts as though he is superior. Such people actually think they are superior to others because they have not learned to accept things as they are. A sense of superiority is like a house of cards that can crumble at the touch of a finger.

Everyone has weaknesses. Wise is he who acknowledges his weaknesses and works steadily to remove them and to replace them with the essential virtues that strengthen him and make him brave, fearless, and truthful. There is always a war between the forces of virtue and vice. Weakness may appear to be strong because it persistently resists accepting and acknowledging its reverse side. Virtue, however, has genuine strength because it is a product of a balanced mind. Weakness arises from imbalance, whereas balance is the true source of strength.

Even though Duryodhana has the most powerful army and the best generals, still he lacks confidence. And when one is not sure of himself, it is difficult for him to be victorious. Confidence comes from inner strength, from the inner conscience that constantly judges one's thoughts, feelings, desires, and motivations. One's conscience protects him from the traps laid by his weaknesses.

अयनेषु च सर्वेषु यथाभागमवस्थिताः।
भीष्ममेवाभिरक्षन्तु भवन्तः सर्व एव हि।। ११

11. Standing according to your assignments in the divisions and at all the major entry points of the battle formation, all of you should surround and protect the commander-in-chief, Bhishma, alone.

Why does Bhishma, the leader of Duryodhana's army, need protection? Because if the commander of the army is lost, the war will be lost. Bhishma, however, has a special power: no man can kill him. It is difficult to believe that anyone who is born is not subject to death, and Bhishma, though very powerful and skillful, is no exception. Among the many fears of Duryodhana is the fear of losing Bhishma, and that fear prompts him to order his army to protect Bhishma with all its might. It is fear that creates defenses and consumes a vital part of one's energy that could be used in positive ways.

Although Bhishma is fighting for Duryodhana, it is not with full-heartedness: Bhishma's and Drona's loyalty to Duryodhana is merely superficial and external. They fight with the knowledge that Duryodhana's cause is unjust. These two great warriors know that Duryodhana will be defeated no matter how much resistance he presents and regardless of the fortifications he is able to create with the help of his brute strength.

Energy and strength exist in many forms and have varied expressions. For example, electricity can be used both for cooling and heating, and a person's energy can likewise be used for either creativity or destruction. It depends on what one chooses and how much skill one has in using his energy. Duryodhana is very powerful, but his power is destructive. The Pandavas, in contrast, represent that stream of energy that is creative and leads one to the source of consciousness.

तस्य सञ्जनयन् हर्षं कुरुवृद्धः पितामहः।
सिंहनादं विनद्योच्चैः शंखं दध्मौ प्रतापवान्।। १२

ततः शंखाश्च भेर्यश्च पणवानकगोमुखाः।
सहसैवाभ्यहन्यन्त स शब्दस्तुमुलोऽभवत्।। १३

ततः श्वेतैर्हयैर्युक्ते महति स्यन्दने स्थितौ।
माधवः पाण्डवश्चैव दिव्यौ शंखौ प्रदध्मतुः।। १४

पांचजन्यं हृषीकेशो देवदत्तं धनंजयः।
पौण्ड्रं दध्मौ महाशंखं भीमकर्मा वृकोदरः।। १५

अनन्तविजयं राजा कुन्तीपुत्रो युधिष्ठिरः।
नकुलः सहदेवश्च सुघोषमणिपुष्पकौ।। १६

काश्यश्च परमेष्वासः शिखण्डी च महारथः।
धृष्टद्युम्नो विराटश्च सात्यकिश्चापराजितः।। १७

द्रुपदो द्रौपदेयाश्च सर्वशः पृथिवीपते।
सौभद्रश्च महाबाहुः शंखान् दध्मुः पृथक् पृथक्।। १८

12. *Causing Duryodhana great joy, the elder of the Kurus, the grand-father Bhishma, a man of splendor, loudly roaring a lion roar, blew the conch.*
13. *Then conches, kettle drums, tabors, drums, and trumpets suddenly blared forth, and that sound was tumultuous.*
14. *Then, standing in a great chariot drawn by white horses, Krishna and Arjuna also blew their celestial conches.*
15. *Krishna, the Lord of Senses, blew his conch, named Panchajanya, and Arjuna, the Winner of Wealth, blew his conch, named Devadatta; Bhima, he of fierce deeds, blew his great conch, named Paundra.*
16. *King Yudhishthira, the son of Kunti, blew the conch Anantavijaya; Nakula and Sahadeva blew their conches, named Sughosha and Mani-pushpaka respectively.*
17. *And the King of Kashi, the excellent archer, as well as Shikhandi, the great charioteer, Dhrishtadyumna, Virata, and the uncon-querable Satyaki*
18. *Drupada and the sons of Draupadi, each and every one, O King, the mighty-armed son of Subhadra—they all blew their conches, each his own.*

The leaders of both armies blow their conches, and the armies beat their drums and blow their trumpets to inspire their own soldiers. First Duryodhana's army creates a fierce sound to terrorize the Pandavas, but the Pandavas' army returns a mighty sound with full confidence. The gestures and sounds that are created to frighten the opposition have two possible origins: fear and confidence. When human beings are frightened, they do not create music but frightful sounds. Sri Krishna and Arjuna, who are confident of their strength, create a melodic sound. In fact, the whole of the Bhagavad Gita is a dialogue between Sri Krishna and Arjuna that creates a beautiful melody, a divine song. The sounds created by Duryodhana's drummers are violent; they are created out of excitement, fear, and anxiety. Their sound does not compose any poetry or song, for it has its origin in the destructive aspect of *Shakti,* the primal force that resides within. That primal force has two aspects: one is merciful, gentle, and kind; the other is cruel, brutal, and annihilating. The war represents the inner conflict between the annihilating and merciful powers within each person.

स घोषो धार्तराष्ट्राणां हृदयानि व्यदारयत्।
नभश्च पृथिवीं चैव तुमुलो व्यनुनादयन्।। १९

19. *The tumultuous, reverberating sound tore the hearts of the sons of Dhritarashtra, echoing all around the heaven and earth.*

The fierce sounds of the Pandavas' conches frighten Duryodhana and magnify his feelings of guilt. Guilty is he who does not acknowledge his mistakes, for he does not believe in being corrected and is not open to helpful suggestions from any quarter. He neither listens to the voice of his conscience nor to the advice of his counselors. He closes all the doors of learning, isolating himself in the fortress of his own egotistical views. He does not want to know anything, and he goes on feeding his ego by creating a false reality for himself.

अथ व्यवस्थितान्दृष्ट्वा धार्तराष्ट्रान् कपिध्वज:।
प्रवृत्ते शस्त्रसम्पाते धनुरुद्यम्य पाण्डव:।।२०

20. *Now, Arjuna, the son of Pandu, who had Hanuman as the emblem on his flag, seeing the sons of Dhritarashtra standing well organized as the weapons had begun to be hurled, raised his bow.*

In the *Ramayana*, a more ancient epic than the Mahabharata, *Hanuman* plays a vital role in defeating the demon, *Ravana*. Hanuman is one of the greatest symbols used by warriors, for he had enormous strength. In the Mahabharata, the symbol of Hanuman also plays a prominent role. The flag that is hoisted on Arjuna's chariot has a monkey, the symbol of Hanuman, on it, and this inspires Arjuna's army and terrifies the army of his enemies. Hanuman was the greatest of all devotees, a sadhaka and a *brahmachari* with single-pointed devotion for Lord Rama. Hanuman's one-pointed devotion gave him unparalleled strength and assurance of attaining his goal. The wise teacher encourages his students to develop such one-pointedness.

Arjuna's devotion is exactly like that of Hanuman. He is with his lord and guide, Sri Krishna, all the time. He is learning to apply all his resources with full sincerity and might. That is why he is called Arjuna, "one who makes sincere efforts." In preparing for the war, the symbol of Hanuman on Arjuna's flag inspires him and helps him to be confident. He knows that he is fighting a just war and that the greatest of yogis is his teacher. His self-confidence is enormous, but as we shall soon see, Arjuna is about to lose all his confidence and become despondent.

How is it possible for one to confidently prepare himself for a fierce battle and then fall into a state of despondency in such a short time? We see here that a human being, no matter how positive he feels, can slip down to the valley of sorrow as a result of a single thought that draws his attention to the body, which is weak.

Even after attaining *samadhi* (a state of transcendent consciousness in which all of one's questions are answered), one comes down from the height of tranquility, for even the practice of samadhi is done in the cage of human limitation. When we study the lives of great spiritual leaders, we find that a moment comes when they are swayed from their heights and become absorbed in body identification. For example, Buddha decided to follow the path of renunciation and left his family. Nonetheless, he soon returned home to see his infant child once more, but then he remembered his resolve and again rushed back toward the Rajgiri forest.

Realistically one should understand that although the highest call of life is the inner urge to know the Ultimate, the call of the charms and temptations of the external world is very powerful and can create obstacles on the path. Therefore, a sadhaka should not be proud or complacent about what he has attained. Even to the last breath of sadhana, attachments to the world and to relationships are prone to disturb the sadhaka.

हृषीकेशं तदा वाक्यमिदमाह महीपते।

अर्जुन उवाच

सेनयोरुभयोर्मध्ये रथं स्थापय मेऽच्युत।। २१

यावदेतान्निरीक्षेऽहं योद्धुकामानवस्थितान्।

कैर्मया सह योद्धव्यमस्मिन् रणसमुद्यमे।। २२

योत्स्यमानानवेक्ष्येऽहं य एतेऽत्र समागताः।।

धार्तराष्ट्रस्य दुर्बुद्धेर्युद्धे प्रियचिकीर्षवः।। २३

संजय उवाच

एवमुक्तो हृषीकेशो गुडाकेशेन भारत।

सेनयोरुभयोर्मध्ये स्थापयित्वा रथोत्तमम्।। २४

भीष्मद्रोणप्रमुखतः सर्वेषां च महीक्षिताम्।

उवाच पार्थ पश्यैतान् समवेतान्कुरूनिति।। २५

21. *That, O King Dhritarashtra, Arjuna addressed these words to Krishna, Lord of the Senses: 'O Steadfast One, place my chariot between both armies,*

22. *While I observe these who are standing here with whom I am about to fight in this battle,*

23. *I would like to see these who have gathered here to fight, who are desirous of doing the wishes of the evil-minded son of Dhritarashtra in battle.'*

24. *Then, O Descendant of Bharata, thus addressed by Arjuna, the Conqueror of Sleep, Krishna, Lord of the Senses, having placed the best of the chariots between both armies,*

25. *In front of Bhishma and Drona and of all the kings, said, 'O Son of Pritha, see all these Kauravas gathered together.'*

Arjuna requests Sri Krishna to drive his chariot between the two armies so that he can observe the strength of the enemy and at the same time estimate the strength of his own army. The aspirant who lacks a keen sense of observation is not aware of his strengths and weaknesses and thus can be swayed by his imbalanced emotions. In the same way that Arjuna prepares for war, the aspirant should prepare himself before he starts to tread the path of sadhana. If the sadhaka is not prepared to tread the path of sadhana, disease, despair, fear, and depression will create obstacles for him.

In the Katha Upanishad the chariot is likened to the body, and the horses pulling the chariot to the senses. As the metaphor is applied here, Arjuna represents the mind, and the driver represents the higher buddhi. The prime nature of the mind is to consider: shall I do it or not? When the mind learns to seek the advice of buddhi, the student ceases to be fickle minded, learning instead to make proper determinations and decisions in all circumstances.

In this verse Sri Krishna is referred to as Achyuta, and the name Gudakesha is used for Arjuna. Achyuta means one who is not fickle, and Gudakesha means the conqueror of sleep. These words denote that the teacher should be firm and consistent and the student should never allow himself to be subject to sloth, inertia, or laziness. Arjuna is an embodiment of a good sadhaka, and Sri Krishna a competent teacher. For lack of decisiveness one becomes fickle, and for lack of awareness one is caught by inertia and sloth. These are serious obstacles that do not allow the student to progress.

तत्रापश्यत् स्थितान् पार्थः पितृनथ पितामहान्।
आचार्यान्मातुलान्भातृन् पुत्रान्पौत्रान्सखींस्तथा।। २६
श्वशुरान् सुहृदश्चैव सेनयोरुभयोरपि।
तान् समीक्ष्य स कौन्तेयः सर्वान्बन्धूनवस्थितान्।। २७
कृपया परयाऽऽविष्टो विषीदन्निदमब्रवीत्।
    अर्जुन उवाच
दृष्ट्वेमं स्वजनं कृष्ण युयुत्सुं समुपस्थितम्।। २८

26. *There the son of Pritha saw those who were like fathers and grand-*
    fathers to him, teachers, uncles, brothers, sons, grandsons, as well
    as companions,
27. *Fathers-in-law, as well as friends in both armies; seeing all those*
    kinsmen standing there, Arjuna the son of Kunti,
28. *Possessed by a pitiful mood, feeling very sad, said these words: I*
    see these kinsmen present here with the intent to fight.

When Arjuna inspects the opposing army, he sees that among its leaders are his teachers, cousins, fathers-in-law, and other close relatives and friends. He suddenly becomes affected by his attachment to his relatives, sinks into a self-created pool of sorrow, and forgets his purpose. Attachment is the greatest source of misery. The strands of attachment bind the sadhaka and weaken his determination, will, and inner strength. He forgets the ultimate goal of life and becomes a victim of mundane and transitory relationships.

In such situations, aspirants may begin to argue with their teachers. Such an exchange can be helpful on the path of sadhana, for it becomes a process of learning if it occurs between a sincere student and a wise preceptor. The dialogue helps one to confront and analyze his weaknesses. Sri Krishna, a perfect yogi, is aware of Arjuna's inner turmoil and allows him to express himself.

When one experiences the grief and sorrow that arise from attachment, he does not remain wise, and the unwise cannot discriminate right from wrong. Because of his involvement and attachment, Arjuna becomes confused and loses his objectivity. Thus, he cannot reach impartial conclusions and act justly. One who is enveloped in attachment is incapable of knowing or deciding things correctly. One who is attached to the mundane life argues irrationally and is unable to understand the consequences of his actions.

सीदन्ति मम गात्राणि मुखं च परिशुष्यति।
वेपथुश्च शरीरे मे रोमहर्षश्च जायते।। २९

गाण्डीवं स्रंसते हस्तात्त्वक्चैव परिदह्यते।
न च शक्नोम्यवस्थातुं भ्रमतीव च मे मनः।। ३०

29. *My limbs are frozen, my mouth is drying up, my body trembles*
and hairs stand on end.
30. *Gandiva, the great bow, is slipping from my hand, and my skin is*
burning. Nor can I stand up; my mind is, as it were, whirling;

Even the finest among men can sink into the depths of sorrow. There are many examples of great seekers on the path of light who experienced moments of grief and sorrow during which they lost touch with the higher reality and became overwhelmed by the strong power of mundane attachment. For instance, the sage Vashishtha became despondent when he lost his son, even though birth and death had already revealed their secrets to him. The nervous system cannot handle such a flood of negative energy. Thus, the body starts trembling, shaking, and jerking, and one loses all control of the body. It is sorrow, anger, and fear that create such symptoms.

Sorrow, infatuation, and other emotions weaken the body and sap the physical strength of even a healthy man. A black bee has tremendous power, enabling it to bore a hole through wood, but when the bee becomes infatuated with the fragrance of the lotus blossom, it is unable to escape from the closing lotus petals that hold it captive after the sun sets. The history of mankind is a testimony to the fact that infatuation for alcohol, an imbalanced attitude toward sexuality, and other addictions weaken human strength. The sorrow that comes as a result of being addicted to objects of the world has power to change the tissues of the body and can turn a trim and taut figure into a flabby one.

The endocrine glands react instantly to stressful situations, and so during a state of anxiety and depression, certain symptoms are noticed. For example, dryness of the mouth occurs because the salivary glands do not secrete sufficiently. If one receives shocking, sorrowful news about someone he loves, that shock may make him cry, and the body may begin to shake and tremble. Evenness of breath and the motion of the lungs, which play a vital role in the regulation of the body, are disturbed. Then the heartbeat becomes irregular, and the blood supply to the brain is inadequate. These are some of the ways that infatuations and emotions interfere with the body's normal responses and have the power to create an imbalance in the body. Because of such emotional imbalances the body starts building up toxins, and the pores lose their capacity to expel the toxic buildup. That disturbs the equilibrium in two systems of the human body: the system that purifies and cleanses the body (the pores, lungs, kidneys, and bowels) and the system that nourishes the body (the liver, spleen, heart, brain, and so on).

Arjuna is agitated and despondent; he is caught up in his attachments and in the emotions that ensue when attachments are threatened. He has lost his mental and emotional equilibrium, and he has lost touch with the source of strength within. That kind of regression is a very serious stumbling block on the forward journey. Human weaknesses are dangerous and destroy human endeavor if they are not put aside and if they are not dealt with using inner strength and pure reason.

If one is addicted to drugs such as heroin and the drugs are suddenly withdrawn, he experiences severe debilitating symptoms. In a similar way when one is strongly attached to an object in the external world and loses or anticipates the loss of that object, he suffers physical symptoms such as those experienced by Arjuna. From the yogic perspective attachment and addiction are equivalent terms: both lead to emotional and physical suffering.

Many mental and physical disorders are the result of attachment to the objects of the world. If the object to which one is attached is threatened, one becomes afraid, and because of the fear of losing the object, he loses mental balance. An imbalanced mind is a source of much misery, and attachment is the cause of all misery. Modern psychologists and physicians are becoming aware that psychological disorders are the main source of many physical diseases and imbalances. Self-created misery is the source from which psychosomatic diseases spring. But that which originates in the mind and is expressed through the body is difficult to cure with medicine. Many of the ills of human life cannot be alleviated by drugs and other physical means.

Modern psychologists need to develop better methods for treating psychosomatic disorders, for analysis remains ineffective and psychological imbalances continue to disturb the physical condition of many clients. Mind and body are in the habit of reacting to one another. Physical pains are recorded, stored, and memorized by the mind. Therefore, the mind is bound to be affected by physical pain. Physical diseases disturb the nervous system and mental life, but the problems that originate in the mind and then reflect on the body are even more serious. When the mind—the center of sensitivity, feeling, thoughts, and desires—is disturbed, the body is tormented and experiences innumerable sorts of pain.

The medicines prescribed to treat mental disorders and diseases caused by mental disturbance do not resolve the underlying disturbance; they merely dull the sensitivity of the nervous system. The pain remains, but for some time one does not experience it. Such medicines are not cures but only temporary means for soothing the sufferer. The body and mind should be thoroughly understood as one unit. Only then will effective means of treatment be developed. One can attain a profound comprehension of mind/body interaction by studying the nature of each from different angles. To understand the body, one should study the body's needs and capacities while eating, sleeping, working, and during times of physical attraction toward others. The inseparable link of these two realities, physical and mental, is *pranic* energy, called the breath of life.

निमित्तानि च पश्यामि विपरीतानि केशव।
न च श्रेयोऽनुपश्यामि हत्वा स्वजनमाहवे।। ३१
न कांक्षे विजयं कृष्ण न च राज्यं सुखानि च।
किं नो राज्येन गोविन्द किं भोगैर्जीवितेन वा।। ३२
येषामर्थे कांक्षितं नो राज्यं भोगाः सुखानि च।
त इमेऽवस्थिता युद्धे प्राणांस्त्यक्त्वा धनानि च।। ३३

आचार्याः पितरः पुत्राः तथैव च पितामहाः।
मातुलाः श्वशुराः पौत्राः श्यालाः संबन्धिनस्तथा।। ३४
एतान्न हन्तुमिच्छामि घ्नतोऽपि मधुसूदन।
अपि त्रैलोक्यराज्यस्य हेतोः किं नु महीकृते।। ३५
निहत्य धार्तराष्ट्रान् नः का प्रीतिः स्याज्जनार्दन।
पापमेवाश्रयेदस्मान् हत्वैतानाततायिनः।। ३६
तस्मान्नार्हा वयं हन्तुं धार्तराष्ट्रान्स्वबान्धवान्।
स्वजनं हि कथं हत्वा सुखिनः स्याम माधव।। ३७
यद्यप्येते न पश्यन्ति लोभोपहतचेतसः।
कुलक्षयकृतं दोषं मित्रद्रोहे च पातकम्।। ३८
कथं न ज्ञेयमस्माभिः पापादस्मान्निवर्तितुम्।
कुलक्षयकृतं दोषं प्रपश्यद्भिर्जनार्दन।। ३९

31. *And I see inauspicious omens, O Krishna; nor do I see any good accruing upon killing my own kinsmen in the battle.*

32. *I do not desire victory, O Krishna, nor kingdom, nor comforts. What use do we have for kingdom, Lord of the Senses, and what to us is enjoyment of pleasures or even life itself?*

33. *They for whose sake we might desire a kingdom, pleasures, and comforts are standing here before us on the battlefield, having abandoned their very lives and wealth.*

34. *Teachers, father-like elders, sons as well as grandfathers, uncles, fathers-in-law, grandsons, brothers-in-law, and other relatives—*

35. *I do not wish to kill them even if they are killing me, O Destroyer of Illusion, not even for the sake of the kingdom of the three worlds. How then could I do so merely for the sake of this earth?*

36. *What pleasure can we derive by killing the sons of Dhritarashtra, O Faultless One? Only sin can accrue to us by killing these felons.*

37. *Therefore, it does not behoove us to kill the sons of Dhritarashtra, our kinsmen. How can we be happy after killing our very own relatives, O Krishna?*
38. *Though the Kauravas' minds are impaired by greed and so are not seeing, the fault accrues by the destruction of the family and the sin in the desire to injure friends.*
39. *How then should we not know enough to turn away from this sin, as we are able to see the fault that accrues upon the destruction of the family, O Krishna?*

It is said that the devil uses scripture for his own convenience. Likewise Duryodhana, the wicked son of an unjust father, applied all possible means to justify his stand. He even exploited religious sentiments so that the kingdom would not have to be returned to the Pandavas. Many political leaders do not hesitate to quote scriptures and in other ways exploit religion in order to attain selfish ends. Many irreligious leaders thus exploit the innocent in the name of God and religion.

Dhritarashtra, the blind father of Duryodhana, asked Sanjaya to persuade the Pandavas not to take up arms. Sanjaya gave a long sermon, saying "O Dharma (Yudhishthira, the eldest brother of the Pandavas), you are the best of men and would never violate the moral law of society. You have the capacity to forgive the sins of the Kauravas. It certainly does not behoove you to be cruel, to fight a fierce war, and to kill your cousins and teachers." Sanjaya advised the Pandavas to become renunciates and suggested that begging would be superior to fighting the war. He gave that religious sermon on renunciation just before the war was about to be fought, and Arjuna's dejection and despondency were brought about by it.

Suggestion creates a hypnotic effect, and hypnosis diminishes the faculty of discrimination. People in general are very much influenced by the suggestions of others, and suggestion is, in fact, the very basis of modern education. It is the wrong method of education, for one loses the ability to inquire and just follows what he has been told without logic and reasoning. If we learn how to free ourselves from the impressions received by suggestive education, we can then independently learn that which is useful, healthy, and valid. There are higher and superior methods of learning and exploring, and there are many dimensions of knowledge that are as yet unexplored by the vast majority of people.

Brahma Vidya (the knowledge of absolute Truth) is the highest knowledge, and direct experience is the best means of gaining that knowledge. Direct experience is by far the finest means to attain knowledge in any dimension of life. One should learn through direct experience, for that alone is valid. All other methods are incomplete and therefore misleading. An aspirant should carefully choose a path for himself by examining his capacities, abilities, and strengths. He should avoid suggestive ideas and thus not become distracted and dissipated. Reading books that dissipate and distract one's mind should be avoided. Conversing with those who are not on the path and living in the company of those who do not practice sadhana also lead to dissipation. One must encourage the faculty of discrimination within in order to counter such negative influences. Seeking advice from a competent teacher is helpful, for a wise teacher is experienced in receiving knowledge directly, and such unalloyed knowledge is free from the fanciful suggestions and influences of ordinary people.

Arjuna is deluded by his attachment and loses sight of his duty and the aim of life. He begins to identify with Duryodhana and imagines that by fighting this righteous war, he will be behaving exactly like Duryodhana. External influences can lead one to think in such an illogical way and thus have a disturbing effect that can change the whole course of one's life. "Not delusion but constant awareness" would be a suitable thought for Arjuna. That would soothe his heart and bring him to the right path.

All of Arjuna's arguments are irrational because they are the outpourings of the influences of the strongest of all enemies: attachment. When one is attached, he isolates himself from the whole and thus deprives himself from listening to the voice of his conscience and to his preceptors. The faculty of discrimination does not then function, and one rationalizes to justify his emotional state. He will then never reach his goal, for he has lost all sense of direction.

In modern life we see most people selling their ideas, trying to prove that they are right. To support their notions, they quote the scriptures or seek other justification. Such a person gives many suggestions to his own mind, for before one can seduce others, he must first seduce himself. Modern man is blind; he does not understand the purpose of life. He sees only the imaginary world that self-suggestion and the suggestions of others have created. He desires quick results and wants to do things in his own way without consideration for others.

There are four types of people: those who are time oriented, those who are goal oriented, those who are life oriented, and those who are purpose oriented. In today's world we find mostly time oriented people. They are selfish, narrow, and conceited. Time oriented people do things to fulfill their selfish ends without purpose or goal and are not aware of the consequences of their actions. Time is fleeting for them. They have no sense of tomorrow, so they demand immediate gratification. They react impulsively to external stimuli to fulfill their desires for sensory gratification. They take advantage of others; they cannot think beyond their own concerns. Slightly higher are those whose lives are directed toward certain goals. Those goals, however, are related to the pleasures of the mundane and temporal world. But at least those people have goals and do not act impulsively like time oriented people. Higher still is the life of those who try to remain in peace and to live in harmony. They believe in co-existence as a way of life, so they do not like to disturb the equilibrium of others nor do they desire to possess unlawfully the wealth and property of others. But the highest path is followed by those who are purpose oriented and who direct all their energies and use all their resources to fulfill their single purpose: Self-realization. Duryodhana is time oriented and is not at all conscious of the purposefully oriented life. Arjuna, by contrast, is expected to be an embodiment of a purposefully oriented life, but he slips from the highest to the lowest level because of the influences of attachment.

The physical and psychological symptoms that are experienced by Arjuna make it clear that his objection to fighting is not based on non-attachment and renunciation but on intense emotional reactions due to his attachment. A student sometimes talks as though he has the wisdom of a great master, whereas his behavior shows that he is under serious strain and stress and that his mind is imbalanced. Such "wisdom" is not part of any knowledge but is described by Patanjali as false knowledge. Many people are capable of delivering a sermon full of wondrous statements of wisdom, but one has to examine through which channel that wisdom is coming. Wisdom of speech is not the same as true wisdom. When the body is in a state of equilibrium, real wisdom finds its way. Mind and body are the instruments that create melodies that help one to be tranquil and enable him to sing the eternal song of life. But when there is disharmony and the mind and body are not tuned in a coordinated way, they create a cacophony that is unpleasant to the human ear and distracting to the mind. Listening to the "words of wisdom" from the mouth of Arjuna, Sri Krishna knows that this "wisdom" is mere escapism and not the wisdom that inspires one to tread the path of life and light.

कुलक्षये प्रणश्यन्ति कुलधर्माः सनातनाः।
धर्मे नष्टे कुलं कृत्स्नं अधर्मोऽभिभवत्युत।। ४०

अधर्माभिभवात् कृष्ण प्रदुष्यन्ति कुलस्त्रियः।
स्त्रीषु दुष्टासु वार्ष्णेय जायते वर्णसंकरः।। ४१

संकरो नरकायैव कुलघ्नानां कुलस्य च।
पतन्ति पितरो ह्येषां लुप्तपिण्डोदकक्रियाः।। ४२

दोषैरेतैः कुलघ्नानां वर्णसंकरकारकैः।
उत्साद्यन्ते जातिधर्माः कुलधर्माश्च शाश्वताः।। ४३

उत्सन्नकुलधर्माणां मनुष्याणां जनार्दन।
नरकेऽनियतं वासो भवतीत्यनुशुश्रुम।। ४४

अहो बत महत् पापं कर्तुं व्यवसिता वयम्।
यद्राज्यसुखलोभेन हन्तुं स्वजनमुद्यताः।। ४५

40. *Upon the disappearance of family traditions and rules of conduct, vice and unrighteousness subdue the entire family.*
41. *When subdued by vice, O Krishna, the women of the family become corrupted; when the women are corrupted, O Ruler of your clan,*

there occurs confusion of the social structure.

42. *Such confusion leads only to hell for the whole family, including those who have destroyed the family. Even the ancestors fall into hell, since the rites and observances for preventing them from doing so are no longer performed.*

43. *Because of these faults of the destroyers of the family, which cause the confusion of the social structure, the perennial national traditions as well as the family traditions are uprooted.*

44. *When the family traditions of human beings are thus uprooted, O Krishna, these human beings have to dwell in hell indefinitely—so have we heard in the tradition.*

45. *Oh, alas, we are embarking upon committing a great sin as we are preparing to kill our own kinsmen out of greed for kingdom and comfort.*

Woman is the builder of society. The institution of family life is her original idea; she is its architect, and she has remained the custodian of the cultural heritage. Even today in Hindu, Jewish, Irish, and several other cultures, the woman is the center and organizer of the family. It is she who plans the disciplinary program for the children. A society that does not give due place to women goes toward degeneration and disintegration, and if a society starts acting in an irresponsible manner, it is because the family institution has become disturbed.

Arjuna, a brilliant thinker and warrior, plunges into grief when he foresees that the heroes killed in the war will leave innumerable widows. When the population becomes imbalanced, having more females than males, it is difficult to maintain loyalty toward one mate. And if the mind gets involved outside of the marriage, it becomes distracted. The whole course of the individual's life is then altered. Arjuna has the insight to bring that problem to his consciousness. Of all Arjuna's arguments, this one makes the most sense.

Perfect understanding between marriage partners is important, and fidelity plays a significant part in that. If fidelity is lost, the values on which the society is erected crumble, and the progeny are weakened.

Purity in a marital relationship is a significant factor in sharing a harmonious life together and in giving birth to and raising healthy children. In today's society fidelity may seem to be a foolish idea. Some Westerners think that fidelity is merely an Eastern more, but that is simply a justification to support irresponsibility.

Arjuna's prediction clearly reflects what is taking place in modern society. There does not seem to be harmony between individuals either within the family or in society. The construction of society is the profound responsibility of its individual members. That responsibility can be fulfilled only when the members of society practice discipline and self-control. For lack of these arise many mental, emotional, and physiological disorders that consume considerable time and energy. To cure these problems is one of the reasons modern therapy came into existence, but Eastern teachers and therapists believe that prevention is better than cure.

One must understand the difference between human civilization and animal life. If a human being runs around irresponsibly like an animal, it shows that discipline and self-control have not been cultivated in his life. Without practicing discipline, one cannot gather his scattered energy, and all his goals will remain dreams that never materialize. Discipline is not a punishment but a part of growth, without which mental and physical health cannot be maintained.

यदि मामप्रतीकारं अशस्त्रं शस्त्रपाणयः।
धार्तराष्ट्रा रणे हन्युः तन्मे क्षेमतरं भवेत्।। ४६
संजय उवाच
एवमुक्त्वार्जुनः संख्ये रथोपस्थ उपाविशत्।
विसृज्य सशरं चापं शोकसंविग्नमानसः।। ४७

46. *If the sons of Dhritarashtra, with weapons in hand, kill me in the battle while I am unarmed and unavenging, that will be more beneficial to me.*

Sanjaya said

47. Having spoken thus, in the middle of the battle Arjuna sat down on the seat of the chariot, putting away the bow together with the arrows, his mind agitated with grief.

The teachings of the Bhagavad Gita are imparted by Sri Krishna in response to the confusion and despondency of Arjuna. As we have seen, there are many factors that cause Arjuna's despair: (1) He is about to become involved in a heinous war that could destroy the best of men from both camps; (2) The war is between two groups of the same family; (3) Arjuna is fighting against his teachers and elders; (4) He is fighting a fierce battle to regain his and his brothers' rights in the mundane world; and (5) Arjuna is afraid of the destruction of the prevailing order of society and its noble traditions. At the crucial moment when the battle is beginning, these thoughts create a serious dilemma in Arjuna's mind. He is so confused that he cannot discriminate and judge what is right and wrong, what is lawful and unlawful.

Arjuna's mind is so affected that he completely forgets who he is and what his duties are. Confused and dejected, he sinks into grief and casts his bow and arrow aside. Thus, the first chapter has been called *Vishada* yoga, the yoga of dejection or sorrow. The word yoga comes from the Sanskrit root *yuj,* meaning to unite or to join. Here the word yoga has been used in a negative way because Arjuna joins with grief and sorrow rather than with the divine. Patanjali, the codifier of yoga science, describes two kinds of knowledge: right knowledge and wrong knowledge. Right knowledge leads one to positive thinking and experience, whereas wrong knowledge leads one to negativity. Sanjaya's sermon created a negative train of thought in Arjuna's mind. A teacher, counselor, or therapist who is not sincere can misguide and mislead his students.

It is important to carefully study the literature, follow the teachings, and practice the methods of a system for self-transformation. If the methods of sadhana are not well organized, systematized, and methodical, one's mental state can become disturbed. One can then sink into the pool of sorrow instead of reaching the garden of perennial joy. Fortunate are those who are determined to follow the path of Self-realization with sincerity, determination, and a one-pointed mind under the guidance of a preceptor who is selfless, loving, and has already attained Self-realization.

The science of yoga is a scientific and practical exploration of the inner life. It is extremely helpful in self-analysis, self-control, and self-transformation. How can one say that it is not suitable and applicable to modern man? Many are prejudiced against the use of yoga psychology because they have only a superficial knowledge of mental life. Their understanding of the human being is fragmented; they have no insight into higher dimensions of consciousness. It is amazing to note that many contemporary Eastern psychologists have been following in the footsteps of other modern psychologists. That is like forgetting reality and chasing a mirage. Although the system developed by yoga science is thorough and complete, many modern scientists are repelled by the word yoga for no good reason. Mere analytical methods and the study of dreams do not help patients much, for they are not taught how to prevent themselves from becoming victims of external stimuli and internal disorganization. If not properly and systematically guided, an aspirant's mental train is either derailed or runs in a direction contrary to its destination. Arjuna was fortunate to have Yogeshvara Krishna as a guide and counselor to bring him out of that situation.

Here ends the first chapter in which the despondency of Arjuna is described.

Chapter Two
The Way of Self Knowledge

संजय उवाच
तं तथा कृपयाऽऽविष्टमश्रुपूर्णाकुलेक्षणम्।
विषीदन्तमिदं वाक्यमुवाच मधुसूदन:।। १

Sanjaya said

1. *To him who was thus possessed with a pitiful mood, whose eyes were distressed and filled with tears, and who was suffering from sadness, the destroyer of Madhu, Sri Krishna, addressed these words.*

Although Arjuna formerly felt confident of his strength and knew he was capable of destroying his enemy, he lost that awareness when he became overwhelmed with pity. But such pity is merely an outburst of weakness. When one pities others, he identifies himself with those whom he pities, and he is then distracted by the objects of his identification. He identifies with weakness and forgets his true Self. Pity helps neither the one who pities nor the one who is pitied. Arjuna's pity for those on the battlefield led him to pity himself as well.

After making sincere efforts, Arjuna thought there was an

insurmountable barrier in front of him, and he lost his mental balance. Kaṇva Rishi, a sage of the Vedic period, also experienced moments of spiritual turmoil. He had practiced severe austerities and mortifications for many years and had faithfully followed the righteous path of sadhana but was not able to attain his goal. Finally Kaṇva burst into tears and surrendered all human endeavor, thus opening himself to receive the strength that lies beyond the known field of consciousness. When human resources are exhausted, something from beyond comes to one's aid. Sincere efforts and a one-pointed mind with a single desire to know are the keys to attain that experience.

श्री भगवानुवाच

कुतस्त्वा कश्मलमिदं विषमे समुपस्थितम्।
अनार्यजुष्टमस्वर्ग्यम् अकीर्तिकरमर्जुन।। २

क्लैब्यं मा स्म गमः पार्थ नैतत्त्वय्युपपद्यते।
क्षुद्रं हृदयदौर्बल्यं त्यक्त्वोत्तिष्ठ परन्तप।। ३

The Blessed Lord said

2. *From where has this ignominy favored of the ignoble, un-heavenly, and disreputable, entered you at such a troublesome time, O Arjuna?*

3. *Do not lapse into impotency, O Son of Pritha; it does not well behoove you, Abandon this littleness and weakness of the heart and rise, O Scorcher of Enemies.*

On one's journey to self-awakening, he encounters many stumbling blocks and cries for help from the divine or a wise teacher and counselor like Sri Krishna. Arjuna suffers from self-pity and dejection and thus ignores his inner strength, but Sri Krishna makes Arjuna aware of that strength.

A child first learns from his parents and then from his teachers in school, but that education is far from complete. All that he has learned does not bring fulfillment. There is still the role to be played by the spiritual teacher, who is one's greatest friend. Such a friend helps one to overcome the trials and tribulations of life. One purpose of the spiritual teacher is to protect his student with his mighty, tender, and loving arms whenever he is in danger or faces a dilemma.

Responding to Arjuna's state, Sri Krishna, a true friend and great teacher, speaks to him and makes him aware of the need to fulfill his duty. Sri Krishna explains to Arjuna that he has completely forgotten himself and has become a victim of false identification. He says, "A warrior like you should not behave in a cowardly manner. Remember your noble Aryan heritage and perform your duty." The word Arya is a Sanskrit word that means "fully civilized." The Aryans established a most ancient culture that was sustained by a community of individuals who were learned, intellectual, full of wisdom, and who understood life both within and without. The language of the Aryans was Sanskrit, and their vast literature is profound and beautiful. Sri Krishna reminds Arjuna of the glorious past of his ancestors and makes him realize that he is a *kshatriya* (warrior), and not a coward.

Arjuna is in danger, and it is therefore necessary that he immediately assimilate all his scattered energy and overcome his feelings of pity and despondency. All too often the call of one's attachments dissipates the mind, and one forgets the source of power and light that is hidden within. Sri Krishna makes Arjuna aware of the courage that is within him and encourages him to act on the basis of that courage. In the moments of weakness in life, the great ones always restore the courage of their beloved students with their graceful advice.

Three distinct ways of understanding and approaching life are allegorically described in the Bhagavad Gita. First, the Kauravas are dependent on external resources and the physical strength of their army. They represent the materially-oriented perspective, as they are concerned with the external world and are not sensitive to the inner life. Second, Arjuna, a skillful warrior and a true seeker, loses his sense of direction when he forgets the deeper reality and identifies himself with the weak. Because of pity, Arjuna is crippled and unable to use his skills and inner strength. Arjuna is more sensitive and compassionate than the ignorant person who identifies with material existence, but his sensitivity cripples him and makes him ineffective. Third, at the most dangerous period of Arjuna's life, Sri Krishna awakens him to still another level of consciousness, leading him to realize that which will dispel the darkness of his ignorance. In that mode of consciousness one is aware that the immortal Atman is the center of his being. After attaining that awareness, one becomes self-confident and fearless. Understanding these three levels of consciousness makes one aware that compared to inner strength, external strength is of little value. If inner strength is lost or forgotten, one becomes weak, no matter how much external might he possesses.

अर्जुन उवाच
कथं भीष्ममहं संख्ये द्रोणं च मधुसूदन।
इषुभिः प्रतियोत्स्यामि पूजार्हावरिसूदन।। ४

Arjuna said
4. *O Lord Krishna, how can I fight back with arrows against Bhishma and Drona in the battle; they are both worthy of my honor and respect, O Destroyer of Enemies.*

The dialogues between the enlightened ones and their students are revered and recognized as great sources of knowledge. The Upanishads are full of dialogues between the enlightened ones and true seekers. In those dialogues the seeker places all his doubts before his spiritual teacher with profound confidence in him, and the teacher dispels those doubts with his enlightened explanations. Here Arjuna becomes perplexed when he sees face to face his elders and his teachers ready to fight him. He does not understand why those great people should be killed, even though he knows they have lost touch with the higher dimensions of reality and are knowingly supporting an unjust cause simply to prove their loyalty. Upon what should Arjuna act: truth, justice, and dharma; one's so-called self-imposed duty; or attachment, pity, and cowardice? This confusion will be eliminated by the teachings of Sri Krishna.

गुरूनहत्वा हि महानुभावान्
श्रेयो भोक्तुं भैक्ष्यमपीह लोके।
हत्वार्थकामांस्तु गुरूनिहैव
भुञ्जीय भोगान्रुधिरप्रदिग्धान्।। ५

5. *It is indeed better in this world to live by begging than to kill the gurus of great stature. By killing my gurus, I would be attaining only worldly, blood-smeared pleasures and gains, and ignoring righteousness and liberation.*

In this verse Arjuna uses the word *guru* to refer to Bhishma and Drona. Killing a guru or a teacher is the most heinous crime one can imagine. But is he a guru who supports the unjust? In this dialogue it is Sri Krishna alone who is a true guru. Throughout life we learn from many teachers, but there is only one guru. The guru is he who is totally selfless and completely free from greed and the expectation of receiving something from the student. The true guru gives the best he has and never accepts anything from his students. Is there anything that a real guru will not do or has not done selflessly for his students? Selflessness alone is the singular expression of love. Guru is a sacred word that has been misused many times in the past and is completely vulgarized today. To declare that "I am a guru" is a false pronouncement; the modern "guru" is a spiritual joke.

The authentic guru-disciple relationship is the highest of all. The relationship between teacher and student also is worthy of reverence, but in no way can a teacher be called a guru. The actual word that should be used for a guru is *gurudeva,* which means "that bright being who dispels the darkness of ignorance." The gurudeva represents a noble tradition through which flows pure love inseparably mingled with unalloyed knowledge. The Bhagavad Gita is a dialogue in which that profound knowledge is imparted by Sri Krishna, the gurudeva, to his disciple, Arjuna.

Arjuna experiences conflict about whether he should fight the war or follow the path of renunciation. He thinks of abandoning his duty, retiring to a forest dwelling, and living by begging alms. That is a most dangerous tangent for Arjuna, who should prefer to not live than to live in such a condition. Arjuna's thought does not arise out of non-attachment, which is a primary and essential requisite on the path of renunciation. Therefore, he has no right to justify his refusal to fight by using the argument that it would be more appropriate for him to become a renunciate and beg alms. The sort of reasoning that Arjuna offers is not only dangerous to himself but injurious to those innocent students who are just beginning to tread the path and might follow his example. Had Arjuna retired and adopted the life of a renunciate, the noble tradition of renunciation would have been reduced to meaninglessness.

In everyone's life there come such moments when he loses the faculty of discrimination and decisiveness. He wants to escape instead of resolving the conflict. We often see people use spirituality and meditation as means to escape, and many people renounce the world in such a state of uncertainty. But true renunciation is entirely different. It is the highest of all paths trodden by the best of men who have already analyzed the values of life with its currents and cross currents. It is not a path of escapism. Performing one's own actions skillfully is necessary as long as one lives in the world.

न चैतद्विद्मः कतरन्नो गरीयो
यद्वा जयेम यदि वा नो जयेयुः।
यानेव हत्वा न जिजीविषामः
तेऽवस्थिताः प्रमुखे धार्तराष्ट्राः।। ६

6. *Nor do we know which one of us is the more powerful, whether we would win or whether they would win over us. Those, whom upon killing we would have no desire to continue living, the very sons of Dhritarashtra, are standing before us in prominence.*

Arjuna's arguments clearly show his intense uncertainty about whether he should fight or retire. He is obsessed by both the fear of being victorious and the fear of being defeated. Such uncertainty comes when one has lost the sense of discrimination, and such an indecisive person is unable to fight the battle of life.

कार्पण्यदोषोपहतस्वभावः
पृच्छामि त्वां धर्मसम्मूढचेताः।
यच्छ्रेयः स्यान्निश्चितं ब्रूहि तन्मे
शिष्यस्तेऽहं शाधि मां त्वां प्रपन्नम्।। ७
न हि प्रपश्यामि ममापनुद्याद्
यच्छोकमुच्छोषणमिन्द्रियाणाम्।
अवाप्य भूमावसपत्नमृद्धं
राज्यं सुराणामपि चाधिपत्यम्।। ८

7. *My true nature subdued by the fault of miserableness, my mind deluded as to the righteous conduct, I ask you: whatever is definitely better, do tell me that. I am your disciple surrendering to you. Do teach me and guide me.*
8. *I do not see anything that might remove this grief that is drying up my senses—not even a prosperous kingdom without enemies, nor sovereignty over the gods.*

Arjuna admits that his mind is not functioning well; he is full of doubts and is indecisive. One's acknowledgment of his confusion is a step forward, for it shows that he is ready to learn. The student, with full conviction and trust, then places the entire book of his life before his teacher for scrutiny. That is always expected of a good student. If one accepts that he is ignorant, he can be led by a competent teacher because such an aspirant is open to receiving higher knowledge. At that point one has *jigyasa,* which means a strong desire to learn and practice Brahma Vidya. It is an extraordinary moment when one accepts a great teacher as his own, requests the teacher to accept him as a student, and in turn is accepted as a student by the teacher. Sri Krishna, who has always been Arjuna's friend, now becomes his teacher as well. That is a unique relationship.

We learn two lessons from Arjuna's predicament. First, no leader, sadhaka, or hero should take it for granted that he will not slip back to the sorrowful, bewildered state of despondency. Second, in everyone's life there comes a time when he experiences difficulty in deciding that which is right. Great men are great because they do not lose their equanimity in a difficult situation no matter how catastrophic it seems to be. And if there is a temporary state of disturbance or uncertainty, they are able to recover from such a lapse.

One should realize that he can even recover from a serious mental disturbance such as that experienced by Arjuna. Self-confidence can be regained by becoming aware of the deeper dimensions of life. If the system of sadhana is well organized, the sadhaka may stumble, but he will once again tread the path. One finds obstacles in every phase of life, and at times it may seem that one cannot gather his strength. That is only natural in human life. But those like Arjuna who are guided by a great teacher emerge safely from the misery created by the lack of proper perspective.

In his sorrow Arjuna loses his equilibrium and cries plaintively for help. Sri Krishna, possessing perfect knowledge and mastery of all levels and forces of life, brings Arjuna back to the state of equanimity, encouraging Arjuna not to weaken himself, not to be scattered or dissipated.

संजय उवाच
एवमुक्त्वा हृषीकेशं गुडाकेशः परन्तपः ।
न योत्स्य इति गोविन्दं उक्त्वा तूष्णीं बभूव ह ।। ९

Sanjaya said

9. *Arjuna the Master of Sleep, a scorcher of enemies, having uttered this to Krishna, Lord of the Senses, again addressed Govinda (Krishna), saying, 'I shall not fight,' and then lapsed into silence.*

Arjuna asserts that he will not fight, showing that he is not fully prepared to listen to the words of Sri Krishna even though he outwardly professes surrender. Underneath, in the subtle realms, lie lurking seeds of lust, greed, and attachment, the latter being the most powerful. For this reason, the aspirant is unable to follow the advice of his preceptor and enters into arguments with him. Even after a student acknowledges his teacher s spiritual attainment and decides to surrender to him, the surrender is not complete because the student still lacks direct experience. Self-confidence and complete surrender are impossible without direct experience.

Arjuna wants to find a solution to his problem, so he accepts Sri Krishna as his preceptor, although he still has some resistance. In modern psychotherapy, the client also resists. Resistance is a habit that continues to play an important part in the client's life even though he may understand that such a habit is injurious. Resistance occurs because of helplessness and lack of knowledge, so both practice and knowledge are essential.

A disciple is still ignorant even after surrender before the master, for surrender before the teacher is not enlightenment. It is only the primary step. This is essential, but it is far from being complete. At this point Arjuna has not yet received the instructions that will completely free him from his self-created bonds of misery. The darkness is not dispelled by surrendering. Light alone tears the veil of the mist, and that light flows from the eternal stream of knowledge. Accepting a teacher is taking a step toward the light.

A teacher is like a boat that is the essential means to help one cross the mire of delusion. The teacher shares his experiences, making the student aware of the obstacles and stumbling blocks on his journey. A seeker should not delude himself and believe that by accepting someone as a guru or becoming a disciple, he does not have to practice, that he will become enlightened without any effort. Spiritual leaders such as Sri Krishna, Jesus, Moses, and Buddha did not possess the power to enlighten the students who accepted them as their guides but who did not listen, follow, and practice their teachings.

After asserting that he will not fight, Arjuna lapses into silence because of his grief and sorrow. Silence makes the mind one-pointed. So if one is in grief, the grief becomes more intense in silence; if one is in love, silence intensifies the feeling of love; if one is on the path of Self-realization, silence offers no distraction but joy beyond estimation.

Defeatism leads one to retreat to a passive way of being. That is not what is expected of a warrior or aspirant, who should instead set an example for others to follow. Arjuna's refusal to fight is an escape and not a virtue. It is not renunciation, for a renunciate has to burn all mundane desires in the fire of knowledge. Arjuna talks of renunciation without understanding it. In weak moments one may seek an escape and think of renouncing instead of dealing with the issues that are of vital interest to the individual and to society as a whole. One who follows the path of renunciation in such a situation is a coward and an escapist.

Pacifism as it is expressed by Arjuna is an entirely different way of responding to a situation than the philosophy of *ahimsa* (noninjury). In pacifism one has no control over the situation, whereas in ahimsa one expresses the philosophy of love by way of negation: non-injury, non-killing, non-harming, and non-hurting. If one applies the code of ahimsa, an important part of yogic teachings, he will be able to truly love. When one learns how to love with mind, action, and speech, he then starts practicing truth. Love comes first; truth comes afterward. But love and truth are actually synonymous: one is an expression of the truth and the other is truth itself. They are inseparable, like two sides of the same coin.

Mahatma Gandhi, the father of the Indian nation, practiced the teachings of the Bhagavad Gita for more than forty years. He was like a great warrior who set an unparalleled example in the world. Gandhi understood that ahimsa is the law of life and therefore advocated non-violence. But Gandhi was not a pacifist. He actively and assertively led his nation to independence. When one is a failure and is not capable of attaining something, he withdraws. Such pacifism is a product of defeatism and not at all a creative quality. There comes a time in every student's life when he cannot handle a situation, and then he becomes a non-participant. That type of pacifism leads one to inertia and sloth, the greatest of all enemies for the aspirant.

Of course pacifism can arise from an entirely different motivation. To fight a war that is unrighteous, that is not for a just cause, is definitely a heinous crime. Withdrawing from participation in such wars is also a motivation for pacifism. Those who do not wish to fight, kill, or destroy others unjustly have a right to withdraw themselves. That kind of pacifism is healthy.

In the case of Arjuna, war is inevitable, and it is for a just cause. Arjuna is a kshatriya (warrior); his primary duty is to fight. If a renunciate were to join the army and participate in battle, he would not be following his path of dharma (duty). And if a warrior in the midst of a battle were to become a renunciate, it would create great chaos. There would be a serious problem in one's life if the hands and feet were to abandon their respective duties and assume each other's duties. Life would be impossible if the ear tried to see and the eyes to taste. It is important to know one's dharma, to know the right action and the right time. The dharma of Arjuna is to fight and not to retire. Arjuna's thought of renunciation is mere escapism: the thought does not appear until he is on the battlefield. This clearly shows that Arjuna has been unwisely influenced by the counsel of Sanjaya and is unwilling to perform his duties.

तमुवाच हृषीकेशः प्रहसन्निव भारत।
सेनयोरुभयोर्मध्ये विषीदन्तमिदं वचः।। १०

10. To him who was sad, O Descendant of Bharata, there between the two armies, the Lord of the Senses said these words smiling at him:

After Sri Krishna listens attentively to Arjuna, a dignified smile appears on his face. Sri Krishna's smile is like the smile of a father who, even though he sees his child tormented by grief and sorrow, feels confident because he understands that this is only a temporary phase. He knows that after receiving helpful advice, his child will soon come out of his confused emotional state and make great strides toward understanding and balanced action. Sri Krishna does not smile because he pities Arjuna. His smile is a smile of confidence. For Sri Krishna is fully confident that he can bring Arjuna out of his desolation and lead him to Self-realization.

Earlier, Arjuna wanted Sri Krishna to participate in the war, forgetting that he himself is the greatest of all heroes of his time. Sri Krishna, a friend and preceptor, does not want Arjuna to be dependent on the resources of others and encourages him to fight his own battles. Here again the teachings of the Bhagavad Gita are useful to modern man, for modern man tends to be dependent on leaders, teachers, and preceptors. Final emancipation, however, necessitates that one learn to light his own lamp. Sri Krishna agrees to freely advise Arjuna whenever he needs his help, as a selfless teacher lovingly advises his student. He remains with his disciple in the midst of the battlefield, showing him the path and explaining the methods for conquering all the foes that reside in every human mind and heart. A human being is often weak and prone to negative suggestions that are detrimental to his unfoldment, but with determination and selfless advice from a preceptor, one can attain a balanced state of mind.

An important characteristic of both a good teacher and a good psychotherapist is to have empathy for the student's or client's predicament while not identifying with the student or client. It is the responsibility of a guide to lead his student and impart the profound knowledge attained by the guide's own direct experience. In modern psychology the mechanics of therapy focus on solving the obvious problem and on the analysis of certain unconscious conflicts. There is nothing to lead one beyond the conscious and unconscious mind so that he does not repeatedly fall into the trapping tides of the unconscious mind and become overwhelmed by his emotions, thoughts, moods, and reactions. Modern therapists have theoretical knowledge to a certain extent, but they are still caught up in the unresolved issues emanating from their own unconscious. They have not gone through an adequate training program to reach a genuine state of equanimity and tranquility, though they may pose as though they are peaceful and content. Many therapists suffer from the same conflicts and problems as their clients. The Upanishads say, "The blind lead the blind, and there is no hope." In attempting to resolve one's conflicts, it is important to choose the right guide.

The therapy applied by Sri Krishna includes knowledge of the Self, the organization of internal states, the explanation of various methods of sadhana, and the way to perform one's duties skillfully and selflessly. Sri Krishna does not merely deal with the surface problems or the symptoms presented by Arjuna but with Arjuna's whole being from the beginning to its final destiny.

श्री भगवानुवाच
अशोच्यानन्वशोचस्त्वं प्रज्ञावादांश्च भाषसे।
गतासूनगतासूंश्च नानुशोचन्ति पण्डिताः।। ११

The Blessed Lord said
11. *You are grieving about those over whom one should not grieve, and yet you are speaking words of pretended wisdom. The wise do not grieve about those who are yet breathing nor about those who have ceased to breathe.*

Aspirants can be divided into three categories. Students in these three categories have different qualities, and their strengths are on different levels. The first kind of aspirant is like an elephant that is very powerful but is unable to separate sugar from sand. Such an aspirant is unable to distinguish what is helpful from what is harmful to his growth, what is real from what is illusory and binding. Another type of student is like the ant that makes great efforts and is capable of separating sugar from sand but has no capacity to store what it has gained. Such an aspirant repeatedly slips back to the point from which he started. The third type of aspirant may be compared to the bee that is able to collect the sweetness from the flowers and transform it into honey. Such a student comprehends and assimilates the truths that are offered and continues to apply them in his daily life. Arjuna fits within the third category of students. He is open and ready to integrate the teachings of Brahma Vidya into his own life. Thus, Sri Krishna begins to impart that perennial knowledge to Arjuna, and that knowledge leads him to understand that his grief and sorrow are based on his sense of false identity and strong attachment.

Sri Krishna, the teacher of Brahma Vidya, first makes Arjuna aware of the center of consciousness, Atman. He teaches Arjuna that if he constantly remains aware of that center, he will not go back to the grooves of his past habit patterns. Arjuna reasons as though he is a wise man, but in actuality he is mourning and deep in sorrow. Wise is he who has learned to discriminate truth from untruth and who is not disturbed by the past or by what he imagines will occur in the future. Such a man understands that past, present, and future are merely realities created by the human mind, which is frail and weak. A wise man has profound knowledge of all dimensions of life and is free from all conditionings of the mind. He understands the mystery of birth and death. A wise man is he who has attained the knowledge of Atman.

In this verse two words are important and informative: *gatasu* and *agatasu*. *Gatasu* means the dead and comes from two roots: *gata* (gone) and *asu* (breath). *Agatasu* means not dead, literally, "whose breath is not gone." The living are those who are still breathing, and the dead are those whose two breaths, inhalation and exhalation, have abandoned the city of life. Death is just the casting off of one unit of the entire composite that makes up the human being, that part which is considered to be mortal. Death and birth are two strong habits of the body; they have nothing to do with annihilation. Death does not annihilate the essential; it merely brings about a change of the coverings around it. Assuming a new covering is called birth, and casting off the old is called death. There is no death for the Atman because: (1) Atman is eternal; it is never born and never dies; it is a perennial source of knowledge; (2) Atman is self-existent and does not need the support of anything else, for Atman alone exists everywhere; and (3) Atman is formless: although it assumes and casts off forms, it remains unaffected.

The great teachers first make their students aware of two distinct realities. One is called the absolute Reality, and the other is called the apparent reality. They are like light and shadow. With the help of that discriminative knowledge, the student becomes fearless and determines to remove the barrier created by his limited knowledge.

Sri Krishna's first advice to Arjuna is to develop clarity of mind and skill in dealing with the external world while at the same time understanding that the temporal and mundane world is merely the apparent reality. Without comprehensive knowledge of both the absolute and apparent realities, the discriminative faculty is not able to function properly, and strong habit patterns create a network of entanglement that draws the consciousness to external awareness.

In the Indian system of psychology, the student is led beyond mental life. Mind in its totality should be understood, but it is more important to be aware of the source of knowledge, the center of consciousness, Atman. Knowledge of Brahma Vidya is essential for learning the psychology of the East. If one studies only the conscious and unconscious parts of the mind and analyzes only the waking, dreaming, and sleeping states, he will be unable to comprehend the perennial psychology of the Bhagavad Gita.

Ancient psychologists thoroughly studied both psychology and philosophy, which are separate subjects but are essentially connected. The second chapter of the Bhagavad Gita, beginning with this verse and going through Verse 38, teaches *Samkhya* philosophy, the most ancient system of the seven schools of Indian philosophy. The word Samkhya means "that which explains the whole." It is an analysis of all levels of life and the universe and is the very basis of yogic science. *Yoga* is a practical science and is supported by Samkhya philosophy. Samkhya philosophy has given birth to the science of mathematics, the very basis of all sciences. Thus, Samkhya philosophy is the mother of all sciences, and yoga science is its practical side. They are one and the same, but one offers the formulas and conclusions, while the other is experiential and experimental.

न त्वेवाहं जातु नासं न त्वं नेमे जनाधिपाः।

न चैव न भविष्यामः सर्वे वयमतः परम्।। १२

देहिनोऽस्मिन्यथा देहे कौमारं यौवनं जरा।

तथा देहान्तरप्राप्तिर्धीरस्तत्र न मुह्यति।। १३

12. *There never was a time, indeed, when I was not, nor you, nor these rulers of people, nor shall we all from this moment on ever cease to be.*

13. *As in the body of this body-bearer (Atman) there is childhood, youth, and old age, so there occurs the transfer to another body. A wise one does not become confused in this matter.*

There is nothing that loses its existence. Existence is never lost, changed, or subject to destruction. That which changes is the form. After one becomes aware of the center of consciousness, Atman, he understands that at the core of his being, he is unchangeable and indestructible. When Sri Krishna instructs Arjuna not to grieve, he is leading him from the temporal and mundane to the absolute Reality, which alone is truth.

Sri Krishna tells Arjuna that both he and Arjuna have lived before, and that there was never a time that they were not. Life is an eternal wave in the infinite realm of eternity; it is a timeless reality. If one becomes aware of that, he is free from sorrow. Ordinarily human beings have only knowledge and awareness of the mortal part of life. They think and talk within the apparent reality where death and birth are experienced. But when a student becomes conscious of the nontemporal, unchangeable, and timeless reality, he is no longer fearful of death and birth, which are only experienced in the world of names and forms.

The names and forms constantly change: birth and death are two names for the changes of form that one experiences in this world. But Atman never changes. It remains one and the same in birth, death, and in all stages of one's growth. A wise man is not at all perplexed by the death of the body, for he knows that Atman never dies.

मात्रास्पर्शास्तु कौन्तेय शीतोष्णसुखदुःखदाः।
आगमापायिनोऽनित्याः तांस्तितिक्षस्व भारत।। १४
यं हि न व्यथयन्त्येते पुरुषं पुरुषर्षभ।
समदुःखसुखं धीरं सोऽमृतत्वाय कल्पते।। १५

14. *The contacts between the elements, O Son of Kunti, are the causes of heat, cold, pleasure, and pain. Being non-eternal, these come and go; learn to withstand them, O Descendant of Bharata.*
15. *O Bull among Men, the person to whom these do not cause any suffering, the wise man who is alike to pain and pleasure, he alone is ready for the immortal state.*

Birth and death are two of the innumerable pairs of opposites experienced in the phenomenal world. All opposites are illusions, and so is the case with birth and death. All sensory perceptions create pairs of opposites: pain and pleasure, sorrow and joy, heat and cold. When one of the senses contacts an object, a sensation is received that is carried by the nerves to the brain. It is then attended to by the conscious mind and its memory stored in the unconscious. All sense perceptions are filtered by one's conceptualization. So through the senses, the mind receives information in its own way according to the concepts it has created for itself. Perception and conception unite in creating the phenomena that are experienced. The mind functions in the external world with the help of the senses, which are employed by the mind. Arjuna experiences grief and sorrow because he has not learned to master the way in which perceptions and conceptions influence his mind.

Each experience that one has in the phenomenal world has its opposite, and each experience exists only because its opposite exists. Heat is given definition by cold, and pain becomes a distinct experience only when contrasted with its complement, pleasure. If one seeks one of a pair of opposites, he is sure to be equally influenced by the other, for the phenomena always go together as a pair. When one is led to a higher realm of reality from whence he can comprehend how the pairs of opposites arise as a unit, he learns to develop the philosophy of non-attachment and thus is not affected by the influence of opposites.

Sri Krishna makes Arjuna aware that that which is experienced through the senses is transitory and that the cause of his sorrow and grief is his own deluded, unorganized, and disorderly mind. Teachers in the East always insist on the practice of discipline in order for the aspirant to learn to withdraw his senses and thereby to isolate the mind from the effects of perception. It is the objects of the world and the ways one accepts and conceives of them that create the feelings of joy and sorrow. Discipline is a gradual but steady way of self-training that makes the student aware of higher dimensions of life. Without discipline, the dissipated energy of the mind and the unruly behavior of the senses cannot be brought under control.

Many modern psychologists do not understand the importance of discipline. They equate discipline with punishment. Punishment, however, has the opposite effect of discipline: it produces mental strain that in turn creates physical tension. Discipline is self-applied, whereas punishment is imposed on one by others.

Modern students and teachers think that they can accomplish something of significance without practicing discipline, but that is not true. Modern students do not want to discipline themselves, and yet they search out that which is only attainable with discipline. Discipline should not be forced on the student but should be introduced to him. He should understand that discipline is the first prerequisite for organizing one's internal states. Discipline is a leader that helps one verify, analyze, and know the subtler dimensions of life.

Telescopes have immense capacities in the external world to show us countless galaxies. But if one wishes to look inward to study his thoughts, feelings, and desires, the telescope is of no use. An instrument should be used for the purpose it was designed to accomplish. Self-discipline is an instrument for becoming aware of and mastering one's internal states. The discipline that helps one gather the dissipated and scattered forces of mind should be accepted and practiced regularly. Otherwise the human mind deprives itself of the awareness of the higher dimensions of life.

Arjuna has not yet been introduced by his teacher to the discipline that would enable him to remain unaffected by the pairs of opposites. Here the great teacher. Sri Krishna, helps Arjuna understand that the reality created by sense perception and conception is but momentary and superficial, and that he should not build his philosophy of life on the values created by that mind which knows nothing about discipline.

नासतो विद्यते भावो नाभावो विद्यते सतः।
उभयोरपि दृष्टोऽन्तस्त्वनयोस्तत्त्वदर्शिभिः।। १६
अविनाशि तु तद्विद्धि येन सर्वमिदं ततम्।
विनाशमव्ययस्यास्य न कश्चित्कर्तुमर्हति।। १७

16. *That which is nonexistent never comes into being; that which is existent never goes to non-being. The seers of reality have seen the very end of both of these.*
17. *Know that as indestructible by which all this tangible world is permeated No one has the power to bring to destruction this unalterable entity.*

We live in two realities at the same time. One is within the field of ordinary human consciousness; the other is in the unconscious and even beyond. Only that which is nonexistent, temporal, transitory, and changeable is conceivable by the mind. But that which is self-existent cannot be grasped or known by the mind. It will always exist because it is the self-existent, absolute, and unchangeable reality. That which is existent is called *sat*, and that which is nonexistent is called *asat*—the real and the unreal. The wise seers are aware of these two realities and say that that which is not self-existent (here called nonexistent for it is insubstantial) cannot exist in all times. Therefore, Arjuna is told not to grieve for the nonexistent but to remain constantly aware of the self-existent reality.

The aspirant should understand that in principle there are two distinct realities, the eternal and the transitory. He should practice the habit of not identifying himself with the ever-changing objects of the world. Such identification deprives one of awareness of his essential nature as Atman, pure consciousness. The center of consciousness, the source of wisdom, happiness, and bliss, is indestructible. It is the only existence, and it is imperishable.

The minds of modern students are not clear about the distinction between these two realities. Therefore, they have no aim. Instead of going in the right direction, they go in the opposite direction, toward the world of names and forms. Instead of being happy, they become confused and suffer. Unless one has a profound knowledge of his destination, treading the path is a waste of time. But if one prepares himself by practicing discipline and at the same time has the comprehensive knowledge of the ultimate goal of life, he can reach His destination by following the positive signs and symptoms.

अन्तवन्त इमे देहा नित्यस्योक्ताः शरीरिणः।
अनाशिनोऽप्रमेयस्य तस्मादयुद्ध्यस्व भारत।। १८

18. *Belonging to the unmeasurable, imperishable, eternal owner of the body, these bodies are said to be perishable; therefore fight, O Descendant of Bharata.*

Sri Krishna teaches Arjuna about the unchangeable nature of Atman and the temporal and perishable nature of the body and the external world. Atman has the power to assume any form it likes. All of those forms can be destroyed, but the eternal, incomprehensible Atman is not subject to any alteration. It has the power to assume any body, but still it is not the body. It is without beginning or end *(nitya)*, whereas the body is perishable and transient *(anitya)*. It is characteristic of the body to undergo a series of changes between birth and death, and, in actuality, one experiences death many times in the course of the changes that occur during his lifetime. For a seed to sprout it has to die in its form as a seed. Then alone can it sprout. All new forms come about through the death of an old form. Therefore, we should accept death as an essential reality of life, but we do not. We know that things die, but we do not accept death. There is no cause for sorrow, for Atman is imperishable.

Arjuna is a most powerful and skilled warrior, and he wants to know the highest duty, that which needs to be attended to first. "Shall I fight or not? Shall I continue performing my duties or follow the path of renunciation?" That is Arjuna's conflict. Sri Krishna frees Arjuna from the bondage created by his ignorance, self-pity, despondency, and attachment. He makes Arjuna aware that it is his duty to fight, not to retreat to the forest dwellings, escaping from the reality of life. Even in the path of renunciation, one has moments of confusion about that which has the highest priority. In all conditions of life, whether one prefers to follow the path of action or renunciation, he should learn to understand his duties.

After studying this verse, the unwise and the wicked may conclude that the Bhagavad Gita justifies killing. Such a conclusion shows a lack of understanding of the depth of the teachings and the way in which they are applied. The situation of Arjuna is entirely different from that of a person who is controlled by violent emotions and thus wants to justify his act with the help of the scriptures. Violence is not at all the subject matter of the Bhagavad Gita. The Bhagavad Gita does not say "kill anyone you dislike" but teaches that one should not be afraid to die while performing his duties.

When a doctor uses his surgical knife, he has no intention of killing. He just wants to remove the abscess that can disturb or destroy his patient's whole frame of life. However, when a butcher kills a goat, he has a different intention: he wants to use the goat for his own selfish ends. When a warrior fights to establish the good conduct of life and the highest virtues—justice, truth, and harmony, killing is of an entirely different nature. In that situation refusing to fight is an escape, a disease brought about by mental imbalance. And when mental balance is lost, the whole battle of life is lost.

य एनं वेत्ति हन्तारं यश्चैनं मन्यते हतम्।
उभौ तौ न विजानीतो नायं हन्ति न हन्यते।। १९
न जायते म्रियते वा कदाचिन्नायं
भूत्वाऽभविता वा न भूयः।
अजो नित्यः शाश्वतोऽयं पुराणो
न हन्यते हन्यमाने शरीरे।। २०
वेदाविनाशिनं नित्यं य एनमजमव्ययम्।
कथं स पुरुषः पार्थं कं घातयति हन्ति कम्।। २१

19. *He who thinks the embodied One to be a slayer and he who thinks the embodied One to be slain, neither of them knows correctly. The embodied One neither kills nor is he killed.*
20. *He is never born nor does He die, nor having been, does He ever again cease to be. Unborn, eternal, perennial, this ancient One is not killed when the body is killed.*
21. *He who knows this as imperishable, eternal, unborn, unalterable—how can that person, O Son of Pritha, kill, and whom can he kill or cause to be killed?*

The ignorant think that a human being has the capacity to slay, and that he himself can be slain. These two erroneous conceptions rob one of his inner strength. But when one knows the truth, that Atman cannot be slain, he becomes free from the self-created bondage of his ignorance. For a detailed description of how that bondage is created, one can study *kala* (the time factor) in the twenty-fifth chapter, the *Shanti*

Parva, of the Mahabharata. The time factor is the prime conditioner of the human mind. It is the task of the aspirant to release himself from this conditioning and to attain the timeless state in which there is neither fear nor death nor conditioning. That experience is possible if one systematically practices the inward methods that lead him to the Source, instead of going toward the external world and becoming scattered. There are only three known methods explored by the sages: prayer, meditation, and contemplation. There is yet another way: revelation, which is not a method, for it comes through grace. No external method of knowing can lead one to the fountainhead of awareness, where infinite knowledge beyond measure resides. After attaining that infinite knowledge, one understands that the absolute Reality or Truth is never lost, no matter how many deaths one experiences in his physical and mental life.

In the 20th and 21st verses, which are also essentially found in the Katha Upanishad, one is taught that the Atman is never born and never dies, though it apparently seems to be born and to die. That which is eternal always exists, so it cannot be born. It is ancient, but it appears young, for the body repeatedly comes into being anew. The ignorant confuse the changes of the body with the attributeless pure Self, Atman. But despite the changes of the body, the Eternal remains unchanged.

वासांसि जीर्णानि यथा विहाय
नवानि गृह्णाति नरोऽपराणि।
तथा शरीराणि विहाय जीर्णानि
अन्यानि संयाति नवानि देही।। २२

22. As a man taking off worn out garments later puts on new ones, similarly the Owner of the body, abandoning worn out bodies, enters other new ones.

Suppose we put on various colored lenses one by one. We will see the same thing but in a different light. If we go on changing the angles of our vision along with the lenses, things will look entirely different each time. Actually things are not seen as they are; therefore they are not known the way they are. If the objects of the world are not observed and analyzed thoroughly, one's attitude toward objects will be superficial and distorted. So is the case with human relationships. Human relationships create bondage because the human mind is in the habit of identifying itself with the external world, which is conditioned by time and is continually changing. Yet people ignore that fact and become attached to one another. Misery, bondage, and fear spring from the ties of attachment, and attachment prevents one from remaining aware of the realities of human life.

Fear, which is based on the urge for self-preservation, predominates in our emotional life. Its roots are deeply buried in the unconscious mind, which governs one's conscious activities throughout life. The fear of death constantly remains in the mind of every human being. That fear occurs when body consciousness predominates. All the fears in human life spring from an externally-oriented consciousness.

After one fully examines nature and the objects of the world and analyzes man's relationship with man and the creatures of the world, he still finds that his knowledge is incomplete. He is not satisfied and content with knowing life only in the external world. There is still a desire to know the whole. One wants to explore the higher dimensions of life and turns his mind within. There the world seems to be entirely different—full of images, symbols, ideas, fancies, and fantasies, sometimes in distorted and incomplete forms. If during that time a proper and exact method is not devised, one's increasing awareness of the fleeting nature of the objects of the world leads him to become more confused. We use many branches of science and many methods for analyzing the external world. But there are also many fields within, and there are many methods for exploring the inner world. The competent and experienced teacher imparts definite approaches and methods for probing into the subtler aspects of life. No external means whatsoever help in this journey. It is the journey from the known to the unknown.

Arjuna, like any other human being, becomes confused and full of fears that arise from his attachment to relationships. He starts trembling in the midst of a dangerous situation. Sri Krishna makes Arjuna aware of the higher dimensions of life and their relationship to the external world, starting with the body. What is the body to us? Are we only a body, or is there something deeper and more profound for us to comprehend? Examining the body, one observes that it undergoes many changes. Sri Krishna says that the body is like a garment, and the human being is the owner of that garment. When one changes his garment, he continues to exist.

One can easily understand that the center of consciousness, Atman, is overlayed by many coverings. The aspirant should apply the exact scientific methods taught by the ancient scriptures and teachers to attain an understanding of each covering. These methods enable the student to comprehend both the mere self—body, breath, senses, and all the dimensions of mind—and to help him go to the source of consciousness. Before one reaches the fountainhead of life and light from which consciousness flows spontaneously, he has to understand the various realities that exist. He can then conceive of the idea that human beings have many subtle bodies within the physical body.

The dweller within the physical body casts off the worn out external body and has the choice of assuming a new body. He who knows that the center of consciousness is eternal and undiminishable realizes that the ideas of killing and death are merely notions caused by one's long associaton with the body and the objects of the world.

नैनं छिन्दन्ति शस्त्राणि नैनं दहति पावकः।
न चैनं क्लेदयन्त्यापो न शोषयति मारुतः।। २३
अच्छेद्योऽयमदाह्योऽयं अक्लेद्योऽशोष्य एव च।
नित्यः सर्वगतः स्थाणुः अचलोऽयं सनातनः।। २४
अव्यक्तोऽयमचिन्त्योऽयं अविकार्योऽयमुच्यते।
तस्मादेवं विदित्वैनं नानुशोचितुमर्हसि।। २५

23. *Weapons do not cleave Him, fire does not burn Him, the waters do not wet Him, nor does the wind dry Him.*

24. *He is uncleavable, unburnable, cannot be made wet, nor can He be made dry; the Eternal, all-permeating, absolute, and unmoving: He is the ancient One.*

25. *He is unmanifest, is not the subject of thought, and is said to be incorruptible; therefore, knowing Him, it does not behoove you to grieve after anyone.*

The eternal center of consciousness is infinite and all-pervasive. It encompasses all. Therefore, nothing has the power to cut It into pieces. Fire has no power to burn It, and It is impervious to water and wind. The infinite Atman dwells with all its glory and majesty in the innermost chamber of the human being. Knowing this truth, the wise never grieve. Sri Krishna leads Arjuna toward the fountainhead of knowledge of immortality and thereby helps him attain freedom from all fetters.

Certain verses of the Bhagavad Gita are exactly like those of the Upanishads. The student should understand that the knowledge of the Bhagavad Gita is a modified version of the Upanishads and the Vedas. The great teachers throughout human history have modified that knowledge to make it more accessible to the students of their time and culture. The flowers are the same; it is only the vases that change, and the style of arranging the flowers depends upon the ability of the artist. Knowledge is perennial because its source is eternal.

The beauty of a good teacher is in the way he imparts wisdom, but the teacher's effort is only fifty percent. The other fifty percent is the effort sincerely made by the sadhaka. Arjuna is receptive, one-pointed, and sincere, and he is able to comprehend the perennial knowledge Sri Krishna imparts. It is a true statement that when the student is ready, the master will appear. If one is truly desirous to know, then he will know. Truth and knowledge are one and the same, and that tremendous, inconceivable, immeasurable power comes to the aid of the sadhaka when he has learned to have only one burning desire: to know the Truth.

अथ चैनं नित्यजातं नित्यं वा मन्यसे मृतम्।
तथापि त्वं महाबाहो नैनं शोचितुमर्हसि।। २६
जातस्य हि ध्रुवो मृत्युः ध्रुवं जन्म मृतस्य च।
तस्मादपरिहार्येऽर्थे न त्वं शोचितुमर्हसि।। २७
अव्यक्तादीनि भूतानि व्यक्तमध्यानि भारत।
अव्यक्तनिधनान्येव तत्र का परिदेवना।। २८

26. *Now if you believe that this soul is born each time with the birth of a new body, or that it is eternal, or you believe that it dies upon the death of the body, even then, O Mighty-armed One, you should not grieve thus.*
27. *The death of one born is definite, and the (re-)birth of one dead is also definite. Therefore, in such an unavoidable matter you should not grieve.*
28. *O Descendant of Bharata, beings have their beginning in the unmanifest, in the middle they are manifest, and they end in the unmanifest. Indeed, what is there to wail about?*

To strengthen a *bhava* (positive feeling), one makes all possible attempts to reverse his mental state from its ordinary course, and to become aware of the Self, Atman. This fact should be assimilated by the mind: one who is born is sure to die. Death is inevitable. When one grieves for the dead or dying, it is because of his attachment to the temporal and because of lack of awareness of the eternal. That is why an aspirant should direct all his energy–external and internal, gross and subtle—toward transforming himself so that he gives up his identification with the body and the external world and realizes his identity as the eternal and unchanging Consciousness. Self-transformation is not only a possibility or probability but the single goal of life. The purpose of all spiritual paths is to attain that goal. If it is not attained, the highest of all joys cannot be experienced.

We can easily understand and unveil the mystery of death with a simile. In our everyday speech, we use the expression: the sun rises and the sun sets. The rising sun is like birth, and the setting sun is like death. The idea of the sun rising and setting is taught all over the world. But in fact, the sun never rises and never sets. It is always there. Because of the poverty of our sense perception and our limited perspective, we experience the sun as though it rises and sets. So is the case with the two important events of life: birth and death. In actuality, one is never born and never dies. Birth and death are limited conceptions that arise from the limited knowledge of our minds. Sri Krishna continues his teaching, saying that the bodies that are loved and are dear to us are merely a part of the grand illusion created by our limited vision of the whole.

The 28th verse uses the word *bhuta*, which means being born. When something appears in the world, it does not come out of nowhere without any cause. The expression "one is born" means that the same one who existed before has chosen to assume a new garment. In this way one comes from the unseen to the seen, from the unknown to the known, from the invisible to the visible world. That which is hidden behind the curtain comes forward, and that is called *janma* (birth). This law of life is applicable to all. Birth and death is not a mystery to one who has access to travel on all levels of life.

Anything that occurs in the visible world has its roots in the invisible. Life is like a sentence with many commas, semicolons, and exclamations, but it does not have a period. This never-ending sentence composes a manuscript whose beginning and end are lost. But the middle pages of the manuscript remain with us. By thoroughly studying this fragment, one can catch the thread of the infinite and touch the eternal.

आश्चर्यवत्पश्यति कश्चिदेनं
आश्चर्यवद्वदति तथैव चान्यः।
आश्चर्यवच्चैनमन्यः शृणोति
श्रुत्वाप्येनं वेद न चैव कश्चित्।। २९
देही नित्यमवध्योऽयं देहे सर्वस्य भारत।
तस्मात्सर्वाणि भूतानि न त्वं शोचितुमर्हसि।। ३०

29. *One sees it as a wonder, another speaks of it as a wonder, yet another fears it as a wonder, and yet another hears of it as a wonder. But even someone hearing of it does not come to know it.*
30. *This body-bearer in everyone's body is eternally undestroyable, O Descendant of Bharata. Therefore, you should not grieve after any and all beings.*

All beings exist in an invisible state and then come to a state of visibility. Changes occur only on the surface, for the self-existent glory remains unchanged; changing form does not affect the self-existent Reality. Atman, the Self of all, dwells in all that is perishable, yet It remains imperishable. Sri Krishna imparts this knowledge to Arjuna and makes him aware of the great marvel, Atman. Those who experience Atman completely lose awareness of the external and go into deep contemplation. All words are lost to them, for mere words are inadequate to describe the unfathomable glory of Atman.

The wise do not grieve for either the visible or invisible, seen or unseen. Weapons have no power to destroy the Self. Therefore, there is no cause for grief. As the Isha Upanishad states, "The unborn, free from change, decay, and decomposition, Lord of the body, eternal Purusha is not capable of being killed. It is smaller than the smallest and bigger than the biggest." The Katha Upanishad describes it thus: "Many do not have the opportunity to hear about the Self and even after hearing, many are unable to know It. It is a rare opportunity for a teacher to expound that knowledge to one who is fully prepared, for among thousands of aspirants rarely one strives for perfection."

Imparting the knowledge of Brahma Vidya is the most difficult of all tasks for the following reasons: (1) Students cannot organize their internal states due to lack of discipline, and thus their mental energy remains dissipated; (2) The desire to know Truth is only one of many desires of the human mind, and without a single and one-pointed desire, one is not able to direct the course of his life; (3) The modern way of life distracts one with many preoccupations and involvements; (4) One does not find a suitable and quiet environment for sadhana; (5) The aspirant is easily swayed by a variety of philosophical statements and concepts, and so due to lack of experience, he changes his way of sadhana; (6) For lack of true and selfless guidance from a competent teacher, the student does not make the decision that sadhana is his prime duty and that all other duties that he has to fulfill are only means to attain the goal of sadhana. The goal of sadhana should be understood comprehensively both in theory and practice before one treads the path. There are many opportunities, to become lost in the inner jungle of thoughts, feelings, and desires; (7) The further the aspirant advances in his experience of the inner levels of life, the greater are the obstacles he finds. One therefore needs considerable patience.

Unless one follows discipline in all levels of life, regulating the four primitive urges—food, sleep, sex, and self-preservation— sadhana is impossible. And without sadhana there is no experience of the Self. Five or ten minutes of practice may give one a bit of solace, but sadhana that is not motivated toward the attainment of constant consciousness does not lead to experiential knowledge. For lack of direct experience, one knows yet does not know. The Upanishads say, "One who believes that Atman can be comprehended through the knowledge of the mind is ignorant."

Many aspirants acquire superficial knowledge from reading books or listening to scholars and then contend that they have acquired profound knowledge, but they are merely feeding their egos. Thus, they create additional barriers instead of removing those that already exist. The ego maintains a fortress all the time. It loses consciousness of the Self and forgets that it is a representative of the Self. That is the prime source of delusion.

One should not merely acquire intellectual knowledge but should practice self-discipline, which is an essential requisite and not a source of stress and strain. It is impossible to perform one's own duty successfully without being disciplined. It is important to note here that modern teachers and leaders are not disciplined themselves but nonetheless try to discipline others. Thus, they are not successful. One must first discipline himself before he can teach others self-discipline.

स्वधर्ममपि चावेक्ष्य न विकम्पितुमर्हसि।
धर्म्याद्धि युद्धाच्छ्रेयोऽन्यत्क्षत्रियस्य न विद्यते।। ३१
यदृच्छया चोपपन्नं स्वर्गद्वारमपावृतम्।
सुखिनः क्षत्रियाः पार्थ लभन्ते युद्धमीदृशम्।। ३२

31. *Seeing your righteous duty you should not tremble, for there is nothing better for a warrior than a righteous battle.*
32. *Happy are the warriors who find such a battle that has come of its own momentum and is like an open door to heaven.*

Sri Krishna explains to Arjuna that one's duty is of paramount importance, for it is the means to fulfill the purpose of life. That which supports the fulfillment of one's duty is called *dharma*. The word dharma carries a deep and profound meaning. Dharma is not comparable to religion; it encompasses all the dimensions of life both within and without. It is applied in every phase of life, as it refers to duties done harmoniously, skillfully, selflessly, and lovingly. It supports one in fulfilling the purpose of life and helps one to relate to others and to society in a harmonious way.

At some point every human being becomes confused about his dharma or duty. Arjuna, a warrior who specializes in the science and art of war, should learn to practice and perform his duty, so Sri Krishna instructs him not to think of renouncing his dharma. Instead he shows him the path to follow in order to fulfill his dharma. For Arjuna, fighting the war is the only dharma that can open the gate of heaven for him. All the heavenly joys can be experienced if one learns how to perform his dharma. As it is used here, heaven means knowledge of the higher dimensions, which frees one from the apparent reality of the external world. All great traditions of the world conceive of a heaven that one may attain after death. But those who understand the science and art of death and dying can glimpse the life hereafter while still living.

When one learns to study the past, present, and future as different parts of one whole, he can have a vision of life hereafter, for whatever one was before, that he is today, and the way one directs the course of his life today will create his future. After death the individual soul does not go to heaven or hell but remains in the atmosphere created by his habit patterns. Negative habits lead to unpleasant experiences, which are called hell, and positive habits lead to pleasant or heavenly experiences. Heaven is a predetermined factor that one creates in his unconscious where the habit patterns of merit and demerit remain lively. No external agent can force another to go to hell or heaven. Heaven and hell are realities that one creates with his thoughts, deeds, and habit patterns.

अथ चेत्त्वमिमं धर्म्यं संग्रामं न करिष्यसि।
ततः स्वधर्मं कीर्तिं च हित्वा पापमवाप्स्यसि।। ३३

33. *And, if you will not do this righteous battle, then abandoning your duty as well as glory, you will be incurring sin.*

Sri Krishna tells Arjuna that if he casts off his duties, he will incur sin. Although this word is used by orthodox religions all over the world, it has baffled the theologians of all great traditions. The fear of sin is so deeply ingrained that even after long austerities, penance, and confessions, one still has guilt feelings. The belief in sin creates guilt, and guilt creates fear of punishment.

Yoga science understands sin in a different light. It says that that which is called sin is actually a behavior that creates obstacles for oneself, and that behavior can be modified. For example, if I fail to act lovingly 1 am not committing a sin that will be punished by an external agent, but 1 am erecting a barrier to my realization of my unity with all. That in itself is its own punishment, and by changing that behavior my suffering is dissolved. One should, therefore, make sincere efforts rather than focusing on punishment and becoming afraid. According to yoga science, sin arises from ignorance, which is the mother of all problems. One commits sins or creates obstacles because of his negative habits.

When one knows that a particular act will bring disastrous results yet dismisses that truth, he is doing something out of habit that he should not do. Knowledge means one knows and knows that he knows, and he performs his duties in accordance with that knowledge and then does not create obstacles for himself. Sri Krishna tells Arjuna that if he does not perform his duty he will create obstacles that will prevent him from fulfilling the purpose of his life.

अकीर्तिं चापि भूतानि कथयिष्यन्ति तेऽव्ययाम्।
संभावितस्य चाकीर्तिः मरणादतिरिच्यते।। ३४
भयाद्रणादुपरतं मंस्यन्ते त्वां महारथाः।
येषां च त्वं बहुमतो भूत्वा यास्यसि लाघवम्।। ३५
अवाच्यवादांश्च बहून्वदिष्यन्ति तवाहिताः।
निन्दन्तस्तव सामर्थ्यं ततो दुःखतरं नु किम्।। ३६
हतो वा प्राप्स्यसि स्वर्गं जित्वा वा भोक्ष्यसे महीम्।
तस्मादुत्तिष्ठ कौन्तेय युद्धाय कृतनिश्चयः।। ३८

34. *People will be telling unglorious things of you forever, and such ill repute of someone once honored is worse than even death.*
35. *The great commanders of chariots will believe you to have withdrawn from the battle out of fear. Having been much thought of, you will be belittled in their eyes.*
36. *Those who wish you ill will speak much evil of you, despising your capacity. What can be more painful than that?*
37. *Either, having been killed, you will attain heaven, or having won, you will enjoy the earth. Therefore rise, O Son of Kunti, making the decision to do battle.*

Those who fail to perform their duties consciously and skillfully attain nothing and are not respected in society. They are bad examples to others, bringing about the disorganization of society. Sri Krishna leads

Arjuna to the innermost dimensions of life and at the same time makes him aware that his worldly duties should not be ignored. When a person ignores his duties, others think disparagingly of him. Ill fame influences one and creates an inferiority complex. And when one realizes that it is his own mistake that brought ill fame to him, his inner strength is weakened. One begins to condemn himself, and suicidal tendencies may develop. We often see great politicians suffering from such disastrous effects of public opinion. Those who are stung by negative suggestions become disturbed and unsuccessfully try to protect their self-esteem.

In all situations the aspirant should learn to maintain his inner strength, but inner strength cannot be maintained if there is inner conflict and if there is no clarity of mind. When one is decisive, he preserves his inner strength. Sri Krishna therefore instructs Arjuna to resolve his conflicts and to perform his duty. He explains to Arjuna that there is no reason to fear being slain in battle, for he will then attain heaven. And if he is victorious, he will enjoy the kingdom of the earth. Sri Krishna makes Arjuna aware that it is his duty to fight the just war, that his path is the path of righteousness. Arjuna, after all, is a kshatriya, a warrior. The word kshatriya means one who fights for justice and truth and protects others from injury. Sri Krishna's instructions and guidance strengthen Arjuna's inner awareness, lead him to perform his duty, and provide a great lesson for those who have lost their direction because of the fear of killing or being killed.

सुखदुःखे समे कृत्वा लाभालाभौ जयाजयौ।
ततो युद्धाय युज्यस्व नैवं पापमवाप्स्यसि।। ३८

38. *Holding pleasure and pain, gain and loss, victory and defeat to be the same, make ready for battle. Thus you will not incur sin.*

Pain and pleasure are two opposites that we experience in daily life, but they are relative terms. When one sees the horizon through the window, it appears very limited, but when one goes to the roof, he finds a vast horizon around him. In the same way, when one learns to expand his vision, the meaning of pain and pleasure also changes. Pain and pleasure are two concepts created by our mind and senses when they contact the objects of the world. But when the sense of discrimination is applied, they vanish because one's values change. Pain and pleasure change their values when one attains a higher dimension of life. One feels pain and pleasure according to his inner strength, endurance, tolerance, and purpose in life. One's experience of pain and pleasure is dependent on what is important to him. For example, a mother experiences pain when she gives birth to a baby, but she goes through that pain because she wants to accomplish something higher.

Pain and pleasure have the same source. In the absence of one, the other appears. For example, if one loses his pen he feels emotional pain, but finding it gives a pleasant feeling. That which creates pain today can be a source of joy in the future.

Sri Krishna explains to Arjuna that he should transcend both pleasure and pain and attain a state of equilibrium. He urges Arjuna to let go of the pain he is experiencing because of his narrowmindedness. Pleasure and pain, victory and defeat, gain and loss should be regarded with detachment and equanimity. Sri Krishna tells Arjuna to stand and fight with an inner peace based on that understanding.

In the modern world people become confused about what is right, and they are uncertain about which duties should be given the highest priority. The important is always important; therefore it should be attended to first even though it may seem to be painful. In performing one's duty one should learn to go beyond his identification with pleasure and pain, loss and gain, and all the pairs of opposites.

एषा तेऽभिहिता सांख्ये बुद्धिर्योगे त्विमां शृणु।
बुद्ध्या युक्तो यया पार्थ कर्मबन्धं प्रहास्यसि।। ३९
नेहाभिक्रमनाशोऽस्ति प्रत्यवायो न विद्यते।
स्वल्पमप्यस्य धर्मस्य त्रायते महतो भयात्।। ४०

39. *This wisdom I have told you according to the philosophy of Samkhya; now hear it according to Yoga, the wisdom joined with which, O Son of Pritha, you will abandon the bondage of karma.*

40. *There is no loss of initiative on this path nor is there any possibility of failure. Even a little of this discipline protects one from great danger and fear.*

Sri Krishna has taught Arjuna the philosophy of Samkhya, which helps one to know that which is the Self and to distinguish It from the non-Self. Now he begins his teaching of yoga science. Samkhya philosophy teaches that the Self of all is eternal and immortal and that the world of objects is transitory and changeable. Samkhya is a philosophy, whereas yoga is the profound science of sadhana that applies that philosophy. Samkhya and yoga go hand in hand; without sadhana, philosophy remains mere speculation, and without philosophy, sadhana remains without a goal. When Samkhya and yoga are combined, one experiences the philosophical truths directly; they are no longer mere intellectual concepts. By practicing yoga one can apply the philosophical truths of Samkhya in his daily life.

The path of yoga teaches those disciplines of sadhana that help the aspirant in self-unfoldment. Yoga in action means well-disciplined and skillful action done in a non-attached way, without any expectation of the fruits of one's actions. Sri Krishna, the exemplary teacher of yoga science, explains how to develop equanimity and perform actions skillfully. In the Isha Upanishad the Vedic sages advocate the same way of performing actions: "Find delight by renouncing the fruits of your actions. Do not covet. If you wish to live a long life, learn to perform your actions without attachment."

While following the path of dharma and truth, one can temporarily become confused and commit a mistake, but the quest for dharma and truth will in itself lead him back to right understanding. He will once more perform his duties according to his dharma. Following his dharma helps one to be one-pointed in his thoughts and actions, whereas dissipated and endless are the thoughts and actions of the irresolute. Furthermore, the conscious effort one makes to follow his dharma has an enduring effect. It is motivation that is important here. Having a pure motive, one will perform his duty well.

In the path of sadhana no effort is in vain; all sincere efforts bear their fruits in the unconscious mind according to the inevitable law of *karma*. Impressions live in the unconscious, in the storehouse of one's memory. Even a little sadhana practiced with sincere effort leaves deep imprints in the unconscious mind. Those impressions help and guide the sadhaka whenever he goes off the path. The conscious part of the mind is but a small part of the whole. It is helpful in communicating with the external world but has very little use on the inward journey. If the conscious part of the mind is trained not to create further barriers, then sadhana is useful.

Yoga sadhana alone has explored all the unknown levels of life and is thus useful for knowing the levels of the unconscious and for training the totality of the mind. Although modern depth psychology has come a long way in the last one hundred years in its recognition and exploration of a few of the layers of the unconscious mind, there is no training program in any of the educational and therapeutic systems of the world that can help one know the unconscious to the extent that yoga science can. If one does not know himself on all dimensions, how can he understand his relationships in the external world? Sadhana alone is the way of knowing, understanding, and analyzing the internal states and one's relationship to the external world.

While treading the path of the inner world, the sadhaka comes in touch with those potentialities that guide him unconsciously, or sometimes through dreams, and at other times consciously. Fearlessness thus increases, and self-reliance is strengthened. He is fully protected by the finer forces that exist, although he is not aware of them because of his extroverted nature. No danger can ever befall the sincere sadhaka in his exploration of the inner realms. The sadhaka is completely protected if he is fully dedicated to the goal of Self-realization.

व्यवसायात्मिका बुद्धिरेकेह कुरुनन्दन।
बहुशाखा ह्यनन्ताश्च बुद्धयोऽव्यवसायिनाम्।। ४१

41. O Prince of the Kurus, there is only one determinative wisdom, and the intellects of those who do not have such decisive wisdom are unending, with many branches.

Merely knowing what to do without one-pointedness of mind will not lead one to perform his duty accurately. Therefore, the desired results will not be attained. Just as profound knowledge of what to do is essential, so having a one-pointed mind is equally essential. The modern student tends to know intellectually but does not make sincere efforts to develop one-pointedness of mind. Thus, his mind remains scattered and all his actions result in disappointment. For lack of a one-pointed mind, the modern student jumps from one path to another because he does not understand that it is his scattered mind that is creating barriers for him. He thinks the barriers are outside. Assuming that another path or goal will be better is trickery played by the mind. One already knows what is right, but he does not know how to put it into practice. In childhood the fundamentals of all great truths are taught to us. Then we spend energy in trying to apply those truths, but we fail. We do not realize that with systematic practice we can succeed. The key point of practice as well as of success lies in one-pointedness of mind.

Attention is the first step on the ladder to develop one-pointedness of mind. One must pay wholehearted attention to all of the things he does from morning until evening. The aspirant should also understand why he is acting in a particular way. Actions should not be performed as a reaction without understanding why one does them. The human mind is prone to be reactionary if it is not trained, and an untrained mind creates disorder, disease, and confusion. If one does something with full attention, he will increase his awareness and ability to perform his duty. If one forms the habit of attending fully to whatever he is doing, the mind will become trained, and eventually concentration will become effortless. It is a great quality for one to be able to express his knowledge through his speech and action with a one-pointed mind. Thousands of thoughts remain waiting to be entertained. The purpose of sadhana is to attend to those thoughts in a systematic manner so that they do not create unrest in the inner world. Arjuna is instructed to make his mind one-pointed before performing his duty.

यामिमां पुष्पितां वाचं प्रवदन्त्यविपश्चितः।
वेदवादरताः पार्थ नान्यदस्तीतिवादिनः।। ४२
कामात्मानः स्वर्गपराः जन्मकर्मफलप्रदाम्।
क्रियाविशेषबहुलां भोगैश्वर्यगतिं प्रति।। ४३
भोगैश्वर्यप्रसक्तानां तयापहृतचेतसाम्।
व्यवसायात्मिका बुद्धिः समाधौ न विधीयते।। ४४

42. *This is the flowery speech that the unwise speak, absorbed in the discussions of the Vedas, saying 'There is nothing else.'*
43. *Totally identified with their desire, intent upon heaven, uttering the speech that leads to the fruit of karma in the form of rebirth, ample in specific rituals, resulting in pleasure and power;*
44. *Since they are attached to pleasure and power and their minds are plundered by that speech of theirs, their determinative wisdom does not succeed in leading to samadhi.*

Theologians, scholars, and priests theorize and write commentaries on scriptures such as the Vedas. Yet, however profound their theoretical knowledge may be, they cannot assimilate that knowledge and live according to it without sadhana. Intellectualization is easy, but sadhana is difficult. Many scholars make erudite speeches on the Vedic verses, but they themselves have not realized the full meaning of those verses. Therefore, Sri Krishna teaches Arjuna to practice and assimilate the knowledge. He urges him not to be foolish like those who talk on the Vedas but do not practice the teachings of the Vedas. Such scholars and priests are enveloped with self-interest; their actions are directed toward mundane and temporal gains and the attainment of heavenly joys. As a result they become caught in the snare of births and deaths.

Many religious leaders have forgotten the profound meaning of the great scriptures and merely use them for their own convenience. Motivated to attain external pleasures, they involve the innocent in rituals. Much of the misery we find in society is because of unwise teachings spread by such religious teachers. It is an irony of human history that religious leaders often practice religion to achieve selfish ends. In fact, it has become a tradition that unfortunately misleads the vast majority of society.

A rare few are aware of the fallacies and follies of such selfish leaders and thus prefer to isolate themselves and practice sadhana. But how many such people are there in the world, and how much good can they do with their teachings and writings when the vast majority of religionists preach and teach meaningless rituals that rob the intelligent of the wisdom of the great scriptures? The sages who have seen truth face to face and who were able to touch infinity have always warned sadhakas that real knowledge comes from earnest sadhana, which leads to direct experience, and not from mere study of the scriptures. While intellectual knowledge is often used for selfish ends, those sages knew that truth and selflessness are one. Selflessness is an acquired taste. When one finds delight in being selfless he can lead, serve, and love others and even change the course and destiny of nations. Selfishness feeds the ego, but selflessness leads one to higher levels of consciousness.

त्रैगुण्यविषया वेदा निस्त्रैगुण्यो भवार्जुन।
निर्द्वन्द्वो नित्यसत्त्वस्थो निर्योगक्षेम आत्मवान्।। ४५
यावानर्थ उदपाने सर्वतः संप्लुतोदके।
तावान्सर्वेषु वेदेषु ब्राह्मणस्य विजानतः।। ४६

45. *The subject of the Vedas is the world consisting of the three gunas. O Arjuna, be free of the constituent gunas, free of the pairs of opposites; dwell in the eternal essence, disinterested in worldly and other-worldly success, having cultivated the Self.*

46. *The purpose that is served by a small well as compared to water flooding all around—that much is the meaning in all the Vedic rituals for a son of God who has supreme knowledge.*

Sri Krishna is not condemning the Vedas but is advising Arjuna to go beyond the three attributes of the human mind to attain a state of equanimity. The human mind is composed of three *gunas* (qualities): *sattva, rajas,* and *tamas.* The Vedas explain that these three qualities are present in all that exists in the phenomenal world and so are also found in all human beings, though in different grades and degrees. When the sadhaka understands that the animal tendency is destructive, unhelpful, and of a tamasic nature, he increases his awareness of his human potentials. In the next stage of awareness, he realizes the great marvel of marvels: that the essential nature of his being is divine. He then follows the path of upward travel toward divinity. Without realizing his divinity, a human being can be successful in the external world but can never have a tranquil mind, and he is thus unable to catch a glimpse of the Eternal. He longs to be happy, but that dream is not fulfilled.

The divine nature in the human being is the sattvic quality of equilibrium, which gives one freedom from the influences of the pairs of opposites. Equilibrium is a state of mind attained by human effort. The aspirant who understands the three qualities of the human mind always remains vigilant and increases his awareness of sattva. One of the qualities of sattva is expansion; thus the mind, speech, and action of the sattvic aspirant follows the law of expansion and not of contraction. Contraction leads one to feel separate and small, whereas expansion leads one to realize that the Self of all is his very essence. Animals are totally dependent on the laws of nature, but human beings can cross the boundaries of natural law by attaining altered states of consciousness. The human being is independent in many ways: he has the ability to fathom the laws of nature by which animals live and to use those laws for his own ends. The human being alone has enormous capacity to study the various levels of life that have evolved in the universe. He is divine, human, and animal all at the same time, and his behavior depends on which part of him is most developed.

Through direct experience, sages acquire the essential knowledge of the Vedas; they go to the source from which the Vedic knowledge springs. With inward sadhana they reach the highest summit from which they can have profound knowledge of all levels of life and the universe. They find ever-flowing knowledge within and without. One who is thirsty drinks water, but one who has quenched his thirst has no need to stoop down to fetch water from streams and wells. Thus, the sage who has become one with Truth has no need for the incomplete and limited knowledge expressed through words and concepts.

कर्मण्येवाधिकारस्ते मा फलेषु कदाचन।
मा कर्मफलहेतुर्भूर्मा ते सङ्गोऽस्त्वकर्मणि।। ४७

47. *You are entitled only to actions and never to fruits; do not consider yourself to be a cause of the fruits of actions, nor let your attachment be to inaction.*

After one has attained profound knowledge of all levels of life, what is the surest way to apply that knowledge so that life becomes meaningful and fulfilling? Sri Krishna advises Arjuna to become aware of that which is his and that which is not his. He explains that one has the right to perform his duty, but he has no right to expect the fruits received therein. Neither duty performed with the motivation to acquire the fruits of one's action nor attachment towards inaction is helpful. Both tendencies are harmful. If the law of karma is not properly understood, one becomes helpless and inactive, or he performs actions with attachment to the results and thus becomes disappointed. Disappointment is a great enemy of self-reliance. It obstructs the faculty of discrimination, judgment, and decisiveness—the guiding factors within us.

There are two main principles to be followed when doing one's actions: one should not act impulsively but should counsel within before acting, and one should not perform any action motivated by selfishness.

Right action is superior to inaction. Inaction makes one lethargic, and one who becomes lethargic postpones his duties and joys, placing them in the hands of his fate and future. Students are always warned by their teachers not to become victims of sloth and inactivity, for human beings cannot live without thinking and acting.

Because of the lack of real guidance, some people today take drugs. If one takes drugs, he cannot practice sadhana and make his mind one-pointed and inward. The use of drugs leads to inactivity and then to inertia, and one's acts are then prompted by the motivation of tamas. A tamasic person deludes himself: he thinks that he already knows every-thing, that he has no need to learn and to transform himself, and that he therefore does not have to do his sadhana. He should understand that it is the tamasic quality of mind that disturbs his motivation for sadhana. Motivation needs proper organization with the help of steady sadhana and the guidance of a competent preceptor. Motivation is action in a subtle form. It is what motivates one that is important because one's motivation is responsible for molding his thought patterns and for prompting him to do actions. It is a guiding force, which if properly used can make one victorious in the external world as well as in the unfoldment of his inner potentials. There are two kinds of motivation: one prompts the aspirant to perform actions in the external world, and the other helps him to make his mind one-pointed and inward. The motivation that prompts one to perform action with a desire for reward is predominant in the animal kingdom, so reward and punishment are two methods applied in training animals. The human being, though a higher species, is also motivated by reward and punishment. Yet he can go beyond that. Sri Krishna advises Arjuna to go beyond all expecta-tions, for expectation is the cause of despair and disappointment.

The human being alone has the gift of judgment, discrimination, and decision. Every action has its consequent effect, and the fruition of the action is ordinarily perceived as either a reward or a punishment. But one can choose to make a loving offering of the fruits of his actions for the benefit of others. Then one performs his actions skillfully, self-lessly, and lovingly, offering the fruits of his actions for the sake of humanity. Thus he is constantly praying. Such prayer is actual prayer; it is not at all like the prayer of egotistical people.

Most people are motivated to do actions for the sake of receiving rewards. Attachment to rewards is a deep-rooted habit. Most people do not understand how to be selfless. Such human beings are rajasic. Reward-oriented people are very selfish. They suffer and they make others suffer. Perhaps that is one reason that the best of men have retreated to forest dwellings wondering, "Why do human beings still behave like animals?" After intensive self-study those great ones devised practical methods for transforming humanity, and they gave us their wisdom through the scriptures.

Suffering comes when one is interested in reward. If one performs actions expecting rewards, he is bound to receive the fruits of his actions. The fruits then motivate him to do more actions, and in this way he finds himself caught in the whirlpool of life, never content, always seeking more and more for himself and ignoring or using others for his own gain. Actions done for reward thus create bondage. One becomes a slave to rewards in much the same way that the rat in scientific experiments becomes a slave to the pellet box, performing only those actions that bring him a token reinforcement. But there is a way to attain release from such enslavement; perform your duties skillfully and selflessly without attachment to reward. Then you will be free, a *mukta* traveling and singing the songs of joy without cares or fears.

योगस्थः कुरु कर्माणि सङ्गं त्यक्त्वा धनंजय।
सिद्ध्यसिद्ध्योः समो भूत्वा समत्वं योग उच्यते।। ४८

48. *Perform actions dwelling in yoga, abandoning attachment, O Conquerer of Wealth being alike to success and failure. Equanimity is called yoga.*

Verse 48 further explains the way to do one's actions without creating conflict and suffering for oneself and for others: one should maintain equanimity within and harmony between himself and others. Evenness and tranquility are based on constant awareness of one's own essential nature, which is *satyam, shivam, sundaram* (truth, happiness, and bliss). Unless one understands the fleeting nature of the pairs of opposites—pain and pleasure, sorrow and joy—through the help of profound and systematic sadhana, he cannot go beyond those experiences to attain a state of inner peace.

According to Patanjali, the codifier of yoga science, the practical methods that are applied to attain perfect control of the mind and its modifications are called yoga. The yogi who has control of the mind and its modifications maintains balance of mind and inner composure in all situations and under all conditions. Those who do not have control of their minds are lost, for they remain enslaved by the external environment and their reactions to it.

Modern man does not yet understand the importance and necessity of controlling the mind. He thinks that it is impossible to understand anything that cannot be seen with the eyes and touched by the fingers. It has already been said that such an attitude is the cause of much human misery and the source of innumerable psychosomatic diseases. If modern man learns to do some practices that will enable him to understand his internal states and to organize them in an orderly way, he will free himself from a great deal of misery and suffering. He will be able to eliminate mental and emotional turmoil as well as psychosomatic illnesses. One often hears complaints from so-called rich and well-off people that life is burdensome. The rich man says, "We have all the comforts and amenities of life but not peace of mind." Unless one understands life within as well as without and learns to create a bridge between these two aspects of life, he will never find peace of mind no matter how much wealth he possesses. Why do we not learn to spend some time doing practices that will help us analyze and control our thoughts, emotions, desires, and appetites?

Those who live in the contemporary world often say that they are not happy in their present situations, yet they feel compelled to live under the circumstances in which they find themselves. But what are those circumstances, and who created them? If one analyzes his circumstances, he will find that they are actually self-created. The predicaments one experiences are a result of his disorderly mind, which does not know how to adjust itself to the various relationships that he has created for himself. Verily, all miseries are self-created. One should not blame God for one's own incompetencies. But modern man feels delight in blaming others for his own failures. That is merely an escape and only provides temporary relief through an emotional outburst. Such escape does not work for a long time, for the reality within eventually compels one to face the facts of life. Throughout the East and West, individuals and groups suffering from this self-delusion blame others or God for the situations they themselves create. People have to perform their duties, and yet they do not like to perform them. That creates serious conflict and is one of the chief causes of modern illnesses.

When one experiences repeated conflict between his duties and his desires, various forms of neurotic disorders and psychosomatic disturbances result. One who performs his duties grudgingly experiences no happiness in life. Or one may run away from his duties and lead an undisciplined life of self-interest. Many people remain torn by conflict or plagued by guilt because they have avoided their duties. Then they experience anxiety, or the anxiety is expressed in physical symptoms.

Modern psychologists are making futile efforts to probe into the heart of these disorders, and they have not as yet found adequate methods to resolve them. Their results are often long in coming and incomplete. The Bhagavad Gita, however, offers a profound method for removing all such disorders by leading one to a state of inner composure from which he can perform actions skillfully and without negative repercussions for himself or others. To attain this way of being, one must transform himself through sadhana. Harmonious action in the world will follow later. Without sadhana, peaceful living is not possible.

In order to achieve successful outcomes from the actions he performs, one must have a well-balanced mind. When the aspirant understands the importance of equanimity of mind, he pays attention to his inner organization and becomes aware of those finer forces that normally remain in a dormant state. Anything that is within is easily accessible if one follows a definite path of sadhana. Regardless of which path one follows, if he follows it resolutely and steadily, he will attain a balanced state of mind and thus will not commit errors when performing his duties.

When one learns to enjoy the beauty and grandeur of nonattachment, he acquires the ability to love his duties and comes to experience the offering of the fruits of his actions as the highest of all joys. Non-attachment becomes a great delight and the love of his life. Love and non-attachment are synonymous. One may erroneously believe that non-attachment leads to inaction and indifference. On the contrary, when one learns to do his duty with non-attachment, he is performing his dharma with love. Such a yogi need not seek salvation elsewhere, for he is already a mukta, a free man. He lives in the world yet is free from it.

One who has learned to surrender all the fruits of his actions in the service of humanity is constantly praying. He does not create obstacles for himself. How ironic that most human beings create obstacles for themselves and then make efforts to remove them! Is that an enlightened way of living? Many students today waste their time and energy in that sort of folly; although they work hard, they do not attain anything. The true sadhaka, however, always remains vigilant and does not slip back to his past habits. Instead he attains the next level of consciousness.

The yogi should understand two symbols: the lotus, which grows in water though its petals remain untouched by the water; and the sun, which shines eternally and equally for all yet remains above and far away, unaffected by the changes occurring in the world. These are symbols of the yoga of equanimity, which leads one to perfection.

दूरेण ह्यवरं कर्म बुद्धियोगाद्धनंजय।
बुद्धौ शरणमन्विच्छ कृपणाः फलहेतवः।। ४९
बुद्धियुक्तो जहातीह उभे सुकृतदुष्कृते।
तस्माद्योगाय युज्यस्व योगः कर्मसु कौशलम्।। ५०
कर्मजं बुद्धियुक्ता हि फलं त्यक्त्वा मनीषिणः।
जन्मबन्धविनिर्मुक्ताः पदं गच्छन्त्यनामयम्।।५१

49. *Action is by far lower than the yoga of wisdom, O Arjuna. Seek to take refuge in wisdom. Those whose actions are causes of fruits are petty minded.*
50. *One endowed with wisdom relinquishes here both the good deeds as well as the bad ones. Therefore, be directed toward yoga; yoga is skillfulness in actions.*
51. *The wise men endowed with wisdom indeed give up the fruit that arises from action; liberated from the bondage of birth and its attendant cycles, they reach the state of wellness and holiness.*

After describing the negative effects of working for rewards, Sri Krishna explains the importance of performing disciplined action with non-attachment. The term *buddhi yoga* refers to action performed with a mental attitude of non-attachment to the fruits of one's action. Buddhi has the ability to discriminate between the real Self and the non-Self, and with such discrimination one can develop non-attachment to the non-Self.

A person with a dissipated mind is unable to comprehend the limitless joy that is experienced by the aspirant who is tranquil, performing his duties selflessly and skillfully. But when the mind is tranquil, pure reason (buddhi) is able to function. A tranquil mind alone has the capacity to maintain inner poise, which inspires and leads one to perform action skillfully and without attachment to the results. Such actions become a means for fulfilling the purpose of life. Whereas actions performed with selfish desire bind one to the objects of the world, actions done with non-attachment lead to complete freedom.

A disciplined mind and non-attachment are two important requisites for performing skillful action. If these qualities are absent, the mind is continually tossed by preoccupation with gain and loss, success and failure. Such a disturbed and distracted mind is not helpful at all; instead it is repeatedly a source of disappointment and can create misery, grief, and sorrow.

Skilled action is the gift of a disciplined mind, and nonattachment is the gift of buddhi yoga, the yoga of pure reason. Skilled and disciplined action and non-attachment are separated here only to enable one to understand the importance of developing both, but actually the two qualities go hand in hand. Disciplined action is definitely superior to inept and harmful action. This is clear when we examine the fruits of each. Although disciplined action brings positive results, one is still not free because those results prompt him to do more actions. It is not possible through disciplined action alone for one to come out of the whirlpool created by his actions and the fruits he receives from those actions. Only when disciplined action is combined with non-attachment is one free from the bondage of his actions.

The deeds performed by one who has a tranquil mind are totally different from those performed by selfish people who desire to enjoy the fruits arising from their deeds. When the thought of dedicating and surrendering the fruits of one's action is predominant in one's mind, he is indeed selfless. A selfless person is concerned with the needs of others; his focus is on giving rather than on receiving. The family institution helps one to understand the philosophy of giving. When a man learns to give to his wife, children, and other family members, he is taking the first step in learning to give. He can expand that awareness to his neighbor, nation, the whole of humanity, and to all creatures of the world. Learning to love others is one side of a coin; the other side is life itself. Without love, life is impossible, and without life, love is impossible. Love and life are two sides of the same whole; they are inseparable—nay, they are one and the same!

In modern life instead of learning to give, everyone in the family expects to receive without giving. Whereas giving is an expression of selflessness, expectation is an expression of selfishness. A selfish husband and father uses his wife and children to satisfy his ego. He does not know the law of giving. When this way of being is typical, the family institution radiates hatred instead of radiating love, and chaos is created in society.

When one has expectations he is never fulfilled, but giving is a fulfillment in itself. The truth that every action has a reaction is acknowledged equally by philosophers and scientists. Expectation rebounds on the human being, and so does love. When one has expectations the result is dissatisfaction, disappointment, distress, sorrow, and pain. But when one gives there is a feeling of satisfaction and contentment through and through. The reaction received from giving is fulfillment. The wise person gives for another reason as well: he knows that the expectation of receiving rewards brings those rewards, and then he will become caught in the whirlpool of attachment and bondage to those rewards. That leads to a kind of suicide, for one becomes smothered by his accumulated possessions.

The Upanishads say, "Enjoy through renunciation, for that is the way of salvation." But the question arises: How is it possible for one to live in the world and to discharge his duties without becoming attached to the objects of the world? The Bhagavad Gita explains that this can be accomplished by developing the understanding that all things of the world, animate and inanimate, are not ours. We have the right to use and enjoy them but not the right to possess them. This teaching is like a ray of light that tears the veil of false identity and possessiveness, which always creates misery. One should have an exact, profound, and comprehensive attitude toward life. He should understand the law of action and reaction and the importance of giving up possessions. Otherwise the joy of giving and loving is changed into sorrow and misery. But instead of understanding this fact, modern man becomes overwhelmed by the sense of ownership. And when one possesses something that does not really belong to him, he lives as a thief and not as a free man.

Intellectuals raise the question: If one does not desire the fruits of action, will he be motivated to act? In response to this question, the sages who have trodden the path and graciously left their footprints for us to follow have said again and again, "Have a desire so that you perform the action, but do not have a selfish desire, for selfish desire is the very source of misery, but selfless desire brings joy and makes you free." When surrendering the fruits of actions becomes the basis of one's life, he knows nothing but giving. And at that stage further knowledge is not needed, for one has already attained the goal of life. He realizes his oneness with all and lives in that realization. Therefore, give up all the fruits of your actions to others and live in perennial happiness.

यदा ते मोहकलिलं बुद्धिर्व्यतितरिष्यति।
तदा गन्तासि निर्वेदं श्रोतव्यस्य श्रुतस्य च।। ५२
श्रुतिविप्रतिपन्ना ते यदा स्थास्यति निश्चला।
समाधावचला बुद्धिः तदा योगमवाप्स्यसि।। ५३

52. *When your intellect overcomes and crosses the confused mass of delusion, then you will reach the state of dispassion concerning all that you have heard and learned and all that you have yet to hear and learn.*
53. *When your intellect, previously confused by the variety of teachings, remains firm and unmoving in samadhi, then you will attain yoga.*

These verses explain the evolving state of buddhi. When buddhi soars high, tearing the veils of delusion, one rises above all intellectual pursuits. The teachings that may be encountered from outside are already accessible through buddhi and are fully grasped. All knowledge is known to such a one, and he attains the highest state of yoga. When buddhi is fully developed, one has freedom from the mire of delusion, for he has unalloyed knowledge. Pure buddhi is able to unfold all the secrets of the universe, and all the feebleness and conflicts of the mind are resolved.

The lower mind *(manas)* is that part of the mind which functions by employing the senses to receive knowledge from the external world and employing the organs of action to act upon the external world. All sense perceptions are filtered in a system of conceptualization. A disorganized and uncontrolled mind does not have exact perceptions and thus cannot conceptualize or act accurately. A clouded mind that receives its information through untrained senses forms distorted concepts and remains deluded. But the mind that learns to consult and seek the counsel of buddhi and forms the habit of not initiating action without a decision from buddhi is a well-controlled mind, and it can conceptualize and act in a useful, efficient, and harmonious way. When the lower mind, with the help of sadhana, constantly listens to buddhi with one-pointedness, there is no danger of committing errors.

There are two different states of buddhi: lower buddhi and higher buddhi. The lower buddhi gives diverse instructions one after another, but with its pure reason the higher buddhi gives firm instruction for the benefit of the whole being. It is aware of the source of consciousness within and at the same time has discriminatory knowledge of the external world. All the great spiritual leaders like Buddha, Krishna, Jesus, and Moses acted with the help of pure reason, which is called higher buddhi. Pure reason or higher buddhi is completely sattvic without any tinge of rajas or tamas. Those who have complete mastery over their internal states acquire the gift of pure reason, and then no one in any circumstances can ever change the course of their actions. Socrates, even while drinking the goblet of hemlock, did not alter his convictions. Jesus on the cross did not say, "Forgive me. Don't crucify me." With the help of the same pure reason and firm faith, Moses asked the sea to part and create a path. Pure reason, firm faith, and will power function together and make a great force that can perform all manner of wonders. In such a state all the functions of mind work in a unified way, and there is no doubt at all.

According to Eastern psychology, the ego or sense of I-ness is like a rock without buddhi; it is dumb and deaf. But Western psychologists attribute all the qualities of buddhi to the ego because they do not have the comprehensive knowledge of the various faculties of mind. Their way of analysis involves knowing through the intellect, logic, and external observation, whereas the perennial psychology of the East has differentiated various functions of the mind with the help of discipline and the introspective method of inner sadhana. This method is based on direct inward knowledge, whereas the methods of modern psychologists rely on the collection of data from external observation. Western psychologists have begun to realize that the study of the waking state alone is not sufficient, and they are now probing into one level of the unconscious, the dream state. But there are other subtle dimensions of life that are part of the unconscious that are not explored by modern psychology. Modern psychologists do not understand that which is beyond observation and the analysis of thoughts and emotions.

According to Eastern psychology, there are subtle dimensions of life still to be explored by the West. Suppose a mosquito bites someone who is in deep sleep. His fingers reach for the bite, yet he is not aware of it. What is that level of life that remains awake recording such occurrences even during the sleeping state? The perennial psychology of the East has answers to these questions. According to that psychology, it is not the mind that goes through the waking, dreaming, and sleeping states. The mind shares the experiences, but it is actually the individual self *(jiva),* which is quite different from the ego, that experiences the waking, dreaming, and sleeping states. The individual self presents a personality of its own, for it uses a particular vehicle called the unconscious, which is the reservoir of all the past impressions of mind, action, and speech. As long as the self uses the unconscious as a vehicle, it is called jiva, but the moment the Self renounces the vehicle, it is called pure consciousness.

As long as the intellect is clouded, one remains selfish, and as long as he remains selfish, the mind is impure. One then depends on others and loses self-reliance. He collects pleasurable objects and remains deluded and allured by the temptations of the external world. His troubles increase day by day, and sunk in immense sorrow, he struggles for peace. In the course of seeking truth, he may meet a sadhaka or spiritual guide. Then alone does he think of coming out of the mire of delusion created by his selfishness. He begins to cast off his infatuations and to seek practical methods of ridding himself of the impurities of the mind and intellect.

Scriptural knowledge has its importance, for it inspires the aspirant on the path of sadhana; the scriptures constantly remind the sadhaka of the goal of his life. But how did these scriptures come into existence, and why are they accepted as testimony in guiding sadhakas? Sveta Upanishad says that the great sages in deep contemplation and in the highest state of tranquility came in touch with the supernatural power and thus experienced the profound knowledge and wisdom of the timeless and infinite eternal Truth. If the sadhaka systematically practices fathoming all the levels of life and goes to the source from which the wisdom of the Vedas flows, he will experience the direct knowledge that is higher than the knowledge received by hearing the Vedic scriptures and their interpretations.

The knowledge attained through sadhana is higher than any other source of knowledge. There are three accepted methods of attaining this wisdom, and there are three aspects of one's being that need to be controlled and disciplined. Numerous paths are described in various traditions, but among these paths prayer, meditation, and contemplation have been universally accepted and verified by the ancients. Discipline of mind, action, and speech are auxiliary, preliminary, and essential steps in each of these three different approaches. Let us explain and understand each of these distinct approaches separately.

Prayer purifies the way of the soul; it is a means to expand one's consciousness within. It is not a mere petition but makes the mind aware of the dimension of life that is the very source of one's being. Prayer has immense power and can lead one to the highest state of ecstasy. It is the way of using emotional power by awakening, evoking, and transforming it. History reveals that constant prayer can transform human beings. There is no doubt that if prayer is properly practiced, positive results are imminent.

There are two types of prayer. The inferior type of prayer is egocentric prayer. It is used by the selfish person who merely desires to fulfill his wants. "I" remains the center of such prayer: "O Lord, give me this, do this for me, help me to have this object." This sort of prayer, full of wants, is used just to fulfill one's selfish ends. Though it works, it does not lead one to nearness to the Absolute. Such prayer, regularly conducted in all great religions, reduces the magnanimity of prayer to a selfish petition. It does not lead one to go beyond the mire of delusion created by the ego.

When the aspirant understands that possession of the mundane objects of the world for which selfish people pray does not make one happy, he realizes that egocentric prayers have limited effects with limited gains. He begins thinking, "I am committing a mistake somewhere. Either my method of prayer is incomplete or my motives are not right." Egocentric prayer is thus discarded by the true aspirant, and then he seeks the higher way of prayer: God-centered prayer. God-centered prayer gives immense joy to the human mind. Those who practice this approach believe that God is a being who has full power to fulfill the desires of human beings. Overwhelmed with this idea, they pray to God to give them strength, wisdom, and skill so that they can discharge their duties efficiently and at the same time understand the meaning of life. In God-centered prayer one does not leave all the human responsibilities to God with the expectation that God will take care of those responsibilities, but one prays to God to give him strength so that he can understand and fulfill his duties and serve others selflessly. This type of prayer expands one's consciousness, whereas ego-centered prayer envelops one with selfish words and makes one small, petty minded, greedy, and inconsiderate. The Lord's Prayer is an example of God-centered prayer. It is a glorification of God and has no selfish motivation; it is like a stream crying to meet the ocean. In God-centered prayer, the individual accepts God in his life as a guide, leader, and judge of his actions and speech.

Prayer is very useful, but at the same time it advocates and promotes the philosophy of dualism, which asserts that man and God remain forever distinct. The individual always remains an individual, and there is no union with God, only a nearness to God. Dualism is an acceptance of two separate existences. There has been a great deal of debate by scholars about whether dualism is a valid philosophy. The validity of the dualistic approach is not a matter to be debated. Dualism should be understood as a stage of sadhana that provides a path that can eventually lead to the higher realm of knowledge, that of complete unity. It is valid as a preliminary stage of sadhana, as an experience on the way to the realization of the Absolute.

The next approach is deeper, more profound and systematic, and is suitable to explorers and yogis. It is called meditation. Meditation is an inward method in which a systematic study is conducted to gain knowledge of the Absolute. It goes beyond prayer to help one realize the higher dimensions of life. In this approach it is believed that the human being is a dweller in two worlds, the world within himself and the world outside. One develops profound self-mastery so that he is able to go to the Source of consciousness through a meditative method and to simultaneously develop the ability to perform his duties skillfully, selflessly, and lovingly. Meditation thus has two aspects: meditation in silence and meditation in action. The Bhagavad Gita teaches both. Many scholars, however, do not know how to practice meditation and do not understand how the meditative mind can be capable of performing skillful actions. But karma yoga (the yoga of action) and *dhyana yoga* (the yoga of meditation) cannot be separated. One who has the ability and capacity to meditate in silence also has the capacity to perform his duties skillfully. Sincerity, truthfulness, and purity of heart are prerequisites for the method of prayer, but in meditation, stillness, even breathing, withdrawal of the senses, calming down the conscious mind, going beyond the unconscious, and finally attaining the state of tranquility or samadhi are the systematic steps one has to follow.

Many incomplete methods are practiced these days, and according to their advocates these methods are the only way. Such claims by bogus teachers are laughable. Meditation as taught by Patanjali's method is a systematic approach, like climbing a ladder and finally reaching the highest rung, the state of samadhi. It is not at all religious, and to give it religious color, as some mistakenly do, is to vulgarize a purely scientific and methodical way of attaining samadhi, a state in which all of one's questions are resolved. Samadhi is the goal of the meditator. In that supreme state, which bestows serenity in all conditions, the individual unites himself with the self-existent Reality. There are no short cuts such as those taught by many modern teachers. Meditation is a discipline that must be resolutely practiced if one is to be transported from the physical to the subtlest aspect of his being and finally to that fountainhead of life and light where the purest consciousness perennially resides in all its glory.

Marvelous results can be observed when the method of meditation is introduced gradually, step-by-step. Meditational therapy is the highest of all therapies, providing that the therapist is competent and knows how to apply this form of therapy systematically.* All other methods of

---

* See *Psychotherapy East and West*, Swami Ajaya. Honesdale, PA: Himalayan Institute, 1984, pgs. 218-222.

therapy offer only momentary relief, and often one becomes dependent on the therapist. In meditational therapy, however, the student is led toward self-reliance, self-examination, self-verification, self-analysis, and self-attainment.

Modern students often ask the question, "How many days, months, or years must we train ourselves?" That depends upon the aspirant's sincerity, determination, and one-pointedness of mind and on how regularly he practices. The Bhagavad Gita teaches meditation in action, meditation in life, and Arjuna learns this method and becomes enlightened. The teachings of the Bhagavad Gita last for only eighteen days, and these eighteen days of teaching encompass the entire knowledge that one needs in order to have a comprehensive knowledge of Atman, the Self, which is the Self of all. In meditation itself, the time factor is annihilated because meditation is a state of mind beyond the prime conditionings of time, space, and causation. Ordinarily the student should first learn to rid himself of his old habits and the stains of the *samskaras* and impressions of his past deeds, which create a setback in his inward journey. The time factor totally depends on the individual. If the student is like Arjuna and if his teacher is like Sri Krishna, enlightenment will come very fast, but if he does not meditate and follow the other practices regularly with full determination, progress can be very slow.

The third approach, that of contemplation, is practiced by a fortunate few. To perform skillful action with non-attachment, one must sharpen his faculty of discrimination, judgment, and decisiveness. Knowledge flows from within, and the external world is the field of expression of that knowledge through various avenues that are available to us—mainly mind, action, and speech. Contemplation is not an unorganized way of thinking; it is a precise method. For contemplation one must train buddhi in all its aspects. A trained buddhi has pure reason, and pure reason has immense power to lead the aspirant to the door of liberation. First the student listens to the scriptures and studies them under the guidance of a competent teacher, an enlightened one who has gained direct knowledge and who is able to understand the subtleties of the teachings of the great ones. Then, like a humming bee, with great joy he collects fragrances from different flowers and converts them into honey. The first step is called *sravana,* and the second is called *manana.* One then attains the third step, called *nididhyasana,* which means assimilating the knowledge one has gained and living according to it. After attaining that step, *sakshatkara,* in which the knowledge of the whole is revealed, occurs.

We have described three approaches in brief. Now we will explain the importance of discipline, without which one cannot be successful in any of these approaches. Discipline should be practiced on three levels: mind, action, and speech. The human being knows everything that he ought to know about how to live in the world and how to relate to others. He has been taught, for example, the importance of being kind and gentle. But one does not know how to put those principles into practice. The emphasis of this commentary is therefore on practice. As our gurudeva used to say, "Do not waste your time thinking and planning to follow the path. Decide and just follow."

Spiritual sadhana requires the discipline of mind, action, and speech. Even preliminary discipline of mind, action, and speech can lead one to the experience of supernatural phenomena not ordinarily experienced by students who collect information but do not practice. Sometimes the great *swamis,* sages, and yogis who have practiced discipline speak with profound certainty, and whatever they say happens exactly as they said it would. They do not care to debate about what truth is; they simply say that when one practices nonlying, he speaks the truth. We have recorded many instances in which a sage has said something that seems impossible, yet it happens just as he said. By following samyama (discipline), one can perform such miracles. A miracle is a miracle only as long as one does not know how it came about; the moment that is known, it is no longer a miracle. If one wastes his power of speech indulging in useless discussions, talking nonsense, lying intentionally, hurting others through his speech, condemning others, or speaking against another's religion, *vak shakti* (the power of words) does not find effective expression through his speech. But if one conserves his power of speech and does not lie, his speech can become so powerful that whatever he says will come to pass.

If one also disciplines his actions by not doing what is not to be done, he will find that he is doing his actions more efficiently and more accurately than before. The question may arise: How can one know what is not right? The answer is that one's conscience already knows what is right and wrong, good and bad, helpful and unhelpful. One simply has to tune into his inner conscience, which guides him all the time. That is called seeking counsel within before performing action. It has already been explained that one already knows—he simply has to practice. In the course of practicing not doing that which is not to be done, one will find that he is being guided from within. Then he can learn to develop a dialogue with his conscience, which is not polluted by the fickleness and feebleness of the mind. Experimenting in this way leads one to understand that the real counselor is within each person.

The first and foremost duty of a true and selfless teacher is to introduce his student to that inner guide which leads one during the waking, dreaming, and sleeping states. When one takes a few moments from his busy life and learns to sit calmly in a quiet place, the inner counselor begins counseling. It would be helpful if modern therapists and psychologists, as well as priests and spiritual teachers, would learn to listen to the inner counselor and then introduce that inner guide to their clients and students.

After practicing disciplined action and speech and studying their marvelous effects, one should learn to understand and practice mental discipline. When one does not allow his mind to think that which is negative and which makes him depressed and sad, his mind begins forming new habits of joy. Slowly he begins discriminating between helpful thoughts and those unhelpful thoughts that consume more human energy than anything else. This introspective (inspecting within) method leads one to the next step: witnessing. Here one learns to witness all that happens, both in the external and internal worlds, without becoming involved in it. While one is still learning, he must be patient and not become disappointed if at times he fails to remain a witness but instead becomes emotionally caught up in what is taking place. In pursuing such a self-training program, one should make a commitment to himself for the sake of his growth that he will practice regularly and faithfully no matter what. This is not the same as following a commandment or a blind injunction. Many people are afraid to make commitments because they believe that by not making commitments they will be free, but lack of commitment is merely irresponsibility and does not bring about true freedom. When one is afraid to make a commitment, it is because he is fearful of accepting responsibility, but real freedom is attained only when one is no longer a slave of his emotions and mental life. To be responsible is to be strong. With the help of mental discipline, one's internal organization can be arranged in a way that prevents emotional disturbances and physical maladies.

After understanding the importance of the discipline of mind, speech, and action and after practicing that discipline regularly for some time, one experiences certain extraordinary phenomena that are based on those realities that cannot be understood by the conscious mind. In each approach, whether it be prayer, meditation, or contemplation, discipline plays a role, like that of a father who protects his loving child with his tender arms and loving teachings.

अर्जुन उवाच
स्थितप्रज्ञस्य का भाषा समाधिस्थस्य केशव।
स्थितधीः किं प्रभाषेत किमासीत व्रजेत किम्।। ५४

Arjuna said
54. What is the description of a person of steady insight who remains in samadhi, O Krishna? How does a person of stable wisdom speak forth? How does he sit? How does he walk?

The path of equanimity does not promise that one will attain godhood, but it will lead one to attain a state of tranquility, a state of perfection free of misery and pain. In this verse the word *sthita-prajna* (steady insight) carries deep meaning. Arjuna asks his revered teacher to describe the man of perfectly poised discernment who has established himself in his essential nature. How does he speak? How does he sit? How does he walk, and how does he carry out his duties? How can one know that a person has attained an equable state of perfection?

Arjuna's question carries great meaning and is equally valuable to modern man. He wants to know the definite signs and symptoms that denote that one has attained a state of equanimity. Since all human beings express themselves through speech and actions in much the same manner, how does the behavior of the great man differ from that of the ordinary man? How does the great man express his thoughts, emotions, and desires? How is his mind, action, and speech guided by his inner attainment of tranquility? The ancients developed a behavioral psychology of considerable breadth. They not only studied the motivations of one's behavior but also the behavioral signs and symptoms of various internal states and the means for modifying behavior. In many cases, signs and symptoms help one to analyze the behavior of a human being but not in all cases. For example, a person may cry because of intense unhappiness, because he is touched by an expression of love or beauty, or because he identifies with someone who is suffering. Therefore, we cannot know the reason by merely observing the behavior. In order to analyze human behavior, one must also probe into the deeper level from whence all emotions spring.

The signs and symptoms of one who has inner balance and poise—the way such a one speaks, acts, and sits—are different from those of the human being who has not disciplined himself and has not attained a state of equanimity. Having a tranquil mind, the man of equanimity sits in a calm, still posture. He walks with full confidence, without any fear or uncertainty. He speaks with clarity of mind in a straightforward way.

All men can be divided into two categories: there is the man of equanimity and the man of disharmony. The man of equanimity is the ideal man of the Bhagavad Gita. He remains undisturbed, unattached, happy, and joyous in all external circumstances, but the man of disharmony is completely uncoordinated and suffers from lack of discipline and awareness. The majority of individuals in society are of the latter type; they do not practice any self-discipline. Therefore, their behavior is uncoordinated, and for lack of coordination, unity is not attained. We see this confusion all over in the East and West. The highest method of education known so far is self-education and self-training, but without discipline it is not possible to educate oneself.

The Bhagavad Gita, and this verse in particular, is closely related to the Mandukya Upanishad, one of the best and perhaps most thought-provoking books in the library of man today. The Mandukya Upanishad thoroughly explains three states of mind: waking, dreaming, and sleeping.* The explanation of these states has been expanded in the Mandukya *karika* (commentary) by Gaudapada, the great grandmaster of Shankara. The man who has attained equanimity can survey each of these three states of human experience at once, while at the same time maintaining his position in the state beyond, called *turiya*. Deep sleep is very close to the state of turiya, but in deep sleep one is not aware, while in turiya unbroken consciousness exists. The purpose of the teachings of the Bhagavad Gita is to lead Arjuna and all the Arjunas of the world to attain the state of turiya. That state is the highest that can ever be experienced. One who experiences turiya is called a man of equanimity.

For the ordinary man, waking, dreaming, and sleeping are three different realities, and he is not at all aware of the fourth. However, one who has attained the timeless state of equanimity has gone beyond all conditionings of time—past, present, and future—and for him everything is here and now. The words "here and now" are commonly used, but only a few accomplished ones have experiential access to this reality, for it is a part of eternity. When past and future are available to be experienced here and now, one has attained a timeless state and thus has become an inseparable part of infinity. Infinite knowledge then remains at his disposal.

Ordinary people experience the reality of the waking, dreaming, and sleeping states separately, but one who has gone beyond and has attained the summit can clearly observe the functionings of consciousness in these three spheres of human experience as a single line that is

---

* See *Enlightenment Without God,* Swami Rama. Honesdale, PA: Himalayan Institute, 1982.

continuous rather than broken into three parts. For the man of equanimity the three phases are one and the same conscious and continuous reality, just as morning, noon, and evening are each aspects of a single day. The man of partial and limited knowledge remains in doubt and confusion about the meaning and purpose of his life because he knows only a part and does not have a profound knowledge of the whole. But the great man remains undisturbed and in perfect poise even on the battlefield, for he has discovered the mysteries of both the known and unknown, the eternal and the non-eternal. Such a warrior is victorious in all times, conditions, and states.

The dreaming state is a state of unfulfillment. But that state of mind does have some therapeutic value, for it gives one the opportunity to express all his unfulfilled and suppressed desires. A study of dreams can help one to understand the two lives that we live. One is the conscious life, and the other is that which is forgotten. We think that our forgotten life does not influence our waking life, but that is not true. Dreams are evidence that forgotten, suspended, undealt with, and unfulfilled desires remain sleeping in the unconscious and rise again when there is sufficient reason.

The waking state is experienced by a very small part of the mind and is in no way capable of comprehending the meaning of the whole. Our modern methods of education and training are imperfect because they focus only on that small aspect of the totality of our internal organization. Here lies the tragedy and bankruptcy of the modern way of life and education, that which is the cause of misery in the world today. Why haven't we devised inner methods and made them available for all so that everyone has access to all the states of one's being? Such education was available in ancient times, but it has been largely forgotten today. Modern therapists and psychologists have started probing into the dreaming state, but their exploration is still in an infant stage and needs different methods. They do not have a practical training program to explore the many aspects of the unconscious mind. The Bhagavad Gita, however, offers the knowledge that can help the modern therapist to know the unknown dimensions of life.

Arjuna's questions show that he has come out of his state of despondency. He now intently follows Sri Krishna's teachings and is eager to know more about the state of inner discrimination. Sri Krishna has led Arjuna from the most despondent state of consciousness to the state of balance and inner poise. By analyzing Arjuna's thoughts, actions, and speech, one can clearly understand the differences between these two states. In his former state Arjuna was ignorant, depressed, weak, and full of fear and anxiety. But his questions show that he is now on the path of wisdom and in the process of self-transformation. He is an entirely different person.

When one practices sadhana, a transformation takes place, and the thoughts and behavior of the aspirant change drastically. The power of self-transformation is our most important human resource. If the individual can be transformed, the whole of humanity can be transformed. Will there be a day when human society makes good use of this self-transformation process? That will be possible when the educational system includes those methods of self-discipline by which one can attain the free spirit of the man of equanimity.

श्री भगवानुवाच
प्रजहाति यदा कामान् सर्वान् पार्थ मनोगतान्।
आत्मन्येवात्मना तुष्टः स्थितप्रज्ञस्तदोच्यते।। ५५
दुःखेष्वनुद्विग्नमनाः सुखेषु विगतस्पृहः।
वीतरागभयक्रोधः स्थितधीर्मुनिरुच्यते।। ५६
यः सर्वत्रानभिस्नेहस्तत्तत्प्राप्य शुभाशुभम्।
नाभिनन्दति न द्वेष्टि तस्य प्रज्ञा प्रतिष्ठिता।। ५७

The Blessed Lord said

55. When one entirely abandons all the desires that come into the mind, O Son of Pritha, satisfied within the Self by the Self, then he is called a person of stable wisdom.

56. *One whose mind is not agitated in sorrows, who has no attraction toward pleasures, he from whom attraction, fear, and anger have disappeared, such a meditator is called a person of stable wisdom.*
57. *He who has no attachment directed toward anything, or upon attaining anything good or bad, who neither greets it nor hates it, his wisdom is established.*

When the aspirant realizes that the external world is but a reflection of the ultimate Reality and that although the reflection appears to be real, it is not actually so, the objects of the world lose their value for him. He thus experiences the first important step of freedom in the journey to the timeless infinity. Such a one, following the way of inward experiences, finally attains contentment, for he knows the Self. The Self is known by the Self, and not through any other means. When one makes practical use of this knowledge, he attains a state of non-attachment and is no longer bound by likes, dislikes, hatred, or lust. Then one is free from all emotions, desires, and appetites, and this freedom is very valuable in the path to perfection. There is no power that can take this awareness away from him.

Only a skilled and disciplined aspirant can understand the expressions, ideas, speech, and actions of the realized one who has attained the state of equanimity. The first and foremost sign one notices in such a person is the tranquility of his mind, which is totally without desire. Such a person is an example to others: he lives as though he were in a glass house from which he can see everyone and everyone can see him. That way of living and being is attained through a gradual sadhana in which the aspirant first learns to choose helpful thoughts, emotions, and desires and to abandon those that are not helpful. In the next stage he learns to abandon both good and bad and to witness all of the happenings in the external world, whether they spring from nature or from human society.

Desires have their origin in the primitive fountains of food, sex, sleep, and self-preservation. When one learns to regulate those primitive fountains, desires lose their power over him, and he is no longer a slave but a master. Many naive students think that the worldly objects one possesses must be surrendered or abandoned, but the implication here is entirely different. Surrender has nothing to do with the objects of the world but with the desires that create limitations and conditionings of the mind.

The play of desires exists only in the waking and dreaming states. Desires remain dormant in the state of deep sleep, but one is not conscious in that state. When one is in samadhi, however, he is beyond the states of waking, dreaming, and deep sleep and remains in a perfect state of consciousness in which desires are completely absent. The consciousness of samadhi is not at all like the consciousness of the waking state, which is just a fragment of the totality of consciousness. The consciousness of samadhi is as wide as infinite space; it is all-inclusive and is an unlimited and perennial source of knowledge. The three lower states—waking, dreaming, and sleeping—are experienced by all creatures. But the fourth state, the highest state of equilibrium, is attained only by the true aspirant.

यदा संहरते चायं कूर्मोऽङ्गानीव सर्वशः।
इन्द्रियाणीन्द्रियार्थेभ्यस्तस्य प्रज्ञा प्रतिष्ठिता।। ५८

58. *When, like a tortoise withdrawing his limbs, one withdraws each and all of the senses from their objects, his wisdom is established.*

When one gives up his desires, a new horizon of awareness opens to him. But those who hold on to their desires are not able to experience the higher dimensions of life. Fulfilling desires gives birth to many more desires, and there is no end to that cycle. When one learns to give up desires, however, he is elevated to the next step of experience. There is a mental law that if you give up what you have, you receive something new. That principle sustains life. If we do not give up the carbon dioxide and used up gases by exhaling, we cannot survive at all; we must exhale in order to inhale. In order to survive and to receive, we have to give up. Give up first; only then will you receive. This law continues to help one until the last breath of life. The student is always afraid and hesitant about giving up, for he is attached to all of the things that he thinks belong to him. His false sense of possessiveness is a great enemy on the path of unfoldment. One must learn to have courage and give up what he has in order to receive that which is glorious and beautiful, limitless and infinite.

One of the most important things to be given up is attachment to sensory experience. Withdrawal of the mind from the senses (*pratyahara*) is given a great deal of importance in the path of meditation, but no book specifically describes this process. Students think it is something that will make them passive, but that is incorrect. It is a skill to have complete control and command over the senses, which are employed by the mind to go to the external world and perceive things. The senses create a serious disturbance, for it is their inherent nature to jump from one object to another, compelled by the charms and temptations of the external world. The mind is disturbed and dissipated by such input and is unable to conceive of things as they are. Furthermore, the perceived objects are a source of distraction and dissipation; they create serious obstacles and obstructions for the sadhaka in his attempts to fathom higher levels of consciousness. Therefore, it is important to withdraw one's senses from the world of objects. This is not withdrawal from the world or from one's duties. It is learning to gather one's scattered energy. Withdrawal of the senses is an essential part of sadhana.

There is a very serious problem with the habitual way of perception: the senses have no capacity or ability to know things as they are. They can only have a partial glimpse of an object. That partial view of the object is charming and compelling, and it disorganizes and distorts the human mind. It only gives an inkling of delight and is not able to provide long-lasting joy because the senses have limited powers to know objects as they are.

There are three serious obstacles that interfere with one's ability to have a comprehensive view of the objects of the world: (1) The mind remains clouded; (2) The clouded mind uses incompetent senses to know the objects of the world; (3) The objects of the world change continually. These three problems lead to self-delusion, and one's ignorance regarding the objects of the world is not dispelled. There is an inborn desire in the human mind and heart to know what is real and what is illusory. But ordinarily the mind does not know how to do that. No matter how much training is given to the senses, the senses do not have the capacity to see things as they are. With the desire to experience the whole as it really is, the mind searches for a different approach, one that does not rely on the senses. It is only with pure reason that the mind can know the nature of the objects of the world, for due to their shallow nature, the senses can never peep into the secrets of the unknown side of the objects. No matter how powerful are the instruments used to see the objects as they are, they fail, for they have no power to reveal the true nature of the objects of the world.

There is a systematic method that one can apply to purify the mind so that there is clarity in his knowing. One can focus the mind on one single object—it can be concrete or abstract, large or small—so that the mind withdraws itself from the senses. When the mind is voluntarily isolated and under perfect control, it attains one-pointedness. And if that one-pointedness is turned inward, it becomes a useful means on one's inward journey to another way of knowing. The human being is like a miniature world, so by turning inward and examining himself, one can examine the nature of the universe. The natural tendency of the senses is to lead the mind to the objects of the world. The method that we are explaining is a very beneficial and useful voluntary effort that enables one to see, examine, and verify the nature of the objects of the world. And at the same time it makes one realize that the objects of the world do not hold any quality to charm and tempt the mind, for temptations and charms are created by the false input of the limited senses.

The concentrated power of mind has the ability to know without the help of the senses. In the inner world, the mind does not even need the help of the brain. The brain is only a medium for the energy called mind. It is a powerhouse, not the power; it is a distribution center but not the energy. Many modern physicists do not accept this theory, for they know only one method: applying sophisticated instruments to amplify sensory experiences. When one uses such instruments to study mental functions, they fail, for these instruments can only measure the superficial workings of the brain. Those who follow this method nevertheless contend that the brain is the mind, and that if they can develop the instruments to study the brain's functioning they will be able to understand the mind. They are like the blind man who holds the tail of an elephant and contends that an elephant is like a snake because its tail feels like one.

Modern technology and scientific knowledge are valid as far as the external world is concerned. But there is another exact science that helps one know the unknown dimensions of life. The Samkhya system of philosophy has given birth to yogic science. It is far more advanced and methodical than modern technology and the scientific method that is being used to probe into the microscopic and macroscopic levels of the physical universe.

Because of the limited nature of the senses and the foibles of the mind, one builds his own concepts, which offer a distorted picture of the world. The mind is a huge catalog of conceptions, and it uses these to create a philosophy that is neither reliable nor trustworthy. In order to avoid self-delusion, the sadhaka should understand the importance of voluntary withdrawal of the senses, and then he should make the mind one-pointed and turn it inward. There he will find a higher knowledge that is not contaminated by either the senses or the distracted and dissipated mind.

According to yoga philosophy and psychology, the human being goes through two distinct stages in his journey to Self-awakening. The first stage is traditionally referred to as evolution. In this process, consciousness travels from its subtlemost aspect through ever more gross aspects of existence, obscuring all awareness of oneself as pure Consciousness. Finally one becomes completely identified with the external world. In the second stage, which is traditionally referred to as involution, one reverses direction: he turns inward and commences a journey in which he rediscovers and experiences ever more subtle aspects of his being, finally coming to realize himself as pure Consciousness. Sensory withdrawal is one of the first important steps in the process of involution, a voluntary withdrawal in which the human mind is turned within. The sadhaka goes against the process of evolution, and that is just like going against the currents of a river. One needs to be well equipped for such an undertaking, for his habits and past experiences continually pull the mind outward. A method of concentration must be carefully devised that leads one to a meditative state and then finally to the source and center of consciousness. The withdrawal of the senses is a step forward in the path of meditation. Without it, the unknown part of life cannot be revealed to the human being. One-half is already known, but only the knowledge of the glorious missing half makes one's knowledge complete and perfect.

विषया विनिवर्तन्ते निराहारस्य देहिन:।
रसवर्जं रसोऽप्यस्य परं दृष्ट्वा निवर्तते।। ५९
यततो ह्यपि कौन्तेय पुरुषस्य विपश्चित:।
इन्द्रियाणि प्रमाथीनि हरन्ति प्रसभं मन:।। ६०
तानि सर्वाणि संयम्य युक्त आसीत् मत्पर:।
वशे हि यस्येन्द्रियाणि तस्य प्रज्ञा प्रतिष्ठिता। ६१

59. *When this body-bearer desists from food, the senses and their attractions turn away—all except for taste. But taste also ceases upon seeing the supreme One.*
60. *Even though an intelligent man continues to endeavor, yet the turbulent senses forcibly draw his mind away.*
61. *Therefore, controlling them all, joined in yoga, one should remain intent upon Me. He whose senses are under control, his wisdom is established.*

It is the inherent nature of the senses to contact the external world. The senses have tremendous power; only those who know the technique of withdrawing the senses can realize how powerful they are. A little effort is not sufficient to attain withdrawal of the senses. Aspirants often think that by creating distance from the objects of the senses, by not enjoying the objects, the senses can be controlled. But that is not true. Eating food is a sensory experience, and if one does not eat food for some time, the desire to eat becomes more intense and the mind imagines food in many forms. By depriving the senses from experiencing their objects, the desire for enjoyment can actually increase rather than decrease. By fasting one cannot get rid of the *vasana* (desire) to eat. It is only when the aspirant realizes the Self and finds delight in It that he becomes free from the temptations and attractions created by the senses. But the aspirant cannot have knowledge of Atman as long as the charms and temptations are in the mind.

If one follows the nature of the senses and does not understand that the senses are the source of distraction, his mind will be completely dissipated. The sadhaka must make constant effort; regular practice is important. Patanjali, the codifier of yoga science, states in the Yoga Sutras (1:14) that the sadhaka should practice for a long time without any break and with full effort and profound faith. Otherwise sadhana will not be fruitful. Steady-mindedness is possible only after one has controlled the senses.

These verses remind the sadhaka that he should not be disappointed by the results of his sadhana if he fails once, twice, or even many times. Constant effort will help him to attain his goal. When his wants and desires are abandoned, then alone will he experience freedom.

ध्यायतो विषयान्पुंसः सङ्गस्तेषूपजायते।
सङ्गात् सञ्जायते कामः कामात्क्रोधोऽभिजायते।। ६२
क्रोधाद्भवति संमोहः संमोहात्स्मृतिविभ्रमः।
स्मृतिभ्रंशाद्बुद्धिनाशो बुद्धिनाशात्प्रणश्यति।। ६३

62. *As a person contemplates the objects of the senses, there arises in him attachment to them; from attachment arises desire; from desire anger is produced.*

63. *From anger comes delusion; from delusion, the confusion of memory and loss of mindfulness; from the disappearance of memory and mindfulness, the loss of the faculty of discrimination; by loss of the faculty of discrimination, one perishes.*

If one who constantly thinks of satisfying his desires for sensory gratification finds any hindrance or opposition to the fulfillment of his desires, he becomes frustrated. That frustration leads to anger toward that which is frustrating him. Unfulfilled desire or dissatisfaction is thus the cause of anger. When one becomes angry he forgets to use discrimination, and his memory wavers. That leads to the loss of reason, and one's mind becomes completely imbalanced.

The downfall of a human being begins when he becomes preoccupied with the objects of sensory gratification and the enjoyment of those objects. Such a deluded person goes on collecting the objects of sense enjoyment. He becomes dependent on those objects, and gratification becomes the goal of his life, but his pursuit of pleasure creates self-degradation. Such a person is called a hedonist. When for some reason the objects of sense gratification are absent or not available, he becomes frustrated and angry.

If two such people seek the same pleasure and desire the same object, they become enemies. For example, two great friends might kill each other if they are strongly attracted to and fall in love with the same woman. But two friends who are on the path of Self-realization and share the same goal become even closer, because love for sensual objects is quite different from love for Self-enlightenment. The first leads to selfishness and the latter to selflessness. A selfish person is never able to conceive of the idea of selflessness, which is the singular expression of universal love. When we study the lives and sayings of great people, we find in them the quality of selflessness, no matter what their religious or cultural background might be. Ahimsa (noninjury) and selflessness are common characteristics of these great people, whereas selfishness and violence are the symptoms of those who do not remember the Self, who are preoccupied with and engrossed in sense gratification.

रागद्वेषवियुक्तैस्तु विषयानिन्द्रियैश्चरन्।
आत्मवश्यैर्विधेयात्मा प्रसादमधिगच्छति।। ६४
प्रसादे सर्वदुःखानां हानिरस्योपजायते।
प्रसन्नचेतसो ह्याशु बुद्धिः पर्यवतिष्ठते।। ६५

64. *Conducting oneself with the senses, towards the objects of the senses, however, free of attraction and aversion, and under control of the Self, one cultivating the Self attains a healthy and pleasant state of mind.*
65. *Upon attaining such pleasantness of mind, there is a diminution of all sorrows. The intelligence of a person of such a pleased mind attends quickly upon him.*

Samyama (self-discipline) helps the sadhaka all the time. One who does not believe in self-discipline cannot attain profound knowledge of the Self. Sense gratifications are only momentarily pleasurable: the moment the pleasurable object vanishes, the pleasure disappears as well. And when pleasurable objects are absent, one experiences pain. Attachment to the objects of the world is therefore the source of both pleasure and pain. Tranquility is experienced by the mind that is free from desire for sense gratification. The mind is ordinarily the slave of the senses that are employed by it. But when the mind has control over the senses, it has the power to discriminate right from wrong and that which is helpful from that which is distracting. A steady, stable, and equable mind is a peaceful mind. And a peaceful mind alone is free from grief.

The mind that is free from grief and sorrow and from distractions and dissipations creates a forceful will. With the use of that will, one has tremendous success in attaining his goal. A dissipated mind has no will, but a concentrated and one-pointed mind creates will power. A student with a weak and feeble will is not successful in his sadhana because of distractions, but the student whose mind is concentrated and one-pointed has a firm and determined will force that makes him courageous and fearless and able to remove all sorts of obstacles and barriers.

Modern students are afraid of discipline. They fail to understand its meaning and dismiss it. They have the misconception that discipline is a sort of punishment imposed on them by those in authority. Therefore, the moment they hear the word discipline, they leave. But without discipline, control of the mind is impossible, and without control of the mind, one-pointedness is not possible. Therefore, there is no will power, no courage, no fearlessness, for these qualities successively evolve from the practice of self-discipline.

Modern students have a desire to seek, but they constantly bathe in material waters and find delight in the pleasures they experience there. Preoccupied with sense gratification, their desire to know truth is never fulfilled. They think of going in one direction, but all the while they are going the other way. The sadhaka needs to understand that mind, action, and speech should be directed toward one goal. A division should not be created by having a desire to seek the truth while still pursuing the enjoyment of sense gratification. The way one desires is the way one should think, and the way one thinks is the way he should act. Otherwise a serious division is created within.

नास्ति बुद्धिरयुक्तस्य न चायुक्तस्य भावना।
न चाभावयतः शान्तिरशान्तस्य कुतः सुखम्।। ६६
इन्द्रियाणां हि चरतां यन्मनोऽनुविधीयते।
तदस्य हरति प्रज्ञां वायुर्नावमिवाम्भसि।। ६७
तस्माद्यस्य महाबाहो निगृहीतानि सर्वशः।
इन्द्रियाणीन्द्रियार्थेभ्यस्तस्य प्रज्ञा प्रतिष्ठिता।। ६८

66. *There is no discriminating wisdom in one who is not joined in yoga, nor is there any cultivating of contemplativeness for one who is not joined in yoga. One who has not cultivated contemplation has no peace; how can there be happiness for one who is not at peace?*
67. *The mind that is applied to following the wandering senses, indeed such a mind plunders his wisdom as wind blows a boat in the water.*

68. *Therefore, O Mighty-armed One, he whose senses one and all are held in control and held back from their objects, his wisdom is established.*

Pure reason is the essential means to discriminate the truth from the non-truth, the eternal from the non-eternal. That discrimination helps one to become non-attached to the objects of the world. When one resolutely practices sadhana, he attains the power of nonattachment, and when one is non-attached, he has full concentration. One who has full concentration attains a one-pointed mind and can utilize all of his human resources. He is able to experience peace, and peace brings happiness. That happiness is not the same as the pleasure received from the objects of sense gratification. Pleasure is a joy experienced through the senses, whereas happiness is an outcome of the state of tranquility.

The human body is like a chariot in which the individual self is seated. Human intelligence is the charioteer, and the mind is the reins. The senses are the horses leading the chariot toward the objects of sensory enjoyment. The wise man who is able to make his mind tranquil stands firm and leads the chariot on the path to enlightenment, whereas the unwise lack the wisdom of yoga and are unable to control the senses. Untrained horses are unreliable, but trained horses lead the chariot on the path to enlightenment. Thus, the wise man learns to master the senses. He attains freedom, but he who is unwise and uncontrolled is trapped by the snares of births and deaths.

या निशा सर्वभूतानां तस्यां जागर्ति संयमी।
यस्यां जाग्रति भूतानि सा निशा पश्यतो मुनेः।। ६९

69. *That which is night to the ordinary human being is day to the wise, and that in which the ordinary human being remains awake is night to the wise one who sees.*

This verse contains unique wisdom. The behavior of the sadhaka and yogi is explained by saying that that which is night to the ordinary human being is day to the wise, and that which is night to the wise is day to the ignorant. The song of life of the sadhaka is well understood and assimilated in this verse. The song of life is the eternal song, and the entire music of the cosmos forms an orchestra that plays one and the same song with many variations. The wise person is able to hear that song by making his whole being an ear. That song is not heard by the ignorant one, for he is busy listening to the gross jarring, nerve-shattering, and disturbing sounds of contemporary society.

The sadhakas who have experienced the higher dimensions of life, who are able to have a glimpse of the Eternal, and who have touched the Infinite, are awakened to truth. But others remain sleeping, unaware of truth. While the ordinary man identifies himself with the worldly activities of the day, the sage remains unaffected by the mundane happenings and finds his joy in quiet hours late at night. Ordinary people do not know how to utilize the calm, serene stillness of night, but the yogis enjoy this calmness in the practice of samadhi. For them night drops the blossoms of their sadhana, and they pick up those blossoms dropped by night. Such fortunate sadhakas are blessed. Those rare ones sleep in the daytime and remain awake at night. For ordinary and ignorant people, that is an impossibility. Those whose feet walk in light have a peculiar but wonderful way of using the span of life that is not understood by ordinary people. When everyone in the world remains sleeping, sadhakas remain awake. And when the whole world is awake and preoccupied with the pursuit of sensory pleasure and selfish ends, the sadhaka sleeps. He remains unaffected and uninfluenced by the rush and roar and distractions created by the day.

Sri Krishna hints at the differences in the thinking and behavior of these two kinds of people: the enlightened ones, true seekers and sadhakas who are constantly aware of the truth; and the ignorant who are totally unaware, who chew the weed that grows in the water to quench their thirst rather than drinking the water. The external allurements do contain pleasures, but they have no capacity to quench the thirst. The thirst for happiness is the perennial thirst of man. It is only quenched by the knowledge of the real Self.

आपूर्यमाणमचलप्रतिष्ठं
समुद्रमापः प्रविशन्ति यद्वत्।
तद्वत्कामा यं प्रविशन्ति सर्वे
स शान्तिमाप्नोति न कामकामी।। ७०
विहाय कामान् यः सर्वान् पुमांश्चरति निःस्पृहः।
निर्ममो निरहंकारः स शान्तिमधिगच्छति।। ७१
एषा ब्राह्मी स्थितिः पार्थ नैनां प्राप्य विमुह्यति।
स्थित्वास्यामन्तकालेऽपि ब्रह्मनिर्वाणमृच्छति।। ७२

70. *As waters enter the ocean, which is totally full yet whose basin and boundaries remain stable, he whom all the desires enter similarly attains peace, and not one who desires the desires.*
71. *The person who wanders free of attachment, having abandoned all desire, devoid of ego and of the concept of 'mine,' he attains peace.*
72. *This is the godly state, O Son of Pritha; attaining this, one is no longer confused. Remaining in it even at the final hour, one finds absorption into Brahman.*

The aspirant who has attained calmness and serenity is like the infinite sky in which storms, winds, and lightning may rage but which have no power to disturb the serenity of the infinite. Similarly the storms of desires and emotions pass through the mind but are not at all able to disturb the tranquility of the realized yogi. Ironically enough, one who leads a pleasure-oriented life is usually miserable, whereas the yogi who has perfect self control and has attained a state of calmness knows the joyous art of living and being, which enables him to walk on this earth without being affected by the so-called charms and temptations of the world. Sri Krishna teaches Arjuna that this is the state of mind of one who has realized the Self. Such a Self-realized human being is not subject to delusion, dejection, or despondency. Even at the crucial hour he remains undisturbed, for he identifies himself with his essential nature. Brahman, instead of identifying himself with the ego and the objects of the world. The man who is free from egocentric I-ness and my-ness performs his duties skillfully and joyfully.

Such an enlightened one develops an entirely different attitude toward life, relationships, and objects. He does not identify with the objects of the world and therefore lives in the midst of so-called possessions while maintaining his aloofness. The ordinary man, however, is in the habit of identifying himself with the objects of the world; he clings to his possessions and develops an attachment for them. He is not certain that he will attain what he desires and always remains afraid that he might lose what he possesses. The fear of not gaining what he wants and the fear of losing what he possesses makes him miserable. But the yogi who has attained the state of equanimity, tranquility, and equilibrium knows that the objects of the world should be used only as means, without a sense of attachment. They should not be allowed to dissipate the mind. What is there to possess? Great ones are great because they develop will power so that sense gratification and the sense of possessing things completely lose their value. This attitude comes after complete self-transformation. One then lives in the world discharging his normal duties without being affected.

Such a man is always aware of the truth that he has come to this world as a traveler on a long voyage. He is always like a guest in this world. Such a traveling guest does not carry a burden on his back because the traveling would then become a painful experience. He always remembers that life is like a crowded bazaar, and he devises a method of traveling through that bazaar without being hurt or hurting others. As a guest lives in someone's home without disturbing the members of the family, the traveler thinks, "I am a guest here for a brief stay. Nothing belongs to me." With that attitude there are no chances of becoming attached to the things and relationships of the world. For a true traveler the world is a base camp where he can compose and gather his resources for the onward journey. Actually we are all travelers through this world, so let us not become attached to it. As a mountaineer has a base camp where he prepares himself to go to the summit, so is the case with us and our stay in the world. Let us make our journey pleasant and facilitative instead of becoming lost.

A sadhaka who has attained a state of equilibrium knows that death, which is horrifying for the ordinary person, creates a wonderful melody like a mother singing a lullaby to put her tired and weary baby into deep sleep. As a short sleep gives rest to the tired baby who then awakens refreshed, death gives rest to the worn, tired traveler who awakens reclothed in a new garb to continue on his way. Death for a sage is merely a change. He assumes a new garment and comes back to his path to continue his journey to the infinite. Death has no power to deviate the attention of such a great man. He maintains his consciousness of Brahman, here and hereafter.

> *Thus ends the second chapter, in which Sri Krishna awakens Arjuna front his deep anguish. In this chapter the dialogue between Sri Krishna and Arjuna encompasses the philosophy of Samkhya and the practical method of yoga science.*

Chapter Three
The Yoga of Action

अर्जुन उवाच
ज्यायसी चेत्कर्मणस्ते मता बुद्धिर्जनार्दन।
तत्किं कर्मणि घोरे मां नियोजयसि केशव।। १
व्यामिश्रेणेव वाक्येन बुद्धिं मोहयसीव मे।
तदेकं वद निश्चित्य येन श्रेयोऽहमाप्नुयाम्।। २

Arjuna said
1. *O Krishna, if you believe wisdom to be greater than action then why are you urging me toward this terrible action?*
2. *With statements that seem mixed up, you are apparently confusing my intellect; therefore, tell me one definitive thing whereby I may attain beatitude.*

In the second chapter of the Bhagavad Gita, Sri Krishna helped Arjuna to sharpen his faculty of discrimination, judgment, and decisiveness and made him aware of the pure Self within, which is timeless and beyond the world of forms and names. He helped Arjuna understand that the Self is not subject to change, death, or destruction, for the Self is timeless and eternal. He also made Arjuna aware of the transitory nature of the world of objects. No matter how much one tries to maintain outer conditions in a state of steadiness, it is impossible to prevent them from changing.

Arjuna experienced grief because he had adopted the assumptions of ordinary people. A person who is unaware of the eternal nature of the Absolute and whose mind is undisciplined and disorderly lives in the midst of confusion. Forgetting the truth that the nature of the Self is eternal and that the nature of the temporal is changeable, such a person becomes infatuated with objects and relationships and becomes attached to them. But with the help of a teacher, one can develop a profound view of both the eternal and the non-eternal. And with sadhana and discipline he can establish himself in his essential nature, which is eternal Truth. He can then learn to perform his duties in a non-attached way, which means doing duties selflessly, lovingly, and skillfully. He realizes that absolute Truth is infinite and encompasses the whole. Attaining that knowledge, he becomes fearless and goes beyond the *maya* of delusion created by the confusion of the mind. Such a state of mind leads one to the attainment of tranquility and equanimity.

Sri Krishna began by teaching Samkhya philosophy and psychology, which distinguishes between the impermanence of the apparent reality and the eternal nature of the ultimate Reality. He then explained the importance of performing one's duties, and finally he described that yoga in which the development of buddhi appears to take precedence over action. It is natural at this stage that Arjuna's mind is confused, for he does not yet understand that Sri Krishna is not presenting contradictory teachings but complementary facets of the process of self-transformation. Arjuna's confusion will gradually be resolved as the dialogue progresses.

The knowledge of Samkhya philosophy imparted to Arjuna was not sufficient for him to understand that his duty, fighting the war, could be helpful for him as well as for the whole society. He has come out of his serious state of mental depression, anxiety, and anguish and now he wants to be completely free from doubt regarding the duties he has to perform. Arjuna has gained knowledge from Sri Krishna, but he still does not know how to apply that knowledge in his daily life. He also needs methods that will help him discipline his mind and attain that summit which will give him the light of direct knowledge and enable him to attain a state of equanimity.

There are major difficulties encountered by the aspirant at this stage: (1) He has gained theoretical knowledge, but that knowledge is not yet fully assimilated in his mind and heart; (2) Without a definite method of sadhana and discipline of the senses, mind, and its modifications, he cannot direct his energies inward and cannot have a one-pointed mind; (3) Lust for gaining the pleasures of the world creates attachment, which is the source of misery; and (4) Because of attachment, pure reason does not function. But when sadhana and discipline are practiced, will power gives the aspirant the gift of inner strength and self-reliance. Will power makes him determined to come out of his old habits. He thereby becomes capable of understanding that non-attachment is true love. Non-attachment and attachment are the creations of the higher and lower mind respectively. One is a state of identification with truth, whereas the other is identification with the temporal.

In the second chapter of the Bhagavad Gita, buddhi yoga and karma yoga were explained separately though they are actually one and the same. Action or duty performed is visible, but the profound knowledge that helps one perform skillful duties is inner action and is invisible. Long before the action is performed outwardly, it is first performed subtly in the inner world. The source of action in the inner world is the pure reason of buddhi. So mastery of invisible action in the subtle world is called buddhi yoga, and action that is skillfully performed in the external world is called karma yoga. A seed in the palm of one's hand has all the potential to bring forth flowers and fruits, but when the seed is sown in the soil and emerges as a plant, then alone does the full expression of the potential of the seed come to the visible world. One is an invisible and unseen reality, the other a visible and seen reality. Buddhi yoga and karma yoga are thus, two expressions of one and the same existence.

These first two verses of the third chapter show that Arjuna does not want to blindly follow the instructions of his teacher but wants to understand Sri Krishna's instructions before he practices and brings his inner experience to full expression. Even after the aspirant resolves to follow his teacher, his mind cannot comprehend the wisdom imparted because of his lack of direct knowledge and practice. Arjuna's queries are genuine and reflect the problems shared by all students. One should learn to be like Arjuna, who persists in putting questions before Sri Krishna rather than following without understanding. Sri Krishna encourages Arjuna to express his doubt and confusion so they can be dispelled. A real teacher never tires of answering the questions of his beloved students. But most students either follow the instructions of their teacher blindly without understanding them, or they just try to understand the instructions intellectually but do not experiment with them and practice to assimilate them correctly. Arjuna, however, is not seeking mere intellectual clarification. His questions are intended to help him resolve his doubts about his path so that he can practice with full conviction and understanding. Having doubt is a valid state of mind, for before anything is done a doubt arises: Shall 1 do it or not? Here Arjuna is like the mind, and Sri Krishna is the perfect yogi and sage who with his pure reason helps the mind to remove its doubt so that action can be performed. The part of mind that doubts is manas; that which decides is called buddhi.

श्री भगवानुवाच
लोकेऽस्मिन्द्विविधा निष्ठा पुरा प्रोक्ता मयानघ।
ज्ञानयोगेन सांख्यानां कर्मयोगेन योगिनाम्।। ३
न कर्मणामनारम्भान्नैष्कर्म्यं पुरुषोऽश्नुते।
न च संन्यसनादेव सिद्धिं समधिगच्छति।। ४

The Blessed Lord said
3. *O Sinless One, in this world I have taught two kinds of discipline: the yoga of knowledge for those whose path is of discriminating wisdom and the yoga of action for the yogis.*
4. *A person does not attain the state of actionlessness simply by not taking initiative in the matter of actions, nor does one attain perfection by mere renunciation.*

Verses 3 and 4 further explain the fine distinction between the path of jnana yoga (the yoga of knowledge) and karma yoga (the yoga of action). Verse 3 indicates that there are two means for attaining the highest state of tranquility. Both are equally valid; neither one is superior. The word *nishtha* means firm conviction or a well thought out and firm decision free from doubt. A firm adherence to the path of knowledge is called *jnana nishtha,* and a firm commitment to the path of action is called *karma nishtha.* The followers of the path of knowledge have a firm conviction that one can attain the highest state of liberation through knowledge alone. The followers of karma yoga believe in performing their duties with non-attachment as a means of self-unfoldment. In the path of jnana yoga, knowledge, nonattachment, and renunciation are the essential values. In the path of karma yoga performing one's duties skillfully, selflessly, and with non-attachment are the prerequisites. It is interesting to note that the function of the five senses in the human body is to gain knowledge, and the function of the five organs (mouth, hands, feet, the organs of excretion and of procreation) is to help one to do his duties through action. These two sets of organs complement one another in the maintenance of human existence. It is also interesting that Carl Jung, the modern psychologist, classified people into two categories: those with an introverted nature and those with an extroverted nature. Those who look inward and try to understand the internal states are more inclined to follow the path of jnana yoga. Those who are extroverted and committed to do their actions are called karma yogis.

The path of jnana yoga involves far more than renunciation. Traditionally it is based on four means: discrimination, nonattachment, a keen longing for liberation, and the six-fold virtues (control of the mind and senses, endurance, turning away from worldly objects, faith, and tranquility). These qualities are explained in subsequent verses. Verse 4 states that one cannot attain perfection by mere renunciation. Suppose an aspirant suddenly decides to follow the path of renunciation but makes his decision impulsively rather than through real wisdom. He renounces his home and all that he owns, for renunciation to most people means creating a physical distance between a person and his objects. But until one has attained the state of non-attachment, he continues to remember his past and to long for all that he has left behind. In such a situation true renunciation is not accomplished, and the real knowledge that helps in the path of liberation is absent. If one is not able to create the fire of non-attachment in his renunciation of externals, he is not able to dispel the darkness of ignorance. Non-attachment and renunciation go hand in hand. In the path of action non-attachment is also important, and there it is related to the fruits of the actions rather than to the actions themselves. Some commentators translate the word *vairagya* as indifference rather than as non-attachment, but that translation does not convey the true meaning of the word. Nonattachment is love for duty and not indifference or disinterest. One does not attain freedom by not doing his duty.

Non-attachment is the highest virtue; it gives freedom both to one who prefers to perform his duty and yet remain unaffected by worldly turmoils and to one who thinks that duties are self-imposed and believes renunciation to be superior to the path of action. Nonattachment is a virtue that helps in both paths. Actually a renunciate also performs his duties with full sincerity in order to attain his goal of final emancipation. In the path of action one performs his actions skillfully and selflessly by remaining non-attached and thereby attaining final emancipation.

Although the paths of action and renunciation are different, the aim of both is one and the same. In the life of a renunciate there seems to be a *tyaga,* a literal separation of oneself from the objects of desire. The renunciate renounces all objects. His sole desire is to attain the state of freedom, and he has a duty to maintain one single desire: to be one with the Absolute. His wheel of life still rotates but without bearing fruits. In the path of renunciation tyaga and non-attachment are two essentials. In the path of action, however, there is no tyaga, but one learns to perform his duty in the midst of all objects and relationships and to renounce the fruits. The path of action is a path of conquest and love. The path of renunciation is a path of sacrifice.

In the path of action one offers the fruits of his actions to others.

He acknowledges the Absolute in everyone. That is prayer and worship in reality and not a prayer of empty words. If one prays but never realizes the profound meaning of the prayer by practicing it in his daily life, he will not find inner satisfaction. Without inner satisfaction one remains anxious.

न हि कश्चित्क्षणमपि जातु तिष्ठत्यकर्मकृत् ।
कार्यते ह्यवशः कर्म सर्वः प्रकृतिजैर्गुणैः ।। ५

5. *No one can remain without performing actions even for a moment. Every creature is helplessly made to perform action by the gunas born of nature.*

   All living beings have to perform actions. As long as one breathes, he performs actions, even if he does not want to. Even sitting still and sleeping are actions. Since one has to perform actions, he should learn to do them in the best possible way. The human being is responsible for all his actions and the fruits (rewards) obtained by those actions. If one resists his duties, he creates conflict and strife both for himself and others, whereas if he learns to act graciously he creates harmony and joy within and without. Resistance can be positive in many circumstances. For example, if one is asked to do something that is against his conscience, resistance is a force that helps him to follow his inner promptings. But resisting one's duties makes misery out of the inevitable. Sattva, rajas, and tamas are three qualities of the human mind that bind the individual and motivate him to act. They will be explained in depth later.

कर्मेन्द्रियाणि संयम्य य आस्ते मनसा स्मरन् ।
इन्द्रियार्थान्विमूढात्मा मिथ्याचारः स उच्यते ।। ६

6. *One of deluded psyche who, controlling the senses of action, continues to remember with the mind the objects of the senses is said to be a hypocrite.*

There is considerable confusion about the path of renunciation. Many so-called renunciates are hypocrites; outwardly they appear to be austere and to avoid contact with the objects that lead to attachment, but their minds remain thinking of the pleasures of the world. That sort of austerity is false and dishonest. Such hypocrites remain deluded, and such austerities never bear fruit. That sort of behavior weakens the human endeavor and does an injustice to oneself. If one continues to live in that way, he creates guilt in his mind. He neither has peace of mind nor is he able to perform his actions with full attention and skill. A hypocritical person is concerned with outward expression and with following the letter of the law, whereas one who is genuine is more interested in his inner experience than in appearance.

The distinction between an outer show and inner experience is an important one. The former has no positive value and may even be .detrimental to one's growth if it is not a reflection of his inner state of being. It is all too easy for one to make an outer pretense of sincerity and to enjoy praise and accolades though his thoughts and feelings are completely contrary. Jesus taught that one should pray in secret and not as the hypocrites do. If one refrains from making a public show of his sincere inner experiences, those experiences are less likely to be contaminated by egotistical gratification.

External renunciation (tyaga) is a step on the path to Self-realization, but if one does not attain inner renunciation (vairagya) he creates many serious problems for himself. Such a person cannot live as a genuine renunciate. As a result of intense emotion, thousands of people spontaneously decided to follow Buddha and to become renunciates. But they soon found that their worldly desires remained with them. They were afraid that the world would not accept them back, so they corrupted the path of renunciation, indulging in the fulfillment of sensory pleasures while still claiming to be renunciates. That has happened in the spiritual traditions of the West as well.

The hypocrisy of some does not invalidate renunciation, the rare path of the fortunate few, for hypocrites are not renunciates. They may dress like renunciates, but their minds still go to the grooves of their old habit patterns. They are not truthful to themselves so they are not truthful to others. Real renunciates are the most courageous of people. They belong to the heavens though they live on the earth.

Hypocritical behavior is an outward expression of a cleavage within the personality. There is a split between one's innermost feelings and thoughts and his outer expressions. The hypocritical person is afraid that others will not accept him as he is, so he uses a false mask so that others will respect him. Then out of fear of condemnation he goes on building a false front. He condemns himself because he is guilty, and he is afraid that others will discover him. A hypocritical person does not allow anyone to know him as he thinks and feels inside, and he may not even know himself. It is likely that he keeps his innermost feelings secret even from himself and consciously identifies with his insincere behavior. If his sincerity is challenged, such a person will bring all his defenses to bear; he will deny, attack, and feel self-righteous. This type of person always remains unknown and a stranger to himself and has nothing to contribute to society, for if one does not even admit to himself his inner thoughts and feelings, how can he possibly explore deeper dimensions and find that inner Self of all? In the process of self-discovery one must uncover, examine, and gain mastery over each stratum of his existence. And the first stratum to be faced is that of the unacceptable qualities that lie hidden behind the facade one presents to the world. Only by fully acknowledging those qualities can one take them in hand and transform himself.

Modern psychologists have noted that a duplicitous way of being is the hallmark of the neurotic. Some have gone so far as to assert that duplicity is the very basis of neurosis, and that when one's inner feeling and thoughts become one with his outer expression, the neurosis and interpersonal melodramas cease. Such therapists focus on helping one to express himself in a straightforward way. When that is accomplished the considerable energy that is invested in keeping one's inner feelings and thoughts hidden from oneself and from the world is freed up. One then becomes energetic and dynamic.

यस्त्विन्द्रियाणि मनसा नियम्यारभतेऽर्जुन।
कर्मेन्द्रियैः कर्मयोगमसक्तः स विशिष्यते।। ७
नियतं कुरु कर्म त्वं कर्म ज्यायो ह्यकर्मणः।
शरीरयात्रापि च ते न प्रसिद्ध्येदकर्मणः।। ८
यज्ञार्थात्कर्मणोऽन्यत्र लोकोऽयं कर्मबन्धनः।
तदर्थं कर्म कौन्तेय मुक्तसङ्गः समाचर।। ९

7. *He, however, who, controlling the senses with the mind, O Arjuna, initiates the yoga of action with the senses of action, he, unattached, is distinguished.*

8. *Do perform the assigned action; action is greater than inaction. Even the journey of your body cannot be successful if you are inactive.*

9. *This world is the cause of the bondage of karma, except for actions performed for the purpose of sacrifice. Therefore, O Son of Kunti, perform actions for the sake of sacrifice and conduct yourself as free of attachment.*

Sri Krishna shows Arjuna that his thought of renunciation is hypocritical, for it comes from confusion and despondency born of attachment. True renunciation, however, is based on non-attachment. It is also important to perform actions with a completely non-attached mind. That is far superior to not doing action or being afraid to act. One who has practiced with sincerity and honesty by applying full human efforts can attain the wisdom of non-attachment. Thus, he is able to control his senses and perform his duties.

A human being cannot exist on this earth without doing actions. There are three kinds of action that we perform in daily life. Actions such as eating, brushing our teeth, and bathing are helpful to ourselves only; they are not helpful to others. Such actions are essential, and when we regulate our habits and properly perform these self-oriented actions, we maintain our health. There is another kind of action, which we perform for ourselves and others in the context of our relationships, that is performed on the basis of coexistence. Sharing in cooking and shopping are examples of that type of action. But here is a higher kind of action that leads one to liberation. In that action all the fruits are surrendered and offered to others.

Verse 8 can be understood in two ways. The first meaning is that one should do those actions that have been decided by the coordinator of all the faculties of mind with full determination, self-confidence, self-control, non-attachment, and will power. That is the highest of all actions, and it will be described in depth later. The other meaning of the verse is that one should perform his duty according to his nature. The three gunas (qualities of nature) motivate the human being to perform actions. Actions performed as the outcome of one's own primitive nature are definitely inferior to the actions performed by self-determined will.

The message of the Bhagavad Gita is that one should create a sense of responsibility toward his own duty. And he should study his own abilities and potentials to help him understand and skillfully perform his duty. When we analyze the abilities of the masses, we find out that there are four categories of people in the world. The first category, those who are mentally brilliant and have profound control over their senses and minds, should devote more time to unfolding their awareness and should use their brilliance to serve society. Their dharma (duty) is to serve others through their brilliance and intelligence, to teach and impart knowledge. The second category, those who are less inclined toward the path of jnana but are physically strong, should learn to use their physical powers in performing their duties. Third is that category of people who have practical knowledge for living in the world. They can earn and gain and at the same time share their earnings with others generously. Fourth are those who can attend to the needs of others and perform services for others and thus make their livelihood.

These four categories were established for the welfare of society and for the distribution of labor. With the passage of time, that division became the caste system, the greatest of all curses in Indian society. In ancient times that division was accepted for the successful integration of society, so that society as a whole did its dharma for the well-being of all. As time passed selfish leaders and priests rigidified those divisions and thus created a great gulf in the social order. They sought to fulfill their own selfish ends by converting the division of labor into the caste system. That enabled them to use and control others.

In the modern world child psychologists and counselors in schools and colleges study and analyze the student's behavior, intelligence, and predominant habit patterns in order to help him select the subjects that will be most helpful to him. It is important for teachers and counselors to make students aware of their abilities and potentials, for if one is forced to study subjects that are contrary to his abilities and interests, he will not be successful. Despite the availability of counseling in schools as well as aptitude and personality tests, most young people today remain confused about the direction their lives should take. Their problem is perhaps the exact opposite of those caught in a caste system. Free to follow their whims, they often pursue that which excites their fancy at the time and then lose interest and jump to something else. Such experimentation has its value, but it is more helpful if it is guided by an attempt to understand one's propensities, inclinations, and inherent skills and assets as well as one's weaknesses. In these verses the idea of acting according to one's nature refers to potentialities, not to the rigid and useless caste system. One should direct his life so that he can use his assets and work with his weak areas, turning them into strengths as well.

Arjuna, physically healthy, strong, and trained in the art of war, talks of following the path of renunciation and forgets his duty. He is not able to understand his dharma but wants to follow the dharma of others. In such a case calamity ensues. Sri Krishna, a great yogi, already knows Arjuna's potentials and thus recommends the path of action, and not the path of renunciation. After one understands his nature and the course of action he should follow, he has still to understand the way to perform his duties. Sri Krishna teaches Arjuna that the highest of all deeds are those performed with non-attachment, those in which the rewards of the actions are offered as sacrifice.

Many a stupid and ignorant person misunderstands sacrifice and applies it in a very distorted and shameful manner: killing and offering a goat, lamb, or other animal to please his god. Butchering animals is a shameful act, but there are many remote corners of the world where people still practice animal sacrifice as a part of worship. There is no logic that can prove that such a sacrifice will please God. How can He who is the law of love and equality be pleased by such rituals? Correctly understood, the word "sacrifice" means to give away even one's rights for the sake of others, willingly and happily. If one can give the best that he has and willingly offer it to the service of others, that is called sacrifice.

सहयज्ञाः प्रजाः सृष्ट्वा पुरोवाच प्रजापतिः।
अनेन प्रसविष्यध्वमेष वोऽस्त्विष्टकामधुक्।। १०
देवान्भावयतानेन ते देवा भावयन्तु वः।
परस्परं भावयन्तः श्रेयः परमवाप्स्यथ।। ११
इष्टान्भोगान्हि वो देवा दास्यन्ते यज्ञभाविताः।
तैर्दत्तानप्रदायैभ्यो यो भुङ्क्ते स्तेन एव सः।। १२

10. *In the beginning the Progenitor, having created the beings, together with sacrifice, exhorted them: Multiply by this sacrifice. May this be the bearer of the fulfillment of desires for you.*
11. *Cultivate the gods by this, and may those gods nurture you. Nurturing each other, you both will attain the highest beatitude.*
12. *The gods, cultivated by sacrifice, will provide for you the desired pleasures. He who enjoys these pleasures given by them without offering them in return is merely a thief.*

Sri Krishna describes the various ways of performing one's duties. He says that duties performed for the purpose of sacrifice do not create bondage, but duties performed selfishly bind the human being to the results of his actions. Giving up attachment and performing one's actions as a sacrifice is the message given in these verses. The term *yajna* (worship or rite) is not used here in the limited sense of offering oblations. Many kinds of yajna described in the scriptures are performed by householders for various purposes. Some people offer oblations, some do austerities, and some think that studying scriptures in a ritualistic way is also yajna. The control of the senses is also a kind of yajna. Practicing the yoga of non-attachment through the control of senses and mind and sacrificing all the fruits of actions is called *anasakti yoga*. Actually human life itself is a yajna. All action performed from morning until evening—eating, drinking, talking, walking, and sleeping—are yajna, though few people are aware of that. The word yajna, which comes from the root "yaj," refers to three types of action: the worship of gods; giving away gifts; and becoming free from fear by controlling the mind and senses, studying the scriptures, and establishing truth, peace, and compassion for all beings. Each of the three types of yajna is performed with the goal of sacrifice, giving up the fruits that are received from such practices rather than retaining them for one's own use. Actions that involve reverence and bring various elements of society together are also called yajna. Yajna can also be categorized according to whether it is performed externally or internally. Ordinary people offer material oblations, but in internal yajna, only those austerities are performed that are helpful in the control of the senses and mind.

When one has performed yajna, the fruits he reaps therein should be offered to others. Such a yajna is the highest of all duties. The action that is selflessly done to help the poor and needy is another beneficial form of yajna. When one learns to give selflessly of the fruits of his actions for the benefit of others, he is free from the bondage created by the fruits of his actions. Such a sacrifice is revered in society and at the same time gives happiness and freedom to those who perform yajna. All truly great people have sacrificed their lives for the service of humanity. Sacrifice is a noble quality of the human being and one of the expressions of a virtuous life. Sri Krishna teaches Arjuna the importance of yajna, that it is a duty and that it should be performed selflessly, not for selfish ends.

Householders perform yajna, for it is important for them to do such duty regularly in order to attain perfection in the world. Selfless service performed by householders is called yajna, but in the case of a renunciate the term yajna is not used in the same way that it is accepted in the external world, for the renunciate has no worldly duties to perform. Whatever duties he does perform are called *antar yajna* (inner yajna). He learns to light the fire of knowledge and burns all his samskaras in that fire, which is symbolized by his ochre robes, ochre being the color of fire. When an aspirant decides to renounce all his personal interests for the sake of attaining the absolute Truth and is determined to follow the path of knowledge, he performs the last rite of yajna by sacrificing all his personal desires. He then attains freedom and is able to tread the path of renunciation.

Verses 11 and 12 refer to the devas or gods. The ignorant think that gods dwell in celestial worlds and have power to control human destiny. Such gods are merely projections of one's internal organization; the creation of gods in the external world is a projection of the unconscious. The belief in gods was created to help those who are not aware of their internal resources and are in need of an objectification of supernatural powers. They need to believe in gods that will help them fulfill desires that they feel inadequate to fulfill through their own means. It is said that those who have seen gods are fools, for they have seen something of their own self and mistakenly believe that they have seen gods. Externalists have created gods for their own convenience, but in actuality those gods are symbols of unknown phenomena that occur within.

For those aspirants who cannot contemplate on the attributeless Eternal, symbols are recommended by spiritual teachers. In the path of meditation certain symbols are used to make the mind one-pointed. The student is then advised to go beyond the symbol to comprehend its meaning rather than remaining dependent on the symbol forever. Thus, in meditation one leaves the symbol behind and goes forward.

The ignorant worship the symbols without knowing and understanding that which lives behind and beyond the symbol. But if one is capable of exploring that which is being expressed by the symbol, he may eventually discover the existence of the formless archetype that is clothed in the form of the symbol. With further work he may attain direct experience of the archetypes, not as objects but by becoming one with the archetypes themselves.

यज्ञशिष्टाशिनः सन्तो मुच्यन्ते सर्वकिल्बिषैः।
भुञ्जते ते त्वघं पापा ये पचन्त्यात्मकारणात्।। १३

13. *Those who eat only the remainder of the sacrifice are freed from all sins. Those sinful ones who cook only for the sake of themselves eat only sin.*

Sacrifice is an inborn quality. It is the quality of giving freely without any expectation. Self-preservation is also an innate quality, not of human beings alone, but of all creatures. Whether one chooses to devote his life to sacrifice or to self-preservation depends on his environment and his training. Those with whom one grew up and with whom he currently spends his time influence him and promote the development of either self-preservation or giving.

For example, in Aryan culture whenever food is prepared the guest is served first, and other members of the family eat the leftover food. That is one step in learning to give and to love others, which finally leads one to complete selflessness, the singular expression of pure love. In contrast to that, modern society leads one to become insecure. The insecure person looks out for his own needs first; he takes the best for himself.

Western culture and psychology consider the ego to be the center of consciousness, but the perennial psychology of the East disagrees. It regards buddhi, pure reason, as one aspect of the internal state called *antahkarana chatustaya* and ego as another. In the West all the activities of the human being are directed toward strengthening the ego. Such a perspective cannot ever incorporate the idea of sacrifice, learning to give the best one has selflessly. We encountered the same problem in explaining the concept of non-attachment, which also is not understood by Western culture. Because the West believes the ego to be the center of knowledge, the idea of sacrifice is frightening, for the ego is insecure and does not want to give up anything it possesses. One thinks that if he sacrifices, he will not have enough for himself. He thinks that sacrifice is a loss because he is attached to and identified with that which would be given in sacrifice. Thus, he is afraid of sacrifice. Actually what one loses in sacrifice is attachment and fear. If one is not attached to the object, there is no loss in sacrifice. The egocentric person believes that sacrifice means being consumed or even dying, but in fact it is only one's egocentric perspective that dies in sacrifice. The ocean is not used up in giving off moisture through evaporation, and the resources of a human being are not used up in sacrificing. Actually the more one sacrifices, the more one has. In sacrificing one gives up that to which he has been holding on, and he is then open to receive. As long as one is holding on, he is closed off to receiving the sacrifice of the universe. So what the egoistic person considers to be a death is life itself from another perspective. Thus, we say sacrifice is life. In the East sacrifice is a virtue not at all related to a sense of self-depletion or having to give something under duress. The East considers the greatest of all human beings to be those who sacrifice their selfish pleasures for the sake of selfless service and the attainment of eternal wisdom.

The giving human being sacrifices his best for his beloved, but the selfish person uses all his so-called loved ones for the sake of his selfish pleasures. Those who are not aware of the law of expansion do not experience the joy of sacrificing and giving. But those who have practiced to strengthen the quality of giving cannot stop giving, for giving fills one with the highest of joys, whereas expecting and taking only lead to momentary pleasure that later results in disgust, disappointment, and a sorrowful state of mind. Those who do not learn to give or sacrifice the fruits of their actions do not know the art of living and being.

The essence of sacrifice is giving selflessly. It is a complete expression of love in the true sense. Those who learn to be content with only their essential needs fulfilled are truly happy, and they use all their resources in the love and service of others. The little bit that is left over is used for the sustenance of their existence in the world so that they can continue giving. Such individuals live for others. But the selfish are not aware of the law of giving and are doomed.

अन्नाद्भवन्ति भूतानि पर्जन्यादन्नसम्भवः।
यज्ञाद्भवति पर्जन्यो यज्ञः कर्मसमुद्भवः।। १४
कर्म ब्रह्मोद्भवं विद्धि ब्रह्माक्षरसमुद्भवम्।
तस्मात् सर्वगतं ब्रह्म नित्यं यज्ञे प्रतिष्ठितम्।। १५

14. *Beings are born from food; food is produced through the rain god; rain is produced through sacrifice, and sacrifice arises from action.*
15. *Know action to arise from the Vedas and the Vedas to be produced from the indestructible syllable. Therefore, all-pervading knowledge of the Vedas is ever established in sacrifice.*

In the universe every action is a ritual, and the ritual is performed for the sake of sacrifice. The raindrop sacrifices itself to become part of the plant, and the sun gives up its energy to give light and life to all beings. The rain that nourished the plants, herbs, and all sorts of food for human beings is a free gift from Providence. That free gift is called sacrifice. The governing center of the universe itself is full of sacrifice: its nature is to give. This very universe is its gift, and it goes on giving freely of itself to the universe.

Food helps to sustain the body, which is an essential instrument for performing action. The gross body is made out of food that gives vital energy, so without food life is impossible. All the various species of creatures propagated in the world live on food, for food creates and maintains their bodies. Rain is essential to the growth of food, and therefore food is born from rain. The wise know that the showers of rain are the showers of blessings received by the earth. The term "rain god" used here does not mean that rain should be worshipped as a god but taken as a link to that which nourishes and sustains the whole universe. For without rain, food cannot be grown, and without food, the body cannot be maintained. "Rain is produced through sacrifice" means the love of the Eternal flows freely and helps the herbs, trees, plants, and food to grow. That love is called sacrifice.

People sometimes interpret this verse to mean that we should sacrifice to the "rain god," but in actuality it should be understood in the other direction. Rain itself is a sacrifice of the Eternal. This verse teaches us that the human being is born out of selfless love, sacrifice. Thus, if one wants to live in harmony with the law of the universe, he should learn to lead his life by loving all selflessly.

एवं प्रवर्तितं चक्रं नानुवर्तयतीह यः।
अघायुरिन्द्रियारामो मोघं पार्थ स जीवति।। १६

16. *He who does not revolve according to the wheel which is thus set into motion, O Son of Pritha, lives in vain, his entire life span sinful, libidinous through his senses.*

The wheel of life rotates only on the basis of sacrifice; it cannot go forward without it. That process can be understood as an expression of the cosmic will. Every individual is gifted by Providence to do selfless actions and to remain non-attached by constantly maintaining awareness of the real Self. Those who are slaves of the sense organs and just live to enjoy sensory pleasure create obstacles for themselves. They are not fulfilling the purpose of life. Thus, they suffer as a result of their own follies.

यस्त्वात्मरतिरेव स्यादात्मतृप्तश्च मानवः।
आत्मन्येव च संतुष्टस्तस्य कार्यं न विद्यते।। १७
नैव तस्य कृतेनार्थो नाकृतेनेह कश्चन।
न चास्य सर्वभूतेषु कश्चिदर्थव्यपाश्रयः।। १८
तस्मादसक्तः सततं कार्यं कर्म समाचर।
असक्तो ह्याचरन्कर्म परमाप्नोति पूरुषः।। १९

17. *The child of Manu who delights in the Self alone and has satiety in the Self, satisfied in the Self alone, for him there is no action left yet to be performed.*

18. *He has no purpose with the actions already performed nor with those not yet performed. He has no dependence for any purpose on any beings at all*
19. *Therefore, perform your dutiful action incessantly without attachment. The person who performs actions without attachment attains the Supreme.*

One who has realized the Self always takes delight in the Self and is content, for he has accomplished the purpose of life. Therefore, nothing remains to be done. He has no selfish interest in performing any action, and he has no selfish motivation in not performing any action. Those who have trained themselves in the art of performing their duties without attachment or selfishness are neither interested in involving themselves with further action nor with non-action. For such great ones there is no bondage of any sort. Whether one lives in the world or away from the world as a renunciate is immaterial. That which is important is attaining a state of tranquility and remaining non-attached all the time. The teachings in these verses elevate Arjuna so that he is able to perform his duties with an equable mind and remain non-attached.

A human being cannot possibly live without doing actions, and when he performs actions he reaps the fruits of those actions. The reaping of the fruits involves him and leads him to go on doing further actions and reaping the fruits again and again. Then he finds himself caught in the bondage of karma. What is the way of attaining freedom from that cycle? The way of freedom is not attained by not doing actions or by continuing to do actions but by surrendering the fruits of one's actions to others. Karma (action) never binds. It is the fruits of the karma and the desire to reap the fruits that create bondage. The message of the Bhagavad Gita is that one should learn to do his duties lovingly, skillfully, and selflessly by being completely non-attached. Only then will he be free from the bondage of action.

The motivation that prompts one to do action is important. For example, suppose someone does charity. What is his motive? Some people do charity for the sake of name and fame so that others will think they are great, and some do charity motivated by the primitive notion that they will be rewarded after death. Conscientious and wise people, however, do charity because they know that freedom can be attained by giving up the fruits of one's actions, for it is the fruits that are responsible for motivating one to do further actions. In these examples similar actions are performed, but they arise from three different motivations. The motivation to do selfless actions helps one to attain a state of tranquility. Finally one attains the state of perfection in which he has nothing to do, for he has already accomplished the noble purpose of his life.

कर्मणैव हि संसिद्धिमास्थिता जनकादयः।
लोकसंग्रहमेवापि संपश्यन्कर्तुमर्हसि।। २०

20. Janaka and others reached total accomplishment through action alone. Even looking at the needs of gathering worldly success, you ought to act.

There were many scholars in ancient times who tried to prove that the path of renunciation is higher than the path of action. Some scholars, however, say that the path of action is higher than renunciation. Such generalizations are inadequate, for it all depends on one's capacities and inclinations. What is crucial in either path is doing one's duty. Sri Krishna explains that there have been great ones in the past who attained perfection by doing their duties. He teaches Arjuna that one cannot attain perfection without doing his duty.

One should analyze his inner abilities so that he can understand his duty. It is the duty of those on the path of renunciation to follow that path and attain perfection. But the majority of people in the world follow the path of action. By following the path of action, one can also attain perfection. Sri Krishna says, "Arjuna, being a warrior you have to perform your dharma. By abandoning your dharma, you can never become perfect. Therefore, do not escape but fight with all your might and with a one-pointed mind, remaining non-attached and maintaining the state of equilibrium in the midst of the battle of life."

Sri Krishna asks Arjuna to do his duty rather than escaping into sloth and inertia. Doing one's duty is dharma. Dharma means to unify different elements of society. If the leaders and wise men of society abandon their duties and follow the path of inaction or renunciation, they will create serious disturbances and disintegration of the society. Janaka was a sage and king who is always cited as an example of one who had the wisdom to discharge his duties skillfully while remaining in a state of equilibrium and non-attachment.

यद्यदाचरति श्रेष्ठस्तत्तदेवेतरो जनः।
स यत्प्रमाणं कुरुते लोकस्तदनुवर्तते।। २१
न मे पार्थास्ति कर्तव्यं त्रिषु लोकेषु किञ्चन।
नानवाप्तमवाप्तव्यं वर्त एव च कर्मणि।। २२
यदि ह्यहं न वर्तेयं जातु कर्मण्यतन्द्रितः।
मम वर्त्मानुवर्तन्ते मनुष्याः पार्थ सर्वशः।। २३
उत्सीदेयुरिमे लोका न कुर्यां कर्म चेदहम्।
संकरस्य च कर्ता स्यामुपहन्यामिमाः प्रजाः।। २४

21. *In whatever way the senior-most one conducts himself, that very way the other people follow. Whatever authority he establishes, the world conducts itself accordingly.*
22. *O Son of Pritha, in all the three worlds I have nothing that is yet to be done, nothing not attained or yet to be attained; yet I, indeed, continue in action.*
23. *If I were perchance not to continue in action without lassitude, O Son of Pritha, and since all human beings follow my path in every way,*
24. *All these worlds would perish if I were not to perform action; I would be the cause of disorder and would kill all these beings.*

In all great cultures of the world, there has always been the noble tradition of following in the footsteps of the great ones. They are accepted as great because of their selflessness and the sacrifices they made for the people who came in touch with them. Thus, they became examples and ideals for ordinary people. A great man is known by certain signs and symptoms that are not found in ordinary people. Ordinary people are selfish; great men are selfless. The minds of ordinary people are uncontrolled and disturbed, whereas the minds of great men are controlled and tranquil. Ordinary people cannot visualize future events, but great men can have such vision.

There are two kinds of great people that we hold up as ideals. First there are the fortunate ones who completely devote their lives to prayer and meditation. Then there are those who know how to live in the world, doing their duties selflessly and offering the fruits of their actions to others. Both are worthy of our reverence. The action, speech, and behavior of the great ones are observed by ordinary people who then follow such great people without any doubts. If by chance the conduct of a great man is no longer exemplary, there is the chance for such conduct to be magnified by the masses in a horrible and exaggerated way. Those who follow the path of selfless service therefore remain austere so that their image is not distorted and thus does not lead others to disappointment and disgust.

Ordinary people have in their hearts and minds an image of what a great man should be like. If the person who is idealized as a hero, leader, or great man does not live according to the image projected onto him by the masses, the revered symbol that they have created for the great man is also destroyed. Sometimes it is the fault of the idealized person, but many times it is due to the false expectations of his following. For instance, before a student comes to meet a spiritual teacher for the first time, he has already formed ideas and impressions about what a teacher should be like. When he goes to the teacher, it disappoints him if the teacher does not talk, sit, and behave the way he expects. He then searches for another teacher that will meet his ideal, but he is not successful in that endeavor, for the student has created an image within and expects the teacher to live according to the projection of his own inner ideal. A similar process occurs between a patient and his psychotherapist. The distortions projected onto the therapist are called transference.* Teachers also have certain expectations: they want to meet the perfect student. Both teachers and students become disappointed with each other's actual behavior, but when they keep their minds open and free from preconceived ideas they can accept each other as they are.

It is important to distinguish between the image that the student projects onto the teacher and the qualities that are prerequisites of a good teacher. A student should not accept a teacher unless he has the following qualities: (1) A teacher should be selfless. (2) All his expressions should be loving, and there should not be greed of any sort from the teacher's side. (3) A teacher should not use his students to serve him in any way, for that makes the teacher dependent on his students. One who is dependent on someone else's resources is not a genuine teacher and should not be followed. (4) A real teacher is never tired of teaching his students. He teaches in many ways—through his speech, writings, and actions, and at a later stage through silence. If those signs and symptoms are missing in the teacher, one should not waste his time and energy following him. Instead of learning and listening to the teacher's instructions, many students foolishly start adoring and worshipping him as though he were a god. Such teachers and students destroy the noble heritage of the teacher-disciple relationship and create confusion for the real seekers and teachers.

Analyzing and studying symbols is one of the profound ways of knowing the qualities of great men. In ancient times there were no printing presses, tape recorders, or writing paper. Therefore, the ancients left certain symbols for future generations so that they could understand the way the ancients lived. For example, if the pictorial symbol of *Ganapati*, the elephant god, is properly understood and analyzed, it becomes clear that the ancients described the ideal qualities of a leader through that symbol. The head of an elephant symbolizes that a great leader should not be violent, for elephants are very calm. They do not live on the flesh of other beings; elephants are vegetarians, and they are both healthy and

---

* For a thorough explanation of this process as it is understood in both Eastern and Western psychology, see *Psychotherapy East and* West, Swami Ajaya, Honesdale, PA: Himalayan Institute, 1984.

intelligent. Using an elephant as an example dispels the notion that it is necessary to eat meat in order to maintain health and vigor. Ganapati has a big belly, which means the leaders should be able to accept all sorts of suggestions from various quarters for the sake of doing justice and selfless service to society. Ganapati is shown with a mouse, meaning that leaders should have counselors like mice who, with the help of their sharp teeth, can cut the net of entanglements and conspiracy that tend to develop around leaders. There are many other aspects of this symbol, Ganapati, that one can learn from, but today instead of understanding the symbolism, many people worship the symbol without knowing its meaning. There are many other symbols, such as the cross, the star of David, and the lotus that are adored and worshipped without knowing their meanings. That is a serious error. The method of understanding such symbolism is a knowledge in itself, like the method of studying dream symbols. It should be studied if one is to understand the world within and without.

Sri Krishna instructs Arjuna to live up to the estimation of a great man, for he is a leader and warrior, and if he fails in doing his duties the ordinary people will follow his example, and the entire organization of the society will become disintegrated, degenerated, and disturbed. The way great people behave is the very way ordinary people try to behave. The standards laid down by the great men become ideals for laymen to follow. The great ones actually have nothing to do—no action or duty whatsoever. They perform actions only in the service of humanity; they have no selfish motivation.

Sri Krishna declares that in all three worlds there is nothing for him to do. What are those three worlds? The world that is known by the ordinary person is a reality created by the senses and mind when one is in the waking state. In the dreaming state that reality is completely changed, and in the sleeping state it vanishes. The mind functions differently in each of these three states and has different experiences in each. These three states of mind are like three distinct realities. The mind functions even in deep sleep, and that subtle functioning of the mind is beyond the realm of the waking and dreaming states. When the mind is trained to go beyond the spheres of these three states, it experiences a state beyond called turiya, which can be termed sleepless sleep, a fully awakened state from which one can have a profound and comprehensive knowledge of the waking, dreaming, and sleeping realities. A great one who has attained the state beyond has nothing left to be done in any of the three worlds experienced in the waking, dreaming, and sleeping states. Sri Krishna is a traveler through the three worlds, having his permanent abode in the fourth, where both actions and the fruits received therein lose their value and meaning. One is not motivated to do duties or actions when he has already accomplished the purpose of his life, for the desire that motivates him to actions is absent in the state beyond. Here cause and effect, which are inseparably mingled, remain completely absent, for motivation and desire are already fulfilled. Their values and influences are reduced to zero; therefore no duty whatsoever remains to be performed. Sri Krishna is leading Arjuna to fathom all three levels of consciousness—waking, dreaming, and sleeping—and finally to attain the state of tranquility so that he can have a clear and comprehensive view of all three realities.

When consciousness is trapped by the deluded mind, the vision is obscured. Partial vision creates further confusion. The confused mind loses its power and does not have awareness of the other dimensions of life. Arjuna is aware of only one state of mind. Influenced by the dramas taking place in the waking state, he does not have profound knowledge of the whole. Sri Krishna, the lord and master of all the states of consciousness, advises, "Rise and go higher and higher and finally attain the state of tranquility."

After the three worlds are explained, one wonders why a fully realized person, having perfect tranquility and being completely non-attached, wants to perform action. That question is answered in Verse 24. All social institutions function because of the particular order established by the leaders. If the leaders do not perform actions to help the masses, the entire society will be disintegrated and destroyed. Many great civilizations have vanished from the earth because the leaders failed to perform their duties. According to the times and the needs of society, great men have come to guide the masses. Though the great men are free from motivations that prompt them to do their duties, they walk on earth with us exactly like ordinary human beings, but with extraordinary skill in performing actions to lead, help, and educate the masses. It is not because they have a need to do that but because of their love for others. Sri Krishna is implicitly saying, "Oh, Arjuna, you are also a great leader, and if you abandon your duty, that will lead to the destruction of your people. At this critical juncture do not shy away, but fight the battle."

There are three categories of great people. There are those who are great by birth, for they have already accomplished all they ought to have accomplished in their previous births. They come to this world with the desire to serve, love, and give. The second group of great people makes serious efforts to attain greatness. In their human effort and endeavor they sometimes slip, yet they are great compared to ordinary people. The third category of great people is composed of those who are made great by publicity and propaganda. That form of greatness misleads the masses and destroys their human endeavor. Unfortunately in a country like ours every year there comes a *"bhagavan," "guru,"* or self-proclaimed *"avatara"* who gains notoriety though he actually has none of the qualities of a truly great man. Such "bhagavans" mislead others and become a curse to the innocent students who follow them blindly. Arjuna belongs in the second category. Sri Krishna instructs Arjuna to do his duty, for he is a leader, and his behavior will be observed and followed by the masses.

सक्ताः कर्मण्यविद्वांसो यथा कुर्वन्ति भारत।
कुर्याद्विद्वांस्तथासक्तश्चिकीर्षुर्लोकसंग्रहम्।। २५
न बुद्धिभेदं जनयेदज्ञानां कर्मसङ्गिनाम्।
जोषयेत्सर्वकर्माणि विद्वान्युक्तः समाचरन्।। २६

25. *O Descendant of Bharata, whatever the unwise do attached to action, that very thing a wise one, desirous of gathering worldly success, should do without attachment.*
26. *One should not divert the minds of the ignorant who are attached to action; a wise man who conducts himself joined in yoga should let them learn how to perform actions lovingly.*

Ordinary people become attached to their duties and the fruits received therein, but wise is he who selflessly performs his duties for the welfare of humanity. Because of his attachment, the ordinary person has no vision of the horizon of the infinite and suffers on account of that limitation. He is always afraid of giving up what he has, and without giving, one cannot receive. Giving and sacrificing are one and the same act. Great men know only giving, which motivates them to perform their duties for the benefit of mankind.

In all social orders of the world, ordinary people follow the great men. The great man, therefore, should not divert the minds of those who are performing their duties but should help them learn how to do actions skillfully. He should lead them to the level of consciousness in which duties done without attachment lead to emancipation.

Students and clients complain, "My duties make me feel trapped. How can I become free? Shall I remain in the situation that I am in, or shall 1 change the situation?" For example a woman says, "My duties to my husband and children have made me a slave." The answer is that it is necessary to perform one's own duties, but if we do not learn to create love for the duties that we have assumed, we will be doing them mechanically without experiencing joy. For those who learn to love their duties and make all possible efforts, the same duties that once created bondage then begin creating happiness. Love is strengthened by giving and thwarted by expectation. While doing duties, just give and you will receive joy. But if you have the expectation of receiving love in return, and the other person from whom you are expecting also expects, these two expectations will clash, injuring the feelings of both parties. Expectation is not love but the source of misery. If selfless giving is missing in the close relationship between husband and wife, the family institution crumbles because the family is intended to radiate love selflessly. Because selflessness is absent we see misery at home, outside, and all over.

The wise person does not abruptly introduce ideas that are beyond the comprehension of ordinary people, but he lovingly helps them to understand without hurting them and brings them home gently. All profound teachings are imparted by great people with love and gentleness. Forced teachings and instructions abruptly imparted are either ineffective or create aversion. We see that happening all the time between parents and children. Whenever the parents are abrupt, though they have good intentions, they make rebels out of their loving children. And that creates a huge gulf in communication. Higher teachings can be intellectually imparted by anyone with the help of the scriptures, but such teachings are not assimilated in the minds and hearts of the students, for they lack the warmth of love and gentleness. But a good teacher imparts the teachings with love and gentleness in his unique way. Such a skill is rarely found. Those who have patience, tolerance, selfless love, gentleness, and inner strength are careful not to abruptly introduce or impose their ideas on others. It is an art that is not taught through books but learned through experience and interaction. One might meet many intellectuals and scholars who can recite the scriptures by heart, but how often does one meet someone who imparts knowledge through love? Sri Krishna, by his own example and instruction, is teaching Arjuna to perform his duties with selfless love and to be an example for others.

प्रकृतेः क्रियमाणानि गुणैः कर्माणि सर्वशः।
अहंकारविमूढात्मा कर्ताहमिति मन्यते।। २७
तत्त्ववित्तु महाबाहो गुणकर्मविभागयोः।
गुणा गुणेषु वर्तन्त इति मत्वा न सज्जते।। २८

27. *With regard to the actions being performed by the gunas of Prakriti, jointly and severally, one whose nature is confused by ego believes, 'I am the agent of action.'*

28. *He, however, who knows the reality of the divisions of gunas and actions, O Mighty-armed One, knows, 'The gunas are interacting with gunas.' Knowing this he does not become attached.*

Let us examine whether the human being alone is responsible for his actions and their consequences. Human beings are in a position to function more independently and profoundly than the animal and plant kingdoms and the kingdom of inanimate objects. The human being is uniquely privileged to act independently, whereas the animal kingdom is completely controlled by nature. There is no free will for animals. But the human being has free will and intelligence, which make him stand apart from the animal kingdom. Actions like eating, sleeping, procreation, and those stemming from the urge for self-preservation are found equally in both the human and animal kingdoms. Those are the actions performed by nature. However, the human being alone has the inherent capacity to perform actions without being controlled by the basic urges. His will power and intelligence give him the ability to understand, analyze, and control the motivations, desires, thoughts, and emotions that are finally translated into action. He has the power to change the course of the whole chain of events from motivation to desire to thought to action. He can be aware of each aspect of the process that leads him to act, and with proper training he can modify any part of it.

Even though he uses his inherent capacity to regulate and modify his actions, the human being is not really the doer of his actions. All actions are actually performed by the governing nature of the universe, called *Prakriti.* The Self, seated unattached and unaffected in the inner chamber of one's being, always maintains its tranquility with all its glory and majesty. It is only the ego that leads the human being to think and feel that he is the doer, the performer of actions, and that he has the right to reap the fruits of his actions. Here there is a subtle point to be understood: anyone who becomes a doer also becomes the receiver of the fruits of his actions. One's false sense of doing and reaping creates misery for him, and he suffers on account of his self-created misery. The ego thus needs to be purified and trained not to identify itself as the doer but to remain a witness by being conscious of the true Self, which exists eternally with its immortal and splendid nature.

The ego is one of four main functions of our internal organization. Our internal organization is like that of a workshop, and the ego is the representative of the real Self. When the ego forgets the real Self, when it forgets that it is only a representative, it creates serious problems of confusion and delusion within the internal organization. It does not counsel with the other aspects of the internal organization and thus loses control over the aspect of mind (manas) that functions both inside and outside and which is actually the main instrument of both perception and conception. When the ego shakes off its false vanity and remembers its role, then it does not create bondage and barriers that stand between the aspirant and the real Self, the source of consciousness and knowledge.

Egoism creates great suffering for the human being, but the wise person does not allow his ego to create obstacles for his growth. He knows that, in fact, actions are performed by Prakriti, the universal nature. Therefore, he is free from such deluded conceptions as: I have a desire to do, I want to do, I am going to do, or I have done.

Prakriti has three qualities called gunas. Those three gunas— sattva, rajas, and tamas—are distinct from one another yet function together. Actually all actions performed by any aspect of nature are led by these three qualities or gunas. The qualities of each object are different from one another. So when two objects come into contact, there is a confrontation, and as a result they either unite and thereby create something new, or they create conflict. In this way the gunas are the source of action in the universe. These three qualities exist together in the human being as well as in every aspect of nature, but when one of them becomes predominant, one's actions take on the quality of the predominant guna. A deed performed in a state of tranquility is a consequence of sattva guna. The deed in which rajas is predominant is performed with a desire to reap the fruits. Tamas leads one to sloth and thus to inaction. No one can remain without doing action, but when one does action with an inert mind, there is no concentration. Therefore, there is total disintegration and chaos.

By studying and understanding these verses, we can realize that we are mistaken to feed our egos, deluding ourselves that we are doing great deeds or serving humanity. A child plucks a beautiful flower and hands it to his mother saying, "Here, Mommy, I am giving this to you," as though the gift comes from him. But the gift of the flower was created by nature out of the gunas, and the child, also motivated by the gunas, is merely transporting it from one place to another, though claiming that it is his to give. The ego, being the predominant part of the internal organization, is deluded by its false identification with the qualities of the Self: it believes that it (the ego) is all-powerful and all-knowing, and that creates the bondage. But when one shakes loose all the fetters by becoming aware of the Eternal, freedom is attained.

Modern psychologists have also asserted that the human being does not perform actions but acts at the mercy of the forces of nature. In fact that is the great insight of modern psychology, which in part arose as a reaction to the rationalistic popular philosophies that preceeded it. Such philosophies held that man acts out of his own rational choices. The behaviorists, however, believe that the human being is moved by habits that are established by reward and punishment. Freud argued that the conscious mind is just a small part of the mind, and that human beings are predominantly moved by unconscious forces. Jung and the archetypal psychologists go a step further and dramatically assert that man is not the doer of actions. Their view is in agreement with these verses, which are difficult to understand at first, for we consistently think of ourselves as the initiators of our actions even though we see other forms of life at the mercy of and reacting automatically to internal and external forces outside of their control. Jung and archetypal psychologists attempt to show that the archetypes, which exist at deeper layers of the unconscious, are continually engaged in ritualistic dramas that are universal and repeated again and again throughout generations. The conscious person, they say, is merely an onlooker to these grand and glorious dramas rather than the actor.

प्रकृतेर्गुणसंमूढाः सज्जन्ते गुणकर्मसु।
तानकृत्स्नविदो मन्दान्कृत्स्नविन्न विचालयेत्।। २९

29. *Those who are confused by the gunas of Prakriti become attached to the actions of the gunas. One who knows the complete reality should not cause conflict in the minds of dull-witted, little-knowing ones.*

Ordinary people who are deluded by identifying with the qualities of Prakriti vainly conclude that they are the performers and doers of the actions. Such ignorant ones think that way, desiring to enjoy the fruits of their actions. The person who knows and is able to dispel the cloud of ignorance should be very careful not to do anything that would cause conflict in the minds of ordinary people. Sri Krishna advises Arjuna not to be a bad example, deluded by the sense of ego, and not to mislead the masses. A leader who has not disciplined himself is unable to lead the masses in the right direction. A leader should have perfect discipline, otherwise instead of serving the masses he can mislead them.

मयि सर्वाणि कर्माणि सन्यस्याध्यात्मचेतसा।
निराशीर्निर्ममो भूत्वा युध्यस्व विगतज्वरः।। ३०

30. *With your mind centered on the Self, dedicating all actions to Me, free of expectation and free of the thought "mine," fight without the fever of fear and anxiety.*

He alone who has learned to direct all his energies and the power of his thoughts, emotions, and desires to attain knowledge of the Self has freedom. The common man remains conscious only of the world of objects, but those who are conscious of the self-existent Reality direct all their energy inward with a one-pointed desire to attain immortality. Ordinary people are ignorant because of their outward desires. The objects of the external world constantly lead one to identify with the changing phenomena and to forget the nature of the Self, which is unchanging and everlasting.

Sri Krishna therefore says, "O Arjuna, dedicate all of your actions with a one-pointed mind focused on the highest Self with no expectation or attachment whatsoever. Without fear and anxiety, fight the battle of life." This verse talks of dedicated action, which actually is prayer in actron. When we pray but cannot dedicate our actions, that prayer is not of much use. Dedicating all of our actions and the fruits we receive therein is higher than the prayer that is uttered by our lips. The poems and hymns we utter are not as profound or as important as dedication of the fruits of our actions. There are two kinds of people: one praises God all the time, the other remains silent and performs his actions, dedicating all the fruits of his actions to the Lord. It is clear that the latter prayer is superior to the former.

ये मे मतमिदं नित्यमनुतिष्ठन्ति मानवाः।
श्रद्धावन्तोऽनसूयन्तो मुच्यन्ते तेऽपि कर्मभिः।। ३१
ये त्वेतदभ्यसूयन्तो नानुतिष्ठन्ति मे मतम्।
सर्वज्ञानविमूढांस्तान्विद्धि नष्टानचेतसः।। ३२

31. *Those children of Manu who ever steadfastly follow this teaching of mine, filled with faith and without malice, they are even freed through those very actions.*
32. *Those, however, who are critical and do not observe this teaching of mine, know them, confused concerning all knowledge, to be mindless, who perish.*

Sri Krishna teaches that all actions are performed by nature. He says to Arjuna, "Therefore shun the idea that you are a doer. Remain detached from the sense of being a doer and be an example for others, for the ordinary people always follow their leaders." Ignorant are those who perform actions thinking that they are the doers, but those who know that all actions are performed by Prakriti and understand the mystery of all three gunas remain free. In these verses Sri Krishna says, "Those who follow my teachings with full faith rejoice in their life on earth." Faith is a word that has been repeatedly used by religionists. The expression, "Have faith," is a common one, but faith has many meanings. It may mean "do not argue; do not use your mind but just follow me blindly." But here the term faith does not have the same meaning as when it is used by preachers and priests while giving sermons in the temples and churches.

Shraddha (faith) implies that apart from the knowledge received from the mind, there is yet another avenue still undiscussed and unknown. That avenue opens spontaneously if one knows how to keep his mind from intervening in that spontaneity. A sadhaka wants to have faith, but all sorts of doubts created by the mind do not allow him to have faith. Faith is not the product of the mind but something living that is experienced by opening the path of the heart that leads to the dawning of spiritual love and intuition. Many great sages attain a state of ecstasy by using the power of emotion, it being higher than the power of thought. If the power of emotion is directed with full heart, one is able to attain that knowledge which is never experienced by the mind. The mind is like a small ruler, and human beings like to measure the universe with the help of this small measuring stick. The power of emotion, however, opens one to another, higher channel of knowledge, which is called intuition.

There are three main channels of knowledge: intuition, intellect, and instinct. Intuition, the highest channel of knowledge, is self-evident and does not need support of any kind. The door to that knowledge opens with the power of emotion (bhava) and not through mental gymnastics. In Verse 31 the path of faith and devotion is being introduced to Arjuna. Many students who cannot follow the path of selfless action are led to follow the path of faith, love, and devotion.

In these verses Sri Krishna opens that channel of knowledge, stressing that the aspirant must have faith in the wisdom imparted by the great teachers. He declares, "Have faith and follow, for the teachings expounded by me are free from error." Here Sri Krishna for the first time exercises his authority with profound certainty in order to lead his beloved student deeper. Often when a student enters into an argument or debate, he forgets that his teacher is teaching not only on the basis of scriptural knowledge but also from his experience of that knowledge. Though we have many experiences every day, those experiences do not always guide us. But the inner experience that has been attained directly is the best guide and instructor and should be followed with full faith, without any doubt. There are many steps that a disciple must fathom in relating to his competent teacher. The teacher never gives such instructions as are given in these verses at the first instance of the meeting with his disciple, but only when the communication between the teacher and student is well established.

There is a prayer that is used even today before the teacher imparts the knowledge of the divine: "May He protect us both, teacher and student. May He lead us both to enjoy the bliss of liberation. May we both make efforts to realize the truth of the scriptures. May our studies bear fruit. May we never quarrel with each other."

Before this teaching was imparted, Sri Krishna and Arjuna had a long discussion, and, like any other student, Arjuna argued. There comes a stage when one goes through a period of argumentation, and this state of mind should not be shunned until all the doubts are resolved. Then the state free from all doubts leads one to another channel of knowledge: intuition.

We have already said that there are three channels of knowledge. The path of pure reason, buddhi, is followed by the fortunate few. The path of buddhi yoga is used by those aspirants who are intellectually oriented for performing duties in the world and also by yogis to control the senses, turn the mind inward, and to finally resolve all questions. Intellectuals, however, use the mind by employing their senses externally with the desire to enjoy pleasures. They are lost in the world of pleasures, whereas yogis attain the state of equilibrium, remaining non-attached and unaffected by the external world and performing their duties skillfully. But among all the channels of knowledge, intuition is the purest of all. And for receiving that knowledge, the mind is not used. The power of emotion is evoked, and thus intuitive knowledge is received.

The third channel of knowledge is also valid but does not lead the student to the summit. That is instinctual knowledge, which is common to both human beings and animals. It is a gift from nature and has the power to cross the boundaries of past, present, and future. For instance, an animal can sense and record the calamities that are about to happen. Pets sense an earthquake long before it creates a disaster, and they leave their homes and run for safety. Animals remain close to nature and are privileged to utilize this channel of knowledge more than a human being can, because for a human being there is always a choice in how to respond, and his mind is distracted and dissipated. Man is usually lost in the jungle of thoughts, trying to find out what to do through mental exercise alone. Thus, he loses touch with instinctual knowledge. Instinctual knowledge and intuitive knowledge are quite distinct. Instinctual knowledge is the knowledge limited to the boundaries of nature, whereas intuitive knowledge fathoms all the boundaries of nature and leads the sadhaka to the timeless and infinite source of knowledge. Most people do not understand the difference between instinctual knowledge and intuitive knowledge. If someone has a premonition that a close relative is about to die, he is said to be intuitive though he is actually relying on instinctual knowledge. In the modern world the distinction between instinctual and intuitive knowledge has been lost, and we think that many people have access to intuitive knowledge when it is really instinctual knowledge. Truth seekers, aspirants, and sadhakas alone have access to intuitional knowledge.

The word shraddha, which is used in Verse 31, is an ancient word that refers to three qualities that are explained by this formula: reverence plus devotion leads to conviction. It is not a faith dependent on belief but firm faith attained through one-pointed devotion. Shraddha directed toward one's teacher is attained by a disciple after long experience on the path. Those aspirants who follow the instructions of the teacher with full conviction are not lost in the conflicts created by the allurements of the world. Those who do not have shraddha, firm conviction in what they are doing, destroy themselves. The aspirants who understand the importance of the teaching given in the 30th verse learn to dedicate all their actions and the fruits of their actions to the Lord of life and cast off the fetters created by attachment. The ignorant, acting on the basis of fallacious reasoning, remain confused, distracted, and doubtful, and a mind full of doubt causes ruin. Those who are devoid of faith are not fit for sadhana and are therefore unable to attain Truth. Such ignorant people see the dark side of everything and waste time in fault finding. But those who follow their path with full conviction and implicit faith finally attain the highest goal. Such faith is necessary on the path of sadhana. Patanjali, the codifier of yoga science, supports this idea in the Yoga Sutras (1:14). He says that sadhana should be continued for a long time without any break and with full and firm faith. Such faith and conviction are essential; without them treading the path is impossible. Full conviction is attainment in itself. One should be sure that it is not lost. Maintaining and strengthening faith is the highest state of sadhana.

सदृशं चेष्टते स्वस्याः प्रकृतेर्ज्ञानवानपि।

प्रकृतिं यान्ति भूतानि निग्रहः किं करिष्यति।। ३३

33. *Even a person with knowledge acts according to his nature. Beings resort to their nature. What can self control do?*

Sri Krishna further explains the functioning of the three gunas that motivate one to perform action. He says that it is not easy to fathom the barriers created by the gunas. The relative proportions of the three qualities differ from one individual to another. In one person one guna is more predominant while in another a different guna predominates. These differences are a result of ones past.

The words *svabhava prakriti,* used in Verse 33, mean "that which is brought forward by births, the inherent nature of a creature." It compels one to act according to his samskaras (svabhava). Thus, self-transformation becomes difficult, and forced methods of restraint do not help. One should therefore not impose such restraints on himself unless he is fully prepared. First the desire to discipline and transform oneself should be strongly felt. The gunas function no matter how much restraint one practices. That restraint which is practiced by the ignorant and leads to suppression and repression is not real sadhana. Mere restraint will not help one to cross the barriers of Prakriti. But that does not mean one should cease practicing self-control, disciplining himself, and directing the senses in a controlled way. The practices of self-transformation are different from suppression and repression. Through self-discipline one develops his positive qualities, and gradually the sattva guna predominates. Sattva is the inherent quality that alone gives the sadhaka power to have a tranquil mind, and that enables him to cross the mire of delusion created by rajas and tamas.

For treading the path of faith, one should learn to be detached from the confusion and conflicts created by the constant reasoning of the mind. Scriptural knowledge and mere reasoning are not at all helpful in the upliftment and unfoldment of the sadhaka. It is therefore important for a sadhaka to understand his own nature and with firm faith to attain a sattvic state of mind.

इन्द्रियस्येन्द्रियस्यार्थे रागद्वेषौ व्यवस्थितौ।
तयोर्न वशमागच्छेत्तौ ह्यस्य परिपन्थिनौ।। ३४
श्रेयान् स्वधर्मो विगुण: परधर्मात्स्वनुष्ठितात्।
स्वधर्मे निधनं श्रेय: परधर्मो भयावह:।। ३५

34. *There are attractions and aversions already facing each and every sense. One should not come under their control, for they are highwaymen waiting for him on the path.*
35. *Better one's own dharma, even devoid of quality, than the dharma of another, even though well performed. Better to die in one's own dharma; the dharma of another invites danger.*

The senses respond spontaneously to the objects of the world. Each of the five senses—seeing, touching, hearing, tasting, and smelling—has their objects—color, that which can be felt, sound, taste, and odor respectively. Each has a distinct mode of perception. The tongue can taste but cannot hear; the eyes can see but cannot taste. Each sense has its own duty to perform, and in performing its duty it flows to its respective objects. When the senses contact their objects, one experiences like and dislike, attraction and repulsion. Ordinary minds react according to those two feelings. Their positive or negative responses to sensory objects keep them from experiencing objectively. That which one person adores is a matter of repulsion to another. Even a sage recognizes something as bitter and something else as sweet, but he does not react like the ordinary person. The sage realizes that it is not the object that causes like or dislike but one's own prejudices, so he learns to tame both reactions. Sages maintain aloofness. They do not waste precious moments of their life in hating or being attracted to others or the objects of the world. Both lust and hatred obstruct the sadhaka's growth again and again. Once they are known and understood and their value is reduced to nothingness, they lose the power to influence the sadhaka. Arjuna's wish to remove those obstacles is evident. Thus, Sri Krishna introduces disciplines in order to help Arjuna perform his duty without being disturbed by those feelings.

Existence and duty are inseparable not only in human life but in nature as well. The sun shines; that is its duty. Likewise all the modes of nature such as fire, water, and air perform their duties. In the human body all the senses and limbs perform their respective duties. If someone foolishly asks the hearing sense to see, he will be disappointed. Therefore, an individual should learn to perform his duty according to his svabhava, the gifts received from his inherent nature.

A student can progress on the path of unfoldment by learning to study his inner potentials, for the duty that one performs should be according to his dharma. One is born with certain qualities into a particular environment, and if he does not discharge his duties according to his dharma but follows the dharma of another, it could prove dangerous and even fatal. If a professor of cultural studies is sent to the battlefield and a soldier who is trained to be an artillery expert is sent to teach philosophy, both will be unsuccessful, disappointed, and put to shame by others. Therefore, one should learn to follow his own dharma and to discharge his duty and progress as an example for others to follow.

The following is a summary of the several kinds of knowledge that have been described thus far. First there is knowledge that is given to us by our sense perception. On the basis of that, we conceptualize and formulate our conclusions. That is the lowest way of knowing, for the mind remains clouded, and all of the objects perceived by the senses in the external world are ever changing. Thus, sense perception is inaccurate and inexact. Such incomplete perception comes before the mind for conceptualization, and by the time the clouded mind formulates and concludes, one's experience of the external world is even more distorted. Perceptualizaton and conceptualization give only a partial and distorted view of the objective world.

Another source of knowledge is instinctual knowledge. It also crosses the boundaries of time and space and is able to give a glimpse of the future, but it too is limited. Nevertheless, it has some purpose: children and animals that are led by this force know many things that are not known by ordinary people.

Two other sources of knowledge that complement one another are knowledge through the mind and knowledge through emotion. There is always imbalance if we do not understand the importance of both of these powers. The power of emotion can help the sadhaka by inspiring him and can raise his consciousness to higher dimensions. Bhava, emotion, should not be lost. It is a great help, a force in the path of self-control. The knowledge that flows through bhava is a great force, and there are no interruptions in that flow. But the knowledge that flows through the mind creates many stagnant pools if it is not allowed to go through the filtration of pure reason. Many times the answers that cannot be figured out by a well-balanced mind are given by bhava, emotion. The stream of knowledge that flows through the mind moves into many nooks and corners, and because of impurities of the mind, this creates small and big stagnant pools, and thus the stream becomes polluted. The stream of bhava is like a river in flood. It rushes like a beloved running toward her lover who does not care about any obstacles, and is not afraid of being caught or trapped. In the stream of bhava, one does not have an enjoyable experience of the path, for he is suddenly transported. He reaches the summit without experience of the path.

The highest of all streams of knowledge is the flow of intuition, which is perfect. Its knowledge is the purest. That flow becomes evident and visible only after we learn that the stream of knowledge that flows through the mind is very lengthy and is full of obstacles. One can get lost on the way. Thus, the aspirant learns to shut the gate that stops the knowledge flowing through the mind and opens the gate that allows intuitive knowledge to flow to its place.

Both yoga psychology and modern psychology have shown considerable interest in differentiating amongst people according to personality or character types. As we have already noted, ancient psychologists have divided people into four categories according to their propensities, and that division has unfortunately evolved into the caste system of India. It is interesting to note that Carl Jung also considered there to be four fundamental personality types, and that the types he differentiated parallel to a certain extent the ways of knowing that have been described in the Bhagavad Gita. In Jung's schema there is the personality type dominated by sensation, the thinking type, the feeling type, and the intuitive type. However, there are some interesting differences between Jung's categorization and the ways of knowing that have been described. For instance, Jung's feeling type is not at all equivalent to knowledge through emotion, as some might think. Rather it is closely related to the experience of like and dislike as described in Verse 34. The feeling type relates to the world primarily along the dimension of liking or disliking what he experiences. From the perspective of yoga psychology Jung's intuitive type is a misnomer. What Jung is actually describing is the personality that functions primarily through instinctive knowledge. As we have noted, intuition according to the yogic perspective is a mode of knowledge that is beyond the ken of the ordinary human being.

Carl Jung also observed that if one does not live in accord with his personality type but tries to be that which he is not, a neurosis is created. For instance, if a sensation type is forced by external circumstances to live as an intellectual, a severe disturbance will be created in his psyche, Jung's conception parallels the yogic concept of living according to one's dharma.

अर्जुन उवाच

अथ केन प्रयुक्तोऽयं पापं चरति पूरुषः।

अनिच्छन्नपि वार्ष्णेय बलादिव नियोजितः।। ३६

श्री भगवानुवाच

काम एष क्रोध एष रजोगुणसमुद्भवः।

महाशनो महापाप्मा विद्ध्येनमिह वैरिणम्।। ३७

धूमेनाव्रियते वह्निर्यथादर्शो मलेन च।

यथोल्बेनावृतो गर्भस्तथा तेनेदमावृतम्।। ३८

आवृतं ज्ञानमेतेन ज्ञानिनो नित्यवैरिणा।

कामरूपेण कौन्तेय दुष्पूरेणानलेन च।। ३९

इन्द्रियाणि मनोबुद्धिरस्याधिष्ठानमुच्यते।

एतैर्विमोहयत्येष ज्ञानमावृत्य देहिनम्।। ४०

Arjuna said

36. *Now, propelled by whom does this person commit sin even not wanting to, O Krishna, as though impelled by force?*

The Blessed Lord said

37. *This is desire, this is anger, born of the guna called rajas, consumer of much, very evil; know it to be your enemy here in the world.*

38. *As fire is veiled by smoke or a mirror is by dust, as a fetus is covered with placenta, so is this world of activities covered by desire.*

39. *It is by this eternal enemy of the wise that knowledge is covered, the insatiable fire in the form of desire, O Son of Kunti.*

40. *The senses, mind, and intellect are its resort; it is by these that it covers knowledge and confuses the body-bearing one.*

Human beings do not intentionally want to create obstacles for themselves, yet they create them. What instigates the human being to create obstacles to his growth? Why can't he live life free of harmful acts? What is that which compels him to do that which is not to be done? When Arjuna asks these questions, Sri Krishna replies that the knowledge of the three gunas has already been imparted to him. It is rajas, one of the qualities of human nature, that prompts one to commit harmful or evil actions. Rajas leads the human being to be active and to do actions motivated by certain desires. Rajas has the quality of projecting itself onto the external world and thus creates a mirage, delusion, confusion, and conflicts. One's projections become the charms, attractions, and temptations. Those tempting forms are actually part and parcel of oneself, but those alluring qualities have been projected outward by rajas, and one foolishly chases after those mirages taking them to be real.

When one's desire is fulfilled he becomes proud, and when it is not fulfilled he gets angry. Pride and anger are two enemies of man. As the clouds hide the sun, as smoke hides the fire, desire obscures the faculty of discrimination and thereby obscures knowledge and controls the mind, intelligence, and senses. Whether the desire is fulfilled or unfulfilled, the mind remains in a state of imbalance and abnormality.

A man of desires becomes self-centered and isolates himself from the reality of the phenomenal world. That leads him to create his own reality. No matter how many sensory pleasures he experiences, the desires of the selfish man are never fulfilled. The more desires one has, the more discontent he becomes. For when one desire is fulfilled, it gives birth to other desires. For example, if the desire to own a house is fulfilled, the fulfillment of that desire gives birth to many other desires, such as having a better house than one's neighbors, a nice garden, new furniture, and a swimming pool. Desires are endless; desire is a canine hunger that is never satisfied or pacified no matter how much one tries to fulfill it. If one puts fuel into the fire, the fire is not quenched but burns more fiercely. Similarly, if one devotes his energy to the fulfillment of sensory desires, instead of experiencing fulfillment his desires only increase.

The wise man understands that desire, which creates misery for him, is produced by rajas. Therefore, he practices to attain sattvic virtues and thus achieve a state of tranquility, which is the nature of sattva. Ordinary people are infatuated with sensual desire, *kama*. Kama is the prime desire that gives birth to anger, greed, attachment, jealousy, and pride. Wherever desire dwells, one suffers from these other evils as well.

The sage knows this and thus always remains vigilant, for desire is such a powerful motivation that it is even capable of blinding the reason of good sadhakas.

The senses, mind, and intelligence of ordinary people are controlled by their desires, for when one desires to enjoy sensory pleasures, his intelligence, mind, and senses are externalized, turned outward toward the objects of desire. Sense, mind, and intelligence are the abodes in which the parasite desire dwells. If one's intelligence, mind, and senses are not trained, they feed the parasite in the same way that fuel feeds the fire. Desire robs the senses, mind, and intelligence of their energy. But that which is the enemy can also become a friend. When one realizes the grand game being played by the gunas, he strengthens only one desire: the desire to attain the state of equilibrium. Then instead of being an enemy, that desire is a necessary means. When a sadhaka has a burning desire to attain freedom, he learns to light the fire of knowledge. He bathes in that fire, and all his worldly desires are burned to ashes. The desire for tranquility alone remains.

तस्मात्त्वमिन्द्रियाण्यादौ नियम्य भरतर्षभ।
पाप्मानं प्रजहि ह्येनं ज्ञानविज्ञाननाशनम्।। ४१

41. *Therefore, first control the senses, O Arjuna. Abandon this evil that destroys knowledge and the experience of spiritual realities.*

It is important to understand here that the battle of Kurukshetra is a battle that is fought in every human heart and mind. Therefore, the historical authenticity of the battle is of no significance for us. Our concern is with the message of the Bhagavad Gita and the way modern man can benefit from its great teachings. We are in search of certain specifics, and this verse explains what the battle is really about, where it takes place, and why it should be fought. Sri Krishna says that desire clouds human intelligence and controls the mind and senses. Therefore, one must learn to have full control of his desires, which are the prime enemy. We have already explained that this refers to the desires that distract and dissipate the energy of the sadhaka. Sri Krishna tells Arjuna to kill that evil desire with the sword of discrimination.

इन्द्रियाणि पराण्याहुरिन्द्रियेभ्यः परं मनः।
मनसस्तु परा बुद्धियों बुद्धेः परतस्तु सः।। ४२
एवं बुद्धेः परं बुद्ध्वा संस्तभ्यात्मानमात्मना।
जहि शत्रुं महाबाहो कामरूपं दुरासदम्।। ४३

42. *The senses are said to be powerful; beyond the senses is the mind; beyond the mind is intellect. The one beyond the intellect, however, is the Self.*
43. *Thus, awakening to the One who is beyond intellect, holding and supporting self by the Self, destroy this elusive enemy in the form of desire, O Mighty-armed One.*

The methods of controlling the senses are concentration and meditation. When the sadhaka desires to attain the highest state of tranquility and to have profound knowledge of the Absolute, his worldly desires are assimilated into that one desire. Thus, the outgoing tendency of the senses is controlled, and the mind becomes one-pointed. From here starts the inward journey.

The flow of perennial knowledge has its source beyond the body, senses, mind, and intellect. The word *para,* which means beyond, is used here. Through mere scriptural knowledge the meaning of para cannot be comprehended, but the sadhaka can easily grasp its meaning through direct experience. The knowledge of the inward journey, which leads the sadhaka from the gross level of consciousness to the subtlemost level, is essential. The word *para* means the beyond within, not outside. Many seekers interpret the word *para* in an external sense, but actually it is used here to indicate the levels of consciousness that already exist within us.

Beyond the body consciousness is the field created by sense perception, and beyond the field of sense perception is another higher and subtler realm of mind, and then there lies the vast field of the unconscious. But subtlemost is the center of consciousness that lies beyond the unconscious. It is called Atman. The senses command and control the body; all the physical movements remain under the control of the senses. The senses, however, are employed by the mind and are directed by the intellect. Over and above all, the Self governs the intellect, mind, senses, and body. Having knowledge of the truth that the self is ruled by the Self, one learns to follow the path of discipline, which helps him to attain the center of pure consciousness.

Verses 42 and 43 are especially important to understand from the viewpoint of sadhana. They show that disciplining the body, breath, senses, and mind is an important requisite that helps one to redirect the flow of energy, consciousness, to its fountainhead instead of allowing it to flow to the objects of the external world and to create more distractions. Worldly desires and an undisciplined mind and senses are great enemies. Worldly desire endlessly breeds more desires. Therefore, such desires should be completely shunned.

Here ends the third chapter, in which the message of doing actions skillfully is explained.

Chapter Four
Knowledge of Renouncing Fruits

श्री भगवानुवाच

इमं विवस्वते योगं प्रोक्तवानहमव्ययम्।
विवस्वान्मनवे प्राह मनुरिक्ष्वाकवेऽब्रवीत्।। १

एवं परम्पराप्राप्तमिमं राजर्षयो विदुः।
स कालेनेह महता योगो नष्टः परंतप।। २

स एवायं मया तेऽद्य योगः प्रोक्तः पुरातनः।
भक्तोऽसि मे सखा चेति रहस्यं ह्येतदुत्तमम्।। ३

The Blessed Lord said

1. *I taught this immutable yoga to Vivasvat; Vivasvat taught it to Manu; Manu taught it to Ikshvaku.*
2. *Royal sages knew this yoga as it was handed down in the lineage of the tradition. Then over a long period of time this yoga disappeared, O Scorcher of Enemies.*
3. *That very ancient yoga I have taught you today, as you are My devotee as well as My friend. This is the highest secret.*

Yoga science is as eternal as human existence. This noble tradition is a perennial stream of knowledge that flows from eternity to eternity. It is knowledge that is not subject to destruction. The knowledge so far imparted by Sri Krishna is jnana yoga of the Samkhya system and karma yoga. Both of these aspects of eternal knowledge, one containing the profound philosophy of life and the other the way of living according to that philosophy, together make life a beautifully poetic song. Such knowledge remains ever young and ever fresh in all conditions. That is why the message of the Bhagavad Gita is called the perennial song. This song carries the all-encompassing and profound knowledge of the individual and the universe, of the world within and without. Knowledge was never born and therefore never dies. It is not possessed by anyone, for it is always there in all times—past, present, and future—for all seekers.

When Sri Krishna states with all certainty that he had expounded this knowledge to Vivasvat, who then had communicated it to Manu and others, he is saying that karma yoga is as ancient as any other path. All the kings in ancient times followed this path that finally leads one to perfection. Sri Krishna is instructing Arjuna to follow the same path that was followed by his ancestors. With the passage of time, this knowledge was lost. For when a nation reveres and preserves the records of the ancients but ignores its application, knowledge is reduced to theoretical conclusions. Sri Krishna is imparting the forgotten knowledge of both theory and practice to Arjuna. Such supreme secrets are imparted by great teachers only to the deserving ones.

All the kings preceding Arjuna for many centuries, as well as Sri Krishna and Arjuna, were from the same ancient tradition. In ancient times in the kingdom of Bharata there lived two traditions. One was called the solar race and the other the lunar race, for they identified themselves with the sun and moon respectively. The solar tradition of Sri Krishna is considered to be the highest of all traditions. It is the tradition of light and knowledge. The sun is the symbol of light: it radiates for all without any selfish motivation yet remains above, unattached, and never tires of radiating its light. The sun is known by its own light, whereas all other things are known by the light of the sun. Sri Krishna, a great sage of the solar tradition, reminds Arjuna of his connection with that tradition. In the third chapter the example of Janaka, the king and sage, was given by Sri Krishna to remind Arjuna that Janaka is a link in that unbroken chain of sages and that Arjuna also comes from that same tradition.

There are many streams of knowledge all coming from one and the same source. When we study the history of the great traditions without bias, we come to know that the unbroken ancient traditions continue to offer something of value to modern man. For example, despite a series of persecutions, the Jewish tradition is still as lively as before because that race follows its tradition today as it did in ancient times. Such traditions have something special in their culture and character that helps them to live with the hope of building their rising generations around the same principles followed by their ancients.

Sri Krishna has the ability to see the past, present, and future. That is a yogic ability attained by going beyond the time factor to the timeless infinite and eternal. When Sri Krishna says that he taught the ancients the same knowledge, it means that he is talking to Arjuna in a state of oneness with the Eternal, which is never born and therefore never dies. The great sages have access to the past and future, and they can connect the missing links. That helps one to study past, present, and future at one glance. For Sri Krishna all happenings are happenings of here and now.

Sri Krishna states that Arjuna is both his devotee and friend. That is an unusual relationship. A sense of devotion exists between God and his servant, but friendship is a term used for two equals. The student often does not communicate with his teacher because of his awe and devotion. For lack of communication, he does not understand the profound meaning of the words imparted by the teacher. The student is a devotee, but the teacher treats him like a friend so that in a friendly atmosphere the law of love and equality can reveal itself to the devotee. Between a lover and the beloved there will always be a huge gulf if the sense of equality and compassion is not shared without reservation. A teacher is a friend, yet such a friend deserves reverence. It is said that in the ladder of love, the first rung is reverence, and devotion is reverence indeed. Love and reverence establish a perfect way of communication. The higher secrets can only be imparted by a friend to a friend. Sri Krishna has so far imparted the knowledge of jnana and karma yoga. Now he is imparting the secrets of attaining happiness by renouncing the fruits of one's actions. Higher knowledge is only imparted to the beloved students, for such knowledge cannot be understood by ordinary people.

अर्जुन उवाच
अपरं भवतो जन्म परं जन्म विवस्वतः।
कथमेतद्विजानीयां त्वमादौ प्रोक्तवानिति।। ४
श्री भगवानुवाच
बहूनि मे व्यतीतानि जन्मानि तव चार्जुन।
तान्यहं वेद सर्वाणि न त्वं वेत्थ परंतप।। ५
अजोऽपि सन्नव्ययात्मा भूतानामीश्वरोऽपि सन्।
प्रकृतिं स्वामधिष्ठाय संभवाम्यात्ममायया।। ६

Arjuna said
4. *Your birth was later and the birth of Vivasvat much earlier;
   how shall I understand this, that you taught it in the beginning?*
   The Blessed Lord said
5. *Many births of Mine have passed and so have yours, O Arjuna. I
   know them all, but you do not know them, O Scorcher of Enemies.*
6. *Though unborn, the immutable Self, being even the Lord of beings,
   yet I incarnate with my own power, having perfect control over my
   Prakriti.*

Arjuna now understands that the instructions that Sri Krishna is
imparting are a profound part of that which was handed down by a long
tradition. But Arjuna's mind rambles in the garden of confusion when
he hears Sri Krishna say that he had also imparted that knowledge to
Vivasvat. He wonders, "My master and teacher is standing before me.
How could he possibly have taught Vivasvat who lived thousands of years
ago?" Arjuna becomes confused, and his doubts are very genuine. He
says, "O Lord, later is your birth, much earlier the birth of Vivasvat. How
shall I understand this?" In order to dispel ignorance the master, referring
to past incarnations, says, "For you know them not, and I know them all.
Atman is eternal; it is never born and never destroyed. I, as Atman, am
the cause of the universe and the Lord of all beings. I have perfect control over my Prakriti; I incarnate with my own power and not because
of the chain of cause and effect." Birth and death cannot be attributed to

the birthless Atman, yet it has the power to incarnate. Ordinary minds cannot grasp this truth, but sages have no difficulty in understanding it.

The sages understand that the past, present, and future are mere moments in the unbroken chain of life. These moments are synchronous; therefore, to the realized ones past and future are the same as the here and now. The ordinary mind has no capacity to uncover the secrets of death and birth, past and future; but those who have attained knowledge of the timeless can easily comprehend the philosophy of reincarnation.

Most of the spiritual traditions of the world believe in the philosophy of reincarnation. Non-believing poses more serious questions than believing, such as why are we forced to be born? Is birth just an accident without any cause? Is birth the total responsibility of Providence, a choice of the Lord who is considered to be the creator of this world? The traditions that do not believe in rebirth or dismiss the issue do not satisfactorily answer these questions. Ordinary people follow the injunctions of the religious scriptures blindly, but it is a demand of an intellectual and inquiring mind to resolve conflicts created by unanswered questions such as: From where have I come? Why have I come? What is the purpose of my life? Where will I go? The philosophy of rebirth and reincarnation alone provides satisfactory answers to these questions.

Many Westerners react defensively when they encounter the philosophy of reincarnation. They dismiss it as a primitive, spooky, or fanciful conception. They are not at all able to consider the merits or deficiencies of this view in an objective way. They are repulsed by the idea of reincarnation and do not want to hear anything about it. It is a clear sign of egotism when one refuses to examine an issue objectively and to expand the horizon of his vision. Most Westerners are afraid of the unknown, though they are equally dissatisfied with the known. Their insecurity leads them to fortify their egos. It is a vicious cycle.

Many Western philosophers such as Plato, Schopenhauer, Kant, and Hegel believed in the philosophy of reincarnation. And there are many people able to recall their pasts verbatim. The validity of reincarnation cannot be decided by debates; it is subject to Self-realization. When one attains a more evolved state of consciousness, his latent memories from his long past unfold themselves before his consciousness.

There are millions of people in today's world who are infatuated with the external and temporal. But there are only a few great and enlightened teachers. For the most part, the blind are leading the blind. Death and birth do not reveal their secrets to ordinary people. Only sages or yogis know these secrets. Ordinary people experience the pangs of death and birth, but divine incarnations such as Sri Krishna do not. These great ones consciously assume various garbs in order to give the message according to the needs of the masses. This type of incarnation is a rebirth of that great man who has already attained the highest, but the ordinary person's death and birth results from the desire to enjoy the world and its pleasures. The minds of ordinary people are entangled by mundane and temporal desires, but the great ones are beyond the influences of the gunas and are thus free from desire.

Death is but a habit of the body, a change—not complete annihilation. It is like passing through an exit in a fortress and then coming back in from another entrance. The pangs of death disturb those who cling to life and to the temptations of the mundane world, but death is not at all terrifying and never a painful experience. It is the fear of death that is the source of the pain that one experiences. Such a fear has no basis, but it remains unexamined by ordinary minds. When one thoroughly examines his fear of death, he realizes that that which is inevitable should be accepted. There is no need for any fear. Fear of not gaining what one wants, fear of losing what one already has, fear of separation, fear of death, fear of the unknown, and all the various kinds of fears dwell within weak minds and defeat the purpose of life. The ancients knew that the sense of self-preservation creates fear. They led their students to encounter their fears, to remove them, and to attain the state of fearlessness. Fear is a self-created suffering that does not allow one to enjoy any object of the world. It mars the joys of life from the sense level to the mental level, and even in the unconscious. Once fear makes the unconscious its permanent abode, it is difficult to get rid of it. Arjuna suffered on account of fear, but Sri Krishna, a master and Lord of life, helps Arjuna by sharing the supreme wisdom.

When a teacher imparts the knowledge of the three bodies (the gross, subtle, and causal), the student understands that the gross material body lives only for a short time between the two events of birth and death. The subtle body is the possessor of the impressions in the unconscious. It is composed of samskaras, impressions of all sorts, both merits and demerits from one's past. The subtle body lives as long as those impressions exist. The causal body, however, lasts for a long time. It is composed of the latent part of the impressions or samskaras that live in a quiet and dormant corner of the unconscious. Those who do not have knowledge of these three bodies identify only with the biological needs of the gross body. But the aspirant who is conscious of these three bodies knows that the physical body is just a gross covering.

There are yogis who go beyond these three bodies to a timeless state, and the knowledge they attain enables them to know past, present, and future in exactly the way that an ordinary man has awareness of only the recent past. They experience the past, present, and future in the same way that ordinary people experience things of the world during the waking state. Sri Krishna is the knower of that science, whereas Arjuna is only aware of his body and its relationship to the external world. Love for the body and objects of the world is a love of poor quality; it is not dependable. Arjuna is not aware of the more subtle bodies, so it is impossible for him to recall the past. Ignorant people remain deluded and suffer, but a great yogi like Sri Krishna has perfect knowledge, for he knows all the past births.

यदा यदा हि धर्मस्य ग्लानिर्भवति भारत।
अभ्युत्थानमधर्मस्य तदात्मानं सृजाम्यहम्।। ७
परित्राणाय साधूनां विनाशाय च दुष्कृताम्।
धर्मसंस्थापनार्थाय संभवामि युगे युगे।। ८

7. *Whenever there is a diminution of dharma, O Descendant of Bharata, and a rise of unrighteousness, then I incarnate Myself forth.*

**8. *For the protection of the good, for the destruction of the evil doers,
for the purpose of establishing dharma, I incarnate Myself from
age to age.***

When dharma is forgotten and duty is ignored, when those who are
committed to their duties are molested by the wicked and unrighteous,
when the entire social order is taken over by evil-minded people, then
the Lord incarnates Himself to establish dharma once again. The word
bharata means love of knowledge. The Lord also incarnates for the sake
of those who have love for knowledge and righteousness. Some people
misuse this verse; they do not understand that although an incarnation
comes to guide the people, the people also have to make efforts to transform themselves. Such people become dependent on the incarnation to
do it all for them. They do not make efforts to know and understand the
law of karma and how to perform duties skillfully. Thus, they fall prey to
laziness, sloth, and inertia, believing that an incarnation will descend and
they will be redeemed. That kind of thinking can cause the downfall of
both the individual and the nation. It can also give birth to false prophets.

There is a difference between being born and being incarnated.
Ordinary people have no control over birth and death, but He who is
Lord of life has all power under His control and thereby descends by
His own will to bring back those who have forgotten their direction.
Ignorant, misdirected human beings suffer, and the incarnation of
the Lord comes to show them the path of wisdom. This has happened
throughout the history of mankind.

Religionists believe that God incarnates, and religions are in fact
based on this belief. But they believe in only one such incarnation and
follow only that one. They claim that other incarnations are false and
that they mislead the people. This reflects the circumscribed and egocentric view of both those who are responsible for maintaining the religious institutions and their followers as well. Any institution, religious
or otherwise, seeks to perpetuate and expand itself at the expense of
those outside that system. Such an ego-oriented and competitive way of
being narrows one and does not allow knowledge to shine forth.

If God can incarnate once, why can't He incarnate again and again? Western religionists do not accept the philosophy of the reincarnation of God because it threatens their institutions. They repeat, "Have faith, have faith, have faith," but why and how remains unexplained. Their explanation is vague and is mere pacification. It does not satisfy those with inquiring minds. The yogic understanding is that Love and Truth incarnate periodically and become abundantly visible on earth. The same message is given, yet with a different emphasis according to the needs of the times. There is no sectarianism in the Bhagavad Gita. Sri Krishna is not speaking as a particular personality but as the universal source of love and truth.

जन्म कर्म च मे दिव्यमेवं यो वेत्ति तत्त्वतः।
त्यक्त्वा देहं पुनर्जन्म नैति मामेति सोऽर्जुन।। ९
वीतरागभयक्रोधा मन्मया मामुपाश्रिताः।
बहवो ज्ञानतपसा पूता मद्भावमागताः।। १०

9. *He who knows My divine birth and action in its subtlety, after leaving the body, no longer goes to another birth; he comes to Me, O Arjuna.*
10. *They who have freed themselves from attraction, fear, and anger— many, purified by the asceticism of knowledge, absorbed in Me, have come to identification with Me.*

These verses explain that birth and death are not under the control of nature but under the control of the individual self. Life and relationship are inseparable: life externally and internally is relationship. The body is related to the breath, the body and breath to the emotions, the conscious to the unconscious mind, and so on. The two units of the self, the mortal part and the immortal part, separate when one dies. The body, breath, and conscious mind are mortal. But even after death the vehicle that carries and preserves all the subtle impressions, the unconscious mind, remains undecayed, and therein the seeds of desire are preserved. These seeds sprout in search of fulfillment and then grow again and give birth to many new seeds, just as an acorn sprouts and grows into a tree that produces many more acorns. Cause and effect live together; birth and death and an individual's circumstances are therefore determined by the individual and his nature. Beliefs such as "I am created by God, and my miseries are also created by God" are based on fallacious concepts. Such unphilosophical, illogical, and irrational beliefs lead ordinary people to suffer. You are the way you wanted to be, and you will be the way you want to be. Those who have attained the knowledge of the Absolute are released from the bondage of births and deaths, for they have gone beyond the sphere of the gunas; they have given up desire. Therefore, there are no seeds, and therefore there is no tree.

There are three categories of beings; ordinary people who have no control over death and birth; great yogis and sages (muktas) who have attained liberation and have perfect control over death and birth; and incarnations who are forces of the Absolute, free from bondage, who come only to guide and help mankind. Birth and incarnation appear to be alike, but actually they are not. Incarnation is a descending force of the Lord beyond the sphere of the gunas and free from bondage. Birth and incarnation are similar events, but they have two separate causes. When the instructions imparted by the incarnation are faithfully practiced by the sadhaka, his experiential knowledge guides him to the summit where he becomes one with the highest.

Human beings are children of God, and children have the same potential as their parents. They simply need to unfold and grow. Essentially and qualitatively, a single drop of the ocean has all the qualities of the ocean. When a drop meets the ocean, it becomes the ocean. Verse 10 teaches that one can attain more than mere intellectual knowledge of the Absolute. In this verse Sri Krishna is not referring to worship of the Lord as a separate entity, but he is making one aware that the potentials one has are exactly like that of the divine Lord. The entire dialogue between Sri Krishna and Arjuna is a dialogue between the pure absolute I and the relative I of the human being. This verse says that the I of the human being is capable of becoming inseparable from and one with the divine.

Many modern students might conclude that Sri Krishna's teachings are sectarian; that the Bhagavad Gita teaches that one should only take refuge in Sri Krishna and in no other form of God. That is not true. Sri Krishna speaks from the heights of that one universal consciousness that is beyond even divine forms and from which the divine forms come. He is not speaking only as a specific incarnation. He is one with all incarnations, and at the same time he is beyond all incarnations.

Though all incarnations are one in their source, authority, and state of consciousness, each clothes the eternal message in a different wrapping. The aspirant is not able to dive completely into the teachings of all incarnations. He will progress most directly if he absorbs himself in one tradition while respecting all others. When he starts practicing sadhana, the seeker is strictly warned to follow only one path, the path he is taught by his teacher, and not to follow other paths. For if one changes the path he follows every now and then, he will not be able to attain the Absolute. Students often leave the path they have practiced, running here and there, which is a sheer waste of time and energy and above all brings complete dissatisfaction and disappointment. That is the actual sense hidden in this verse.

ये यथा मां प्रपद्यन्ते तांस्तथैव भजाम्यहम्।
मम वर्त्मानुवर्तन्ते मनुष्याः पार्थ सर्वशः।। ११
कांक्षन्तः कर्मणां सिद्धिं यजन्त इह देवताः।
क्षिप्रं हि मानुषे लोके सिद्धिर्भवति कर्मजा।। १२

11. *Whosoever in whatever way submit themselves to Me, I confer grace on them in the very same way. Human beings in all different ways follow My path, O Son of Pritha.*

12. *Desiring fulfillment of actions, many here sacrifice to gods. In the human world, accomplishment comes quickly as a result of action.*

Whatever path one follows up a mountain, he finally reaches the summit. Though the ways are diverse, the goal is one. Sri Krishna explains that although people follow various paths to Self-realization, finally they reach one and the same Absolute. Some seekers waste considerable time trying to know this path and that path. And other seekers are confused by the diversity of spiritual paths. It is important for the seeker to start treading his path and to continue on it instead of being lost in the bewilderment of diversity.

Ordinary men worship various gods with the desire of receiving reward. They undoubtedly receive the fruits of their actions. Those who desire worldly gain receive it; to those who are desirous of knowledge, knowledge is given; and to those who desire *mukti* (liberation), that is given to them. Everyone reaps the fruits of his actions according to the universal law: as you sow, so shall you reap. Instead of realizing that one receives according to his actions and thus paying attention to and doing their duties skillfully, many people believe that God is capriciously rewarding or punishing them. They praise God when they are successful and blame Him when they fail. Their irresponsible attitude leads them toward irresponsible behavior. Such people want to enjoy the fruits of their actions but do not want to take responsibility for discharging their duties. As a result they do not receive the fruits they want. The law of karma is inevitable. Therefore, one should perform his duties skillfully with a one-pointed and tranquil mind.

Modern psychotherapy also helps clients to realize that they are responsible for their own actions. Most clients who enter therapy believe that others are responsible for their misery. They either blame their parents or society for the way they were treated as a child, or they blame their spouses, relatives, friends, or the circumstances in their current life. One of the main tasks of a teacher or psychotherapist is to lead the student or client to recognize that he is responsible for his own predicament; that only he can change his circumstances, his attitude, and his behavior. Here the teachings of the Bhagavad Gita and modern psychotherapy have much in common, although the Bhagavad Gita is more direct and didactic in bringing the student to that realization, whereas modern psychotherapy gradually guides the client in changing his perspective.*

चातुर्वर्ण्यं मया सृष्टं गुणकर्मविभागशः।
तस्य कर्तारमपि मां विद्ध्यकर्तारमव्ययम्।। १३

13. I have created the four-fold division of humanity on the basis of their qualities and actions. Though I am its creator, know Me to be the immutable one who does not become an agent of action.

Every creature acts because of the three gunas or qualities. All three gunas are present in each person but in different proportions. That is why different people have different natures. Some people have tamas as the predominant guna, which leads them toward lethargy and identification with worldly objects; others have rajas predominant leading them to action; and in others, the sattva guna is strongest, and they have the greatest understanding. The actions of ordinary people are guided by the predominance of either rajas or tamas. Because they desire to enjoy worldly pleasures, they do not develop the sattva quality and allow it to become predominant.

It is possible to classify personality types according to the predominance of one guna or another. It is interesting to note that although modern psychologists and physiologists are unaware of this concept of the gunas, they classified people along similar lines. Sheldon studied the body types of numerous people and found that subjects could best be classified according to the relative predominance of these factors. It was found that people who are dominated by fatty tissue tend to enjoy sensory pleasure and to be more passive and lethargic than others. Those who have a predominance of muscle tissue, the mesomorphs, are action oriented. And those in whose bodies the nervous system takes precedence

---

* For a more detailed discussion see *Psychotherapy East and West*, Swami Ajaya, Honesdale, PA: Himalayan Institute, 1984.

over fatty and muscular tissue are more oriented toward understanding than toward sensuality or action. The parallel between the system of the gunas and the body typology of these modern psychologists is striking. According to the system described in the Bhagavad Gita, it is the gunas that lead one to develop one or another body and personality type. They classify people according to the relative proportions of each of the three characteristics. That was also done in ancient India: a fourfold classification was established that later became the caste system.

It is unfortunate that these groupings are taken as separate castes, for that has created a wide gulf in Indian society. As in the Western world where people suffer because of their class system, Indian society suffers as a result of the curses of the caste system. In ancient times that classification helped to organize society: it was meant to facilitate the distribution of labor and was based on the principle that one should work according to his ability and receive according to his need. For example, those in whom rajas was dominant, who were mesomorphs in body type and given to action, became the rulers and warriors in society; and those in whom sattva guna was predominant, who were cerebral and who were interested in understanding, functioned as teachers and priests. But today there is complete confusion because the sense of the distribution of labor is lost, and the caste system has replaced it. Instead of giving people work according to their propensities, they are placed into rigid categories according to the categories of their parents, grandparents, and forefathers. Certainly inheritance has an influence, but unfortunately a serious and rigid division has been created among the people of India because of the caste system. This fourfold distinction was originally made by analyzing the qualities and actions of people. It had an entirely different perspective than the caste system, for its aim was to integrate the society into one whole. In the Bhagavad Gita this fourfold division is referred to as *brahmana, kshatriya, vaishya,* and *shudra.* The dispositions, qualities, and actions represented by each of the four groups are found all over the world in every human society.

We have already explained that no one is the doer of action, that the three gunas are the real doers of all that occurs in the world. Action is born out of one's nature. This means that the gunas are established along with one's physical birth. They prompt people to do actions and to perform their duties accordingly.

One can also put the whole universe into such a fourfold division from the microcosm to the macrocosm. There are four separate worlds: the worlds of human beings, animals, plants, and minerals. That differentiation is made because of the distinct qualities of each. The word "man" has been borrowed by the English language from its Sanskrit root *man*, to think, because of man's higher thinking capacity. The human being who has developed the capacities of his mind and controlled his lower nature is primarily influenced by sattva guna. Animals have no capacity to think as a human being; they can only sense and react. They are more rajasic and tamasic. The vegetable kingdom is even more tamasic. The minerals are the most inert and are dominated by tamas guna.

In modern psychology there has been an ongoing controversy that has evolved out of German and British philosophy. The controversy is over the relative importance of that which is inherited versus that which is learned. German philosophy has emphasized the former, and British philosophy the latter. Those views have led to two distinct perspectives in modern psychology, the proponents of which often clash with one another. Yoga psychology, however, acknowledges the importance of both, but it understands inheritance in a different way than modern psychology. According to this view, one inherits not only the characteristics of his parents and ancestors but inherits those characteristics that he has acquired in a previous life as well. The characteristics that one brings from his previous life result from what had been learned through rewards and punishments experienced by both the individual in his previous life and by his ancient forefathers. One is born with both what he inherits from previous generations and what he carries with him as a result of his own previous learning in past lives.

According to yoga psychology, one's birth is not an abrupt or capricious event but a predetermined event that takes place first in the unconscious, in the realm of desire. One is born in order to fulfill his desires from the past. The question arises, "Why is one born into a particular family?" The law that can be applied to answer that question is "similar attracts similar." Birth into a particular family is a choice of both the parents and the child. Attachment is an intense form of desire. If there was attachment in a previous life between two people, it can cause one's birth into a particular family. That heredity influences one cannot be denied, but one's attachment and desires are also an inheritance. All the hereditary qualities occur because of the law of association, attachment. Therefore, there is not much difference between learning and inheritance.

The inevitable law of karma is a continuous chain of cause and effect: an action is performed and one then reaps the consequences, which lead to ever more actions, more fruits, and still further actions. A chain of reactions is thus created. The samskaras or impressions in the unconscious, which are the results of the deeds performed by a person in his previous lives, are part of this chain and are responsible for his birth in this life. But the cycle of cause and effect need not be endless. True learning can completely change and transform the human being. When one knows how to light the fire of knowledge and then burns all his samskaras, he can attain freedom. Although past impressions have a deep impact on the human personality, the right learning program carried out now and in the future has the power to release one from previous impacts and can thus lead him to an entirely new dimension of life in which the past samskaras do not have any influence.

न मां कर्माणि लिम्पन्ति न मे कर्मफले स्पृहा।
इति मां योऽभिजानाति कर्मभिर्न स बध्यते।। १४
एवं ज्ञात्वा कृतं कर्म पूर्वैरपि मुमुक्षुभिः।
कुरु कर्मैव तस्मात्त्वं पूर्वैः पूर्वतरं कृतम्।। १५

14. *Actions do not smear Me nor do I have an attraction toward the fruits of action. He who recognizes Me thus is not bound by actions.*
15. *Even the ancient ones who desired liberation performed actions with this knowledge; therefore you too should perform the same ancient act as done by your predecessors, the royal sages.*

One who has no attachment to the fruits of his actions yet continues performing actions remains unaffected. That which affects the person is his attachment to the fruits therein, so the wise give up the fruits and thus attain freedom. In ancient times the sages knew this principle and attained liberation, but in today's world human beings do not understand the profound philosophy of non-attachment. We see misery everywhere. Because of one's attachments to the results of his actions, to the people with whom he lives, to prestige, and to all sorts of objects, one becomes the slave of his wants and desires. If modern man learns from the ancient traditions, he will decrease many of the miseries that he repeatedly creates for himself and others.

किं कर्म किमकर्मेति कवयोऽप्यत्र मोहिताः।
तत्ते कर्म प्रवक्ष्यामि यज्ज्ञात्वा मोक्ष्यसेऽशुभात्।। १६
कर्मणो ह्यपि बोद्धव्यं बोद्धव्यं च.विकर्मणः।
अकर्मणश्च बोद्धव्यं गहना कर्मणो गतिः।। १७
कर्मण्यकर्म यः पश्येदकर्मणि च कर्म यः।
स बुद्धिमान्मनुष्येषु स युक्तः कृत्स्नकर्मकृत्।। १८

16. *What is action, what is inaction? Even the wise are confused in this matter. Therefore, I shall teach you concerning action, knowing which you will be freed from the foul world.*
17. *One should learn of action; one should learn of action that is opposed to right action; one should learn of inaction. The reality of action is deep.*
18. *He who sees inaction in action and who sees action in inaction, he is the one endowed with wisdom among human beings. He is joined in yoga, a performer of complete action.*

Even great leaders and heroes sometimes become bewildered in deciding between right action, action that is opposed to right action, and non-action. When faced with a decision, how is one to determine which is the best response? Perhaps the action one chooses will have an effect opposite of what is anticipated and will create conflict, disharmony, or grief. In that case is it better not to act at all? Such questions occur to every person many times each day, although the process of considering these choices is so subtle that one may not be aware of it. If one does not know what the right action is, his mind starts pondering over the possible negative consequences of the actions he is considering. That can result in uncertainty, confusion, and loss of will power. Indecisiveness, delay in deciding, and the fear of making a decision are unhealthy and painful. In such cases it is buddhi that needs training. If one is prone to be hesitant and uncertain in deciding how to act, the decisive factor of one's internal organization (buddhi) should be sharpened so that it can promptly and unhesitatingly advise the mind and enable one to make a timely decision. Right action, of course, is always best. Action performed in a state of tranquility with non-attachment is always the right action. Contrary to that is action committed in a deluded state of mind, but even worse is inaction. A suspicious, doubtful, and deluded state of mind inevitably leads to injurious action. Action that is undertaken without taking the counsel of the decisive faculty of one's internal state is injurious action.

Many people are overly cautious and afraid of taking action, so they become inactive. Inaction makes one inert and is worse than wrong action. During the period of inaction one appears not to be performing actions, but he is actually reacting adversely to the situation he faces. He is in a sort of negative withdrawal that leads to slothful ideas: "Why do I need it; why should I do it; I can live without it; I'm not capable; therefore I should not even make an effort to do it."

Inaction is a result of the influence of tamas. In *vikarma*,* action that is opposed to right action, rajas and tamas join, but rajas is predominant. Rajas makes one active, but without sattva one remains deluded.

---

* Vinoba's commentary provoked a lengthy discussion and investigation of other commentaries to delve more deeply into the meaning of the word vikarma. Vinoba's commentary differs from the commentary of his revered teacher, Mahatma Gandhi. Vinoba says that vikarma is a special type of action, and he speaks of it in a positive sense. Verse sixteen itself says that even the great sages are perplexed about these different forms of action, With due respect to Vinoba, vikarma is to be understood as an action that is opposed to karma and performed in a deluded state.

It is actually the sattva quality that keeps the mind tranquil, and action performed in the state of tranquility is right action.

One who has disciplined himself, trained his senses, and attained a concentrated state of mind that always seeks the counsel of buddhi does not commit mistakes in performing his actions. He surrenders the fruits of his actions willingly for the sake of others. Such selfless action has two benefits: the fruits of one's action do not bind him, and his action becomes a form of worship, meditation in action. The yogi goes on performing actions with a tranquil mind and always remains free from the bondage of action. For him there is no self-interest. All his actions are motivated by selflessness, and he is free.

यस्य सर्वे समारम्भाः कामसंकल्पवर्जिताः।
ज्ञानाग्निदग्धकर्माणं तमाहुः पण्डितं बुधाः।। १९
त्यक्त्वा कर्मफलासङ्गं नित्यतृप्तो निराश्रयः।
कर्मण्यभिप्रवृत्तोऽपि नैव किञ्चित्करोति सः।। २०
निराशीर्यतचित्तात्मा त्यक्तसर्वपरिग्रहः।
शारीरं केवलं कर्म कुर्वन्नाप्नोति किल्बिषम्।। २१
यदृच्छालाभसंतुष्टो द्वन्द्वातीतो विमत्सरः।
समः सिद्धावसिद्धौ च कृत्वापि न निबध्यते।। २२
गतसङ्गस्य मुक्तस्य ज्ञानावस्थितचेतसः।
यज्ञायाचरतः कर्म समग्रं प्रविलीयते।। २३

19. *He whose endeavors are all devoid of desires and attendant volitions, him the wise call a pandit, with all his actions burned by the fire of knowledge.*
20. *Abandoning attachment to the fruits of actions, ever satiated, without dependency, even though involved in action, he never does anything.*
21. *Without expectation, his mind and self controlled, ceasing all intake through the senses, performing the action only physically, he does not gather sin.*

22. *Satisfied with gaining whatever comes without seeking, having transcended all opposites of duality, free of small-mindedness, alike in acomplishment or failure, such a person is not bound even upon performing the action.*
23. *For one whose attachment is gone, who is liberated, whose mind is established in knowledge, who conducts his action only for sacrifice, his entire action is dissolved.*

Actions performed without the desire for enjoyment are considered to be pure actions because they arise from knowledge attained in a state of tranquility. One who has learned the art and science of performing desireless action and whose motivations are burnt by the fire of knowledge is called a knower {pandit). Such a wise man remains content and self-reliant. Although his external behavior may appear to be full of activity, he actually does nothing, for he is not the doer. This man of self-control, abandoning all desire for enjoyment and even the means of enjoyment, performs actions merely to maintain his physical existence. He remains unaffected and uninfluenced by the actions and the fruits received therein. Thus, he never becomes the victim of emotional outbursts. He has attained freedom.

Actions are thoughts that are externalized, and thoughts are often controlled by the power of emotion. Emotion has the power to disturb thought and to distort one's actions. Vikarma is that action performed under the influence of unchecked, uncontrolled emotion. There is a vast difference between emotion and thought. In thought there lingers a doubt, but emotion does not have the sense of discrimination. Emotion has a great power to energize a person that thought does not have. Emotion is like a blind man who has the strength to walk but cannot determine which way to go, whereas thought is like the man who can see which way to go but is lame. Some sadhakas use only mental exercises and do not remain aware of the power of emotion. Others are swayed by emotional power without making use of their mental abilities. But the skilled sadhaka unites emotional force with mental power. He brings these together so that they help one another and make the journey easy. A sadhaka should learn to regulate and use these two distinct forces, mental and emotional, to enable him to create a strong and dynamic will power, which will help him in performing actions and duties. It is not only a tranquil mind and skill that are needed to perform action in a skilled way, but also a will force that replaces the desire for sense gratification. Will power is very important in the performance of action as well as in treading the path of the inward journey. If the mind remains dissipated and unregulated emotionality persists, the will power is weak. But the more one's mind is concentrated, one-pointed, and undisturbed by emotional life, the stronger will be his will power. Will power is higher than the power of thought and emotions. With the help of this power, one can do that which is considered to be impossible.

Among the many potentials one discovers on the inward journey, will power is the highest of all. Determination, courage, and fearlessness, which are important to a sadhaka, result from will power. The psychology of the East is practical, experiential, and applicable, and the path of sadhana, in which the development of will is the central focus, is unique. Sadhakas who have mastered this path are rarely seen. In the East, sadhana is more important than external observations and intellectual conclusions. The study and development of will power is a practical subject that most thinkers and intellectuals do not appreciate. In modern psychology and psychotherapy little attention is given to the development of will power except among the existentialists and in psychosynthesis. In these two schools (the latter being derived from yoga psychology), the development of will power is important. But in most systems of psychotherapy, it is totally neglected. Practical training in the strengthening of will power should be a part of therapeutic and self-development programs.

Ordinarily we associate will power with the desire to attain something worldly. We think of the person with a strong will as aggressive and restless. But that is a will allied with the ego. Here will power is conjoined with such qualities as non-attachment to worldly objects, the abandonment of personal desires, and tranquility. Tranquility is a state of being that is attained by the disciplined and desire-free mind. One who is non-attached attains the height of equanimity; he is free from all temptations, charms, desires, and delusions. Using his powerful will to free himself from attachments and from the allures of the world, he performs his actions just for the sake of action and is liberated here and now.

These verses explain a positive way to remove all the errors that one fears he may commit while performing his actions. They describe a state of being in which there is inaction in action. Here lies a great secret, and in knowing that secret, one is free from bondage, even when action has been performed, as though he had never done the action. The Bhagavad Gita teaches us a unique way of performing action through love: non-attachment.

Verse 23 again refers to the importance of sacrifice in bringing about freedom. Sacrifice means giving all the best that one has. The action performed with the zeal of sacrifice washes off all impurities and errors. Sacrifice is one of the greatest virtues that one can develop; it totally changes the course of actions as well as the way one feels when performing actions. It is as though one consciously becomes the ritual or the archetype and loses his personal motivation and desire. It virtually consumes one's personal motivation and acts of itself, and therefore the fruits are also consumed. The binding effects of the motivation, of the action, and of the fruits are completely destroyed. The sacrifices that can lead one to such total transformation are explained in the following verses.

ब्रह्मार्पणं ब्रह्महविर्ब्रह्माग्नौ ब्रह्मणा हुतम्।
ब्रह्मैव तेन गन्तव्यं ब्रह्मकर्मसमाधिना।। २४
दैवमेवापरे यज्ञं योगिनः पर्युपासते।
ब्रह्माग्नावपरे यज्ञं यज्ञेनैवोपजुह्वति। २५

श्रोत्रादीनीन्द्रियाण्यन्ये संयमाग्निषु जुह्वति।
शब्दादीन्विषयानन्य इन्द्रियाग्निषु जुह्वति।। २६
सर्वाणीन्द्रियकर्माणि प्राणकर्माणि चापरे।
आत्मसंयमयोगाग्नौ जुह्वति ज्ञानदीपिते।। २७
द्रव्ययज्ञास्तपोयज्ञा योगयज्ञास्तथापरे।
स्वाध्यायज्ञानयज्ञाश्च यतयः संशितव्रताः।। २८
अपाने जुह्वति प्राणं प्राणेऽपानं तथापरे।
प्राणापानगती रुद्ध्वा प्राणायामपरायणाः।। २९
अपरे नियताहाराः प्राणान्प्राणेषु जुह्वति।
सर्वेऽप्येते यज्ञविदो यज्ञक्षपितकल्मषाः।। ३०
यज्ञशिष्टामृतभुजो यान्ति ब्रह्म सनातनम्।
नायं लोकोऽस्त्ययज्ञस्य कुतोऽन्यः कुरुसत्तम।। ३१
एवं बहुविधा यज्ञा वितता ब्रह्मणो मुखे।
कर्मजान्विद्धि तान्सर्वानेवं ज्ञात्वा विमोक्ष्यसे।। ३२
श्रेयान्द्रव्यमयाद्यज्ञाज्ज्ञानयज्ञः परंतप।
सर्वं कर्माखिलं पार्थ ज्ञाने परिसमाप्यते।। ३३

24. *The act of offering is Brahman; the oblation is Brahman; into the Brahman fire offered by Brahman, it will reach Brahman alone through the harmony (samadhi) of the actions, which are Brahman.*

25. *Some yogis gather and sit around the sacrifice offered to gods. Yet others offer the sacrifice of self by the sacrificial act into the Brahman fire.*

26. *Others offer the senses, such as that of hearing, into the fires of self-control. Some others offer objects, such as sound, into the fires of the senses.*

27. *Yet others offer all actions of the senses as well as actions of the pranas into the fire of the yoga of self-control kindled by and blazing with knowledge.*

28. *Some sacrifice objects; the sacrifices of some are ascetic practices; the sacrifice of some is yoga. Some ascetics of well-honed vows*

perform the sacrifices of self-study and knowledge.

29. *Some others make an offering of prana into apana and offer apana into prana, seizing the movements of prana and apana, intent on the practice of pranayama.*

30. *Others, eating a measured amount of food, make an offering of pranas into pranas. All of these are experts at sacrifice with their sins destroyed by sacrifice.*

31. *Those who eat only the nectar-like amrita, which is the remainder left after a sacrifice, go to eternal Brahman. Not even this world is available to one who does not perform a sacrifice, let alone the next world, O Best of the Kurus.*

32. *Thus many different kinds of sacrifice are spread out before Brahman; know them all to be products of action. Knowing thus you will be liberated.*

33. *Better than the sacrifice in which objects are offered is the sacrifice of knowledge, O Scorcher of Enemies. All action, O Son of Pritha, reaches its fulfillment in knowledge.*

Sacrifice is an act of offering for the sake of attaining the goal of life: Brahman. One who performs the sacrifice, the fire that is lit to perform the sacrifice, the material that is collected for the oblation, the act of offering, and all the means are verily Brahman. For Brahman is the all-pervading, all-encompassing, omnipresent, and omnipotent power. Everything is Brahman.

Brahman is the timeless, infinite, and eternal self-existent power, the ultimate Truth from which springs the entire universe, which sustains the universe, and by which the universe is finally dissolved. This self-existent glory needs no support from any quarter, for Brahman alone exists without a second. Self and Brahman are two ways of referring to the same all-encompassing One. The word Self (Atman) is used with the sense of the indwelling Lord, and the word Brahman is used without reference to the individual. The Self is the Lord within, and Brahman is the formless One beyond all manifestation. Atman in the individual and Brahman in relation to the universe are one and the same undifferentiated ultimate Reality without a second. These are two connotations of the only one Reality that exists.

Yogis traditionally use Verse 24 as a prayer before their meals. It reminds them that eating food is a sort of prayer in itself, that they are eating for Brahman and not for themselves. Therefore, the sadhaka offers his food to Brahman with the feeling that the food is in fact Brahman, the eater is Brahman, and the offering is to Brahman alone. That helps the sadhaka expand his awareness of Brahman. It makes him aware that there is only one existence and that all separation is illusory. Ordinary people are attached to food and do not like to offer or share with others. But the sadhaka on the path of spirituality understands that he should develop the habit of giving so that he does not become a victim of greed, jealousy, pride, prejudice, or egoism. Some yogis perform sacrifices internally. Instead of using any external means, they use their pleasure senses, just as the materials are used in the external world, to perform the oblation; they use their breath as fire and offer all their thoughts, emotions, and desires as sacrifices in order to attain self-control. All the motivations arising from the gunas and desires are offered as oblations into the fire of knowledge. When all the actions, thoughts, desires, motivations, and gunas are offered as sacrifice in the fire of knowledge, the yogi is liberated.

There is yet another path. Pranas are aspects of the vital force that sustains our life on this earth. The word *prana* means the first unit of energy, and it also refers to inhalation. In this form of sacrifice, the breath is offered to the prana within. Thus, the fire sustains the fire. By means of this offering, all impurities are destroyed, and the yogi realizes the highest of truths. Brahman.

These nine verses explain various kinds of sacrifice and give an overall view of sacrificial acts and the importance of performing sacrifice. The word yajna is used to refer to the performance of sacrifice. That act that is performed for attaining Brahman is one type of yajna. There are *Brahma yajna, jiva atma yajna, jnana yajna, vijnana yajna,* and *moksha jnana yajna.* In order to simplify these terms, we can put them into four categories: (1) yajna performed to fulfill mundane desires; (2) yajna performed as a selfless action to serve and help others; (3) yajna performed to attain freedom from the bondage of karma or action; and (4) yajna performed by yogis to burn their samskaras (latent impressions) in the fire of knowledge.

Yajna performed externally is definitely inferior to yajna performed internally. Internal yajna is a spiritual sadhana called jnana yajna. It leads one inward to the source of knowledge and consciousness, whereas external yajna leads to perfection and skillful action and to liberation from the bondage of action. The wise perform jnana yajna and enjoy eternal peace and bliss. The universe is also performing yajna. All that we see and experience is yajna. That is all there is. The difference between the wise and the ignorant is that the wise person does not resist this grand ceremony, whereas the ignorant person creates barriers and resistance by performing yajna for sense gratification and mundane gains.

Brahma yajna is the highest of all yajnas. It is performed with the motivation to attain ultimate knowledge. Therefore, it is not a source of bondage but a means to liberation. That yajna is performed by the sadhaka internally without using any externals, and it is performed by others in the external world. In the external world all actions, expressions, and the best of materials are put together to light the fire of yajna, and desire becomes the offering. One receives the fruits of that supreme action. The fruit one receives from such yajna is that rare skill that allows one to perform selfless actions that do not create bondage. Both yajnas are performed for attaining Brahman.

तद्विद्धि प्रणिपातेन परिप्रश्नेन सेवया।
उपदेक्ष्यन्ति ते ज्ञानं ज्ञानिनस्तत्त्वदर्शिनः।। ३४

34. *Learn this by prostrating, by asking questions, and through service. The wise ones who have seen the Reality will instruct you in this knowledge.*

Verse 34 explains that the preceptor is also a fire into which the offerings are given. The quality of fire is to transform everything into one element and to finally reduce the values of the offering to ashes. A good preceptor or teacher does not put any demands on or require any offering from the student. The light of the teacher is a self-sustained, eternal light. It is the light of knowledge. Offering anything to this fire is a gesture of reverence and love for the teacher, which teaches the student to let go of his greed.

There is a symbolic ceremony performed by spiritual teachers, and although the outward expression is symbolic of an internal process, the external expression is of great importance. In the first step of initiation, the teacher accepts the student and introduces him to the path he has to tread. In the next step the sadhaka brings dried twigs and offers them to the teacher who lights the fire and burns them one by one. In this symbolic ceremony performed between disciple and master, all the disciple's samskaras are burned in the fire of knowledge lit by the gurudeva.

The teacher needs nothing, but the way one approaches his teacher is important for the sadhaka. To receive knowledge it is essential that the aspirant is humble and that he has one-pointed devotion, love, and reverence. If these qualities are absent in the student, he cannot receive any knowledge. When a student asks a question, not in order to test the teacher's brilliance, but to know and receive knowledge, it is important for him to be humble. He should not ask questions for the sake of argument. Egotistical students close the gates of knowledge. When one is polite and humble, his questions are answered and his conflicts are resolved.

Verse 34 instructs Arjuna to become humble so that the knowledge is received by him. In his questioning, he has been fighting with his teacher instead of fighting the battle. There is still obstinance in his questions. His resistance toward the selfless teachings is a result of arrogance. Sri Krishna is teaching Arjuna not to resist but to become humble. Then clarity of mind is easily attained. This does not contradict previous statements that a student should question. But one should be humble when he puts questions before his teacher, and he should receive the answer without resistance.

As has been already noted, resistance is also one of the greatest barriers to change found in psychotherapy. Therapists find that even though their clients come seeking guidance and solutions to their problems, and sometimes pay a great deal of money for the therapist's guidance, they fail to carry out the advice or directions received from the therapist. The therapist is often in a peculiar position: if he gives advice, the client ignores it. Or realizing that the client will ignore his advice, the therapist can keep his suggestions to himself, thereby helping the client to sort out his confusion and conflict and to come to his own conclusions. But then the client feels cheated and demands that the therapist be more direct in telling him what to do. Many explanations for this sort of interaction have been offered. Some therapists call this struggle between therapist and client "the battle for control," whereas others attribute it to the client's defensiveness. One way or another, it must be dealt with. Therapists have devised various means for responding to the obstinacy of the client including paradoxical therapy, in which the client is encouraged to continue or increase his problematic behavior.

In the beginning of therapy, client and therapist may attempt to out-maneuver one another, and this may even last throughout the therapy. Is it any wonder then that psychotherapy lasts so long and has limited results? If the client comes to therapy with good faith, then rapid and remarkable strides can be made in self-transformation. But that is the exception rather than the rule. Progress occurs only to the extent that one goes beyond his resistance, for resistance is holding onto that which one already is. Unless clients learn to become humble, straightforward, and receptive in relation to the therapist, they are not likely to grow. Yet this is rarely achieved in modern therapy, and much of the therapy is spent directly or indirectly in helping the client to develop these attitudes.

But the responsibility for lack of receptiveness should not be put entirely on the client's shoulders, for how often do we find therapists that are truly selfless, giving, and knowledgeable? In an atmosphere of arrogance and selfishness, how can there be a free exchange? Of course, one cannot expect modern therapists to be as selfless and knowledgeable as Sri Krishna, for they are still growing and Sri Krishna is fully enlightened. But we can and should expect them to sincerely work at transforming themselves and to become a genuine example of that which they are teaching.

The situation in which modern man finds himself is not unique. We see again and again that the Bhagavad Gita deals with issues similar to those faced by seekers and clients in the modern world. All the issues of concern to modern psychology such as motivation, perception, habits, reward and punishment, and the unconscious are considered in great depth in the Bhagavad Gita, and theories of these aspects of human functioning are put forth. But the Bhagavad Gita also goes further than modern therapies: it deals with those finer aspects of the human being that are almost completely neglected in modern psychology. The insights and understandings of the perennial psychology of the Bhagavad Gita can do much to enrich modern psychology and psychotherapy.

यज्ज्ञात्वा न पुनर्मोहमेवं यास्यसि पाण्डव।
येन भूतान्यशेषेण द्रक्ष्यस्यात्मन्यथो मयि।। ३५
अपि चेदसि पापेभ्य: सर्वेभ्य: पापकृत्तम:।
सर्वं ज्ञानप्लवेनैव वृजिनं संतरिष्यसि।। ३६
यथैधांसि समिद्धोऽग्निर्भस्मसात्कुरुतेऽर्जुन।
ज्ञानाग्नि: सर्वकर्माणि भस्मसात्कुरुते तथा। ३७

35. *Knowing which, you will not again come to such delusion, O Pandava, and whereby you will see all beings in their entirety in the Self as well as in Me.*
36. *Even if you are the most sinful, excelling all the sinful ones you will cross this arid ocean with the fleet of knowledge.*
37. *O Arjuna, as a well-kindled fire turns all kindling into ashes, so the fire of knowledge turns all acts, even of past lives, into ashes.*

Once the aspirant attains unalloyed knowledge, he does not slip back to his old habits. Such knowledge liberates one from all weaknesses and gives him freedom from misery. As the fire reduces everything to ashes, so does knowledge. All impurities are removed by knowledge alone. A student should learn to enlighten himself by first disciplining himself and following his sadhana, and then he should learn to expand his consciousness to cosmic consciousness. Sadhana starts from the individual self, and from the center of consciousness in the individual, it expands to cosmic consciousness. The process progresses in stages. First one gains voluntary control in withdrawing the senses from the objects. Then the mind is made free from the sense perceptions. Next one encounters thoughts coming from the unconscious. Then the sadhaka examines and analyzes, and accepts or rejects the thousands of thoughts that come forth. This state of introspection helps one to understand his mind because he learns to know which thoughts are useful and which are not. One then uses the knowledge of discrimination to strengthen his decisive factor and then learns to judge as a witness. At this stage one no longer identifies himself with the objects of the world that are stored in the form of impressions in the unconscious. Now the sadhaka remains vigilant that he does not become affected by the unknown part of his mind, the unconscious, and the mind acquires a keen sense of observation and does not involve itself anymore. This state is like witnessing, and that is why the word "seer" is used for such sadhakas, because they have attained freedom from the deep-rooted habit of identification. When one no longer identifies himself with the objects of the world, he realizes his essential nature. After realizing one's own essential nature, he has yet to practice seeing all things in himself and himself in all things. The state in which one sees himself in all and all in himself is the true state of Self-realization. It can be attained by the method already explained or by the method of contemplation. This entire process, this inward journey, is considered to be the inner way of lighting the fire of knowledge (*antar yoga*). Sri Krishna is instructing Arjuna to light the fire of knowledge which alone has the power of reducing attachment to ashes.

With the help of knowledge even the greatest sinner can cross the mire of delusion, just as a boat has the capacity to take one to the other shore. By the fire of knowledge all impurities are burned, all evil thoughts of the mind are reduced to ashes, and the mind is freed from impurities. With the help of pure knowledge and true guidance, even a most evil type of person can attain the goal of life. There are many examples that can be cited from the scriptures of various traditions: Valmiki in the Indian tradition, Saul in the Christian tradition, and Milarepa in the Tibetan tradition. Modern students should therefore understand that there is no point in condemning themselves. Everyone has the capacity and ability to touch that part of eternity within himself through which he can attain pure knowledge and transform himself. Self-transformation finally leads one to Self- realizaton. In that state one can see himself in all and all in himself.

न हि ज्ञानेन सदृशं पवित्रमिह विद्यते।
तत्स्वयं योगसंसिद्धः कालेनात्मनि विन्दति।। ३८
श्रद्धावाँल्लभते ज्ञानं तत्परः संयतेन्द्रियः।
ज्ञानं लब्ध्वा परां शान्तिमचिरेणाधिगच्छति।। ३९
अज्ञश्चाश्रद्दधानश्च संशयात्मा विनश्यति।
नायं लोकोऽस्ति न परो न सुखं संशयात्मनः।। ४०

38. *There is no purifier in this world equal to knowledge. One who is fully accomplished in yoga finds that knowledge in the Self in due time.*
39. *One who has faith, is intent upon serving the gurus, and has mastered the senses attains knowledge. Upon attaining knowledge he very soon reaches supreme tranquility.*
40. *One without knowledge and without faith, of mind filled with doubt, perishes. One whose mind is filled with doubt has neither this world nor the other world nor happiness.*

Among all branches of knowledge the highest is spiritual knowledge, which is attained by the systematic method of the inward journey. The purest of all knowledge is the knowledge of Atman, the center of consciousness, which completely quenches the thirst for knowing the truth. When the sadhaka has firm faith in the inner dweller, Atman, and when he trusts his teacher and understands the scriptures and teachings of the great ones who have already trodden the path of light, then he is capable of performing his duties without committing any error. He does not waste his time uselessly brooding on concerns that dissipate the mind. Such knowledge purifies the way to the center of consciousness. Firm faith, a one-pointed mind, control of the senses, non-attachment, and regular sadhana are important means for seeing oneself in all and all in oneself. Nothing is higher and purer than the knowledge of Atman. Such knowledge gives one perfect peace. Then all doubts are resolved.

In Verse 39, which is very important for all sadhakas, Sri Krishna states that shraddha, which means single-pointed devotion plus full reverence for the path that one is treading, is very essential. Control of the senses is also important. The senses are employed by the mind, and because of the senses, the mind ordinarily remains dissipated and forms bad habits. Therefore, discipline of the senses is important. With the help of one-pointed devotion and discipline of the senses, the highest peace is realized.

But he who has no faith, love, or devotion toward the inner dweller—the controller, the governor, and the fountain of light and life within—and who doubts the basis of his existence, destroys himself. He can never see the positive side of his mind. A negative mind full of doubts is neither successful in the external world nor on the inward journey. When the yogis refer to a doubtful mind, they mean a mind that is not guided by the higher buddhi. The mind that is not trained to take counsel from the higher buddhi always functions with doubts and indecision. Such a mind is unable to attain anything properly. One who has such a disturbed, distracted mind and who has no faith in his own resources, has no self-confidence. He does not have determination or will power. His life is full of misery, sorrow, and grief, and there is no chance for him to attain happiness. Verse 39 clearly explains that without love, devotion, and self-control, knowledge cannot be attained. We have cited examples showing that even evil-minded people who gain knowledge and faith are capable of attaining the state of tranquility and the final state of Self-realization. But those whose minds are dissipated, who do not make any effort to control the senses, and who have no faith in the existence of the Self or God, are always unhappy and suffer.

Developing the power of concentration by practicing control over the senses can give one tremendous mental power. Control of the senses and development of the power of concentration can be attained by anyone. If a thief and a sadhaka are asked to sit in the same room with a heap of gold and jewels, the thief will be able to concentrate better than the sadhaka. The sadhaka must direct his power of concentration toward the attainment of tranquility and then to Self-realization. Evil is he who has a concentrated mind but has no faith in the existence of the Self. He is not conscious of the self-existent Reality within but is conscious only of the objects that give him pleasure. On the path of spirituality, firm faith becomes a leader, without which the power of concentration and austerities can mislead one. If a wicked person learns to develop faith, transformation and Self-realization become possible to attain.

योगसंन्यस्तकर्माणं ज्ञानसंछिन्नसंशयम्।
आत्मवन्तं न कर्माणि निबध्नन्ति धनंजय।। ४१
तस्मादज्ञानसंभूतं हृत्स्थं ज्ञानासिनात्मनः।
छित्त्वैनं संशयं योगमातिष्ठोत्तिष्ठ भारत।। ४२

41. *He who has renounced actions through yoga, he whose doubts have been sundered by knowledge, he who has cultivated the self, him the actions do not bind, O Conquerer of Wealth.*
42. *Therefore, with the sword of the knowledge of Self, cut this doubt that is born of ignorance and that is dwelling in your heart. Resort to yoga. Rise, O Descendant of Bharata!*

In these verses the word yoga has been used in the sense of actions performed skillfully with full mastery for the sake of *loka sangraha* (actions done only for the sake of others). Such actions do not bind the yogi. Action does not enslave anyone; that which has enslaving power is the desire to receive the fruits of one's actions. Desire is the cause of enslavement. But for those who have attained the knowledge of Atman, desires have no existence, so they are free even though they act.

There are three definite means to attain the highest good. First, when all aspects of mind start functioning harmoniously, one reaches a state of tranquility. A harmonious and tranquil mind enables one to perform his duty without attachment. One can also attain the highest yoga by removal of the doubtful nature of the mind with the help of pure reason, which has the qualities of discrimination, judgment, and decision. And the third means is intuitive knowledge for the realization of Self.

Let us distinguish between buddhi and intuition and their respective powers. The aspirant whose buddhi is sharpened by the knowledge of discrimination is skillful in performing action and offers the fruits of his action for the benefit of others. But one who has acquired profound knowledge directly from the source of intuition, the purest of all forms of knowledge, has firm faith in the self-existent Atman.

Manas, the lower mind, functions only in a doubtful manner. It wonders: Shall I do it or not? Is it good or bad? Is it helpful or not? This particular faculty of mind is not capable of discriminating, judging, or deciding. That is why manas is referred to as *samkalpa vikalpa atmaka* (shall I do it or not?). But when this faculty receives the profound counseling of the higher buddhi, it is no longer ruled by doubt, confusion, and conflict. It then acts decisively.

Higher buddhi helps in discriminating and deciding what is right for one to do, but the knowledge of the pure Self is beyond the sphere of buddhi. Intuitive knowledge alone gives one the power of Self-realization. Pure buddhi can penetrate to the deeper levels of one's being, but the finest and highest level is attained not through the knowledge of buddhi or through the mind but through intuitive knowledge alone. Intuitive knowledge does not dawn bit by bit. It is a spontaneous knowledge received by the sadhaka when he has surrendered even the way of pure reason.

We disagree with the many writers and commentators who claim that pure buddhi can be the means of final emancipation because there are, in fact, two powers that are functioning. One is called the ascending power, and the pure buddhi leads that ascending power to the summit of human knowledge. But without meeting the beloved, the descending power, termed *kripa* or grace, even reaching the summit does not bring complete fulfillment. Fulfillment is the unity of the ascending and descending powers. Pure reason falls within human endeavor, but intuitive knowledge is divine. Intuitive knowledge is entirely different than the knowledge of pure reason or buddhi. With pure buddhi one may fathom many finer levels of consciousness, but without intuitive knowledge one cannot attain the Self-illumined source of consciousness. That intuitive knowledge dawns when human endeavor is completed and exhausted.

Intuitive knowledge has immense power to cast off all the fetters of the sadhaka, for then one's inner strength is directly obtained from the source of all strength and knowledge. That source is Atman, the pure Self. As long as one remains dependent on any other source of strength—wealth, health, mind, and even buddhi—he remains imperfect. Perfection is attained through inner strength. There are limitations in all external strengths. If one uses all of his wealth, all his friends, and those who are intellectually gifted, these will not help him to attain intuitive knowledge.

In Verse 41, Sri Krishna calls Arjuna the conquerer of wealth, which in the context of this verse indicates that real wealth and strength lie within, giving one courage, clarity, fearlessness, and the profound knowledge of discrimination. The day an aspirant begins looking and finding within, he begins the process of becoming aware of his inner strength. If he persists on the path of sadhana, he attains freedom on all levels and finally deserves to receive the intuitive knowledge through which enlightenment is attained.

Here ends the fourth chapter, in which the knowledge of renouncing the fruits of actions is described.

Chapter Five

Knowledge of Renunciation and Action

अर्जुन उवाच

संन्यासं कर्मणां कृष्ण पुनर्योगं च शंससि।
यच्छ्रेय एतयोरेकं तन्मे ब्रूहि सुनिश्चितम्।। १

श्री भगवानुवाच

संन्यासः कर्मयोगश्च निःश्रेयसकरावुभौ।
तयोस्तु कर्मसंन्यासात्कर्मयोगो विशिष्यते।। २

ज्ञेयः स नित्यसंन्यासी यो न द्वेष्टि न कांक्षति।
निर्द्वन्द्वो हि महाबाहो सुखं बन्धात्प्रमुच्यते।। ३

Arjuna said

1. *O Krishna, you advise renunciation of actions and again the yoga of action; whichever is the better one of these two, please tell me definitely.*

The Blessed Lord said

2. *Both the yoga of renunciation and of action lead to supreme beatitude. Between those two, however, the yoga of action excels the renunciation of action.*

3. *Know him to be ever a renunciate who neither hates nor desires; devoid of the opposites of duality, indeed, O Mighty-armed One, he is effortlessly relieved from bondage.*

Sri Krishna explained the path of renunciation in the previous chapter, but further confusion arises in Arjuna's mind. Most of the time students do not follow the advice of their teachers because the student's thinking and understanding are based on a lower level of consciousness. Because the teacher speaks from a height that is beyond the student's level of comprehension, the student does not understand the teachings. Communication is thus poor. But teachers persist in instructing their students and gradually lead them to greater and greater comprehension. Only then can the higher teachings be received. A profound and great teacher like Sri Krishna explains the teachings again and again. That is why in the Bhagavad Gita we find the same teachings explained repeatedly from various angles and perspectives. The teacher does not tire of teaching, and the genuine seeker of truth should persist in asking questions until all his doubts are resolved.

Arjuna wants comprehensive knowledge of each path so he can know which to follow and how. He asks Sri Krishna to show him the path that will lead to the highest bliss. Although Sri Krishna imparts the knowledge of both paths, renunciation and action, he leads Arjuna along the path of action because Arjuna in his despondency has forgotten his duty and thinks of turning to renunciation as an escape. In the path of renunciation both action and fruits are renounced. But in the path of action only the fruits are renounced, and action is performed with non-attachment. Both the path of action and the path of renunciation are valid, but Sri Krishna recommends the path of action for Arjuna for the following reasons: (1) Arjuna is infatuated and full of grief because of attachment to his relatives; (2) He is in a state of confusion yet is talking of renunciation, which is merely an escape for him because he does not have the courage to confront the mental conflict he experiences; (3) He is being selfish, thinking only about himself and his position; (4) Thinking of renouncing is a clear sign of cowardice for a warrior. Refusing to fight a just war and running away from the battlefield have nothing to do with renunciation. It is quite evident that Arjuna is not prepared either to perform his duties or to follow the path of renunciation.

We have already explained that the path of renunciation is only for a fortunate few; the masses are more inclined toward action. The path of action is thus the only path for the people of the world. In the path of renunciation both action and fruits are renounced: the fire of knowledge burns all the actions and the fruits of actions. There is no desire, no action, and therefore no fruits. The actions that the renunciate performs are not the same actions as those performed by the people of the world. The actions performed by the renunciate are preparation for deepening his renunciation so he can attain profound knowledge. The renunciate's actions do not lead him toward worldly attainments but toward the divine.

The student should understand that renunciation is not a path to be followed by just anyone. Following the path of renunciation is like walking on the edge of a razor. It needs strong determination, a one-pointed mind, and complete renunciation of both actions and fruits. It requires immense courage, non-attachment, and one single desire: to attain liberation. The reasons that Arjuna gives to Sri Krishna are not the right reasons for following the path of renunciation.

No aspirant should decide to follow the path of renunciation in a fit of emotion or if he is not successful in the world. Disappointment and frustration create the desire for withdrawal and diversion in ordinary minds. It is a state of confusion—not a preparation for renunciation.

When one genuinely wants to renounce, he has a single desire to attain liberation. The quality of that desire is not like the quality of other desires that motivate one to perform actions and reap the fruits. It is a desire for lighting the fire to burn all the samskaras, all the impressions in the unconscious. The fire of knowledge alone purifies and makes one free. Then that desire to attain knowledge is also renounced. The real renunciate is he who has freed himself from the pairs of opposites such as pleasure and pain, love and hate, for he remains in the state of bliss by being one with the Absolute. He has freed himself from the divisions of the phenomenal world.

Arjuna's path is that of action. That path is valid because: (1) It is the path of the masses; (2) When one cannot live without doing actions, he can still discipline himself and practice non-attachment; (3) Deeds performed with non-attachment are selfless deeds, and selfless deeds lead to emancipation; (4) Performing deeds with a tranquil mind and with non-attachment is worship, for in this path the fruits of one's actions are offered to the Lord.

The aspirant should not forget that here Sri Krishna is not addressing a group of renunciates. He is addressing mankind through Arjuna, who has to constantly fight the battle of life by living in the world. Sri Krishna himself is not a renunciate, and Arjuna is not a renunciate either. Sri Krishna imparts the knowledge of how to perform skillful and selfless action, and at the same time he also explains the path of renunciation. He neither condemns the path of renunciation nor advises all renunciates to change their chosen path and to follow the path of action. Commentators create a tug of war by identifying with one path or the other and interpreting the Bhagavad Gita from that point of view. They are extremists who try to pull others onto their path whether it is right for them or not. Many commentators unjustly condemn the path of renunciation without having practical knowledge of that path. Sri Krishna does not condemn the path of renunciation but recommends that Arjuna and the ordinary people of the world follow the path of action.

सांख्ययोगौ पृथग्बालाः प्रवदन्ति न पण्डिताः।
एकमप्यास्थितः सम्यगुभयोर्विन्दते फलम्।। ४
यत्सांख्यैः प्राप्यते स्थानं तद्योगैरपि गम्यते।
एकं सांख्यं च योगं च यः पश्यति स पश्यति।। ५

4. *Only the childish argue about Samkhya and Yoga as being separate—not so the pandits. Resorting to either one properly, one attains the fruit of both.*

5. *The place that is attained by the followers of Samkhya is also attained by those of Yoga. He who sees Samkhya and Yoga as one, truly sees.*

The great learned ones who understand both the path of Samkhya yoga (the path of knowledge) and karma yoga (the path of action) do not find a huge gulf between these two paths, for they know them to be two aspects of the same pursuit. How can one possibly perform actions without knowledge, and how can the fire of knowledge be kindled without action? Behind the yoga of action stands the profound philosophy of Samkhya, and the science of yoga furnishes the means to practice the goal of life. Thus they are inseparable. Both paths lead the aspirant to the spiritual summit. Learning to perform actions is beneficial for the ordinary person, but for one who is free from the pairs of opposites, it is immaterial whether he follows the path of renunciation or the path of action. To one who has attained the state of tranquility, it makes no difference which path he follows. Therefore, the conflict over following one path or the other does not arise in the mind of the learned. Both paths lead to the same end: liberation, emancipation, fulfillment, and Self-realization.

संन्यासस्तु महाबाहो दुःखमाप्तुमयोगतः।
योगयुक्तो पुनर्ब्रह्म नचिरेणाधिगच्छति।। ६
योगयुक्तो विशुद्धात्मा विजितात्मा जितेन्द्रियः।
सर्वभूतात्मभूतात्मा कुर्वन्नपि न लिप्यते।। ७

6. *Renunciation, however, O Mighty-armed One, is difficult to attain without yoga. The meditator joined in yoga, however, attains Brahman without delay.*
7. *Joined in yoga, of purified self, having conquered the self, having conquered the senses, he whose self has become the Self of all beings, is not defiled even when performing actions.*

One should not follow the path of renunciation without first attaining the profound knowledge of how to perform action. Only the knowledge of performing action selflessly enables one to follow the path of renunciation. The path of action is an essential step in renunciation. Confusion comes when we study two things separately and do not study their relationship.

The path of yoga enables one to attain a state of tranquility without which no path can be trodden except the path of misery and confusion. If the path of renunciation is followed without nonattachment, it is based on fake tyaga (giving up) and leads to misery. The yogi who practices and follows the path of sadhana understands that direct knowledge arising from practice alone brings satisfaction.

The great spiritual leaders and sages of every tradition say one and the same thing. But mere belief in their teachings does not dispel the darkness of ignorance, for one needs more than belief in the sayings of the sages. He needs to experience bliss directly. It is necessary for each person to light his own lamp, to dispel the darkness he himself has created. Though one has the sun, moon, stars, and all the lights to help him walk, he will stumble if he does not light the lamp in his inner chamber, for his clouded mind will blind his vision. Though one may be on a perfect road, the uncertainties created by his clouded mind will create mirages and hallucinations that mislead him. A clouded mind leads one to walk in a circle instead of walking forward on the path that has been trodden by the sages. Inner light is more important than all of the lights that shine outside.

Only those who have accomplished perfection in action have the capacity to follow the path of renunciation. Real perfection comes only through renunciation, and only after attaining perfection in action. Perfection in action is total giving, completely giving up the fruits of action. Pure and selfless giving empties one, and then pure knowledge dawns directly from the source of all knowledge.

In the yoga of action both self-control and purification of the heart are important. One who has attained control of the senses and mind and at the same time has purified his heart remains non-attached and performs his actions in a state of tranquility. The way of the mind is to find solutions through thinking, reasoning, and philosophizing, but the way of the heart is to feel and then react emotionally. Emotion has immense power, but it has no ability to reason. The sadhaka is instructed not to ignore his emotional life, not to intellectualize but to give attention to the purification of the heart and also to the control of senses and mind. Purification of the heart means learning to be sensitive, to understand positive emotion and its use as a means to attain ecstasy. That attainment is a different experience than the experience gained by the control of senses and mind. One's sadhana should be designed to include both discipline of mind and purity of heart. Those who have followed such a sadhana and gained the knowledge of the Eternal see themselves in others and others in themselves—loving all and excluding none, including all and embracing all. They perform their actions selflessly while remaining unaffected.

नैव किञ्चित्करोमीति युक्तो मन्येत तत्त्ववित् ।
पश्यञ्श्रृण्वन्स्पृशञ्जिघ्रन्नश्नन्गच्छन्स्वपञ्श्वसन् ।। ८
प्रलपन्विसृजन्गृह्णन्नुन्मिषन्निमिषन्नपि ।
इन्द्रियाणीन्द्रियार्थेषु वर्तन्त इति धारयन् ।। ९

8. *'I do nothing at all.' Thus should the knower of Reality, joined in yoga, contemplate, even while seeing, hearing, touching, smelling, eating, walking, sleeping, breathing.*
9. *Speaking aloud, eliminating, receiving, opening the eyes and closing the eyes, the knower of Reality holds that 'the senses are operative in the realm of the objects of the senses.'*

These two verses are intertwined; they complement each other and fulfill one and the same purpose. The aspirant should gain knowledge and then practice the application of that knowledge. Practice purifies the ego, which otherwise forgets its direction and creates a strong fortress by continually building boundaries around itself. The yogi who has purified his ego acquires perfect control over the senses. In that case the senses work directly for the mind, and the mind works in conjunction with buddhi for the pure ego. The purified ego is able to represent the pure Self called Atman.

That great man who knows the truth and follows the path of non-attached action while performing his mundane duties—seeing, hearing, sensing, touching, tasting, speaking, being alone, and being with others during the three states of waking, dreaming, and sleeping—remains unaffected because he knows that he is not the doer. The senses function, but the owner of the senses does not become involved. In such a state of mind the yogi does his actions but remains aware that he is not the doer.

ब्रह्मण्याधाय कर्माणि सङ्गं त्यक्त्वा करोति यः।
लिप्यते न स पापेन पद्मपत्रमिवाम्भसा।। १०
कायेन मनसा बुद्ध्या केवलैरिन्द्रियैरपि।
योगिनः कर्म कुर्वन्ति सङ्गं त्यक्त्वात्मशुद्धये।। ११
युक्तः कर्मफलं त्यक्त्वा शान्तिमाप्नोति नैष्ठिकीम्।
अयुक्तः कामकारेण फले सक्तो निबध्यते।। १२

10. *Placing his actions in Brahman, abandoning attachment, he who performs actions is not smeared by sin, any more than a lotus leaf by water.*
11. *With the body, with the mind, with intelligence, or with senses alone the yogis perform their actions, abandoning attachment, for the purification of themselves.*
12. *Joined in yoga, abandoning the fruits of action, one attains the peace of those who have conviction. One not joined in yoga, acting out of desire and attached to fruits becomes bound.*

One needs to control the senses and mind and at the same time to have knowledge of the Ultimate in order to give up attachment. Mere discipline does not help one to attain the virtue of non-attachment. He alone who gives up all the fruits of his actions, offering them to the Lord of life and the universe, is not affected by the evil of attachment. He is like the lotus: though it lives in the water, its petals remain unaffected by the water. The lotus, which is a symbol of yoga, reminds us not to be attached while performing actions.

Many people confuse attachment with love. But in fact it is non-attachment that is love, whereas attachment is merely lust and addiction.

If we learn to practice non-attachment in our relationships, we can create a heaven for ourselves here. We can live in a garden of delight. If in the close relationship between husband and wife, both partners learn to see the presence of divinity in one another and remain conscious of it all the time, the relationship will turn from lust to love, from attachment to non-attachment. But if the consciousness of the body remains only on the level of sense pleasures, lust grows and therefore attachment as well. The spiritualization of a relationship is possible provided both partners have one and the same aim, like two wheels of the same chariot, which can make the path easy and joyful. Any relationship that is worthwhile is an expression of love of the divine.

Sri Krishna teaches that all actions can be performed as worship, dedicating the fruits of actions to the Lord. If every action is taken as a gesture of worship, then how can the fruits of action bind the human being? Bondage comes from action performed selfishly for the purpose of sense gratification. Those who have learned the art of dedicating the fruits of their actions and who remain constantly aware of the Lord of life and of the universe, though they live in the world they remain unaffected, like the lotus in water.

Yogis perform their actions selflessly. Their actions are not directed toward reaping fruits for the sake of pleasure. Such yogis are always in perennial joy, for they do not create attachment. This path is the path of selfless love and service. These great lovers of humanity attain the highest state of peace and tranquility. One who performs his actions with attachment and with selfish motives does not know how to give and give up and suffers from the fruits of his actions, which imprison him.

सर्वकर्माणि मनसा संन्यस्यास्ते सुखं वशी ।
नवद्वारे पुरे देही नैव कुर्वन्न कारयन् ।। १३

13. *Renouncing all actions with the mind, the self-controlled one sits happily in the city with nine gates; the body-bearer neither doing anything nor causing anything to be done.*

The nine gates referred to in this verse are the nine openings in the body: two nostrils, two ears, two eyes, the mouth, and the organs of excretion and generation. It is beautifully said in the Ramayana that these nine gates are guarded by guards who are so evil that, instead of protecting the city of life, they always keep these gates open to all pleasurable sensations, for they do not know any other way. But the yogis, having perfect mastery of the nine portals or openings in the body, are not trapped by sense gratification. The yogis control these gates and remain free from the sense pleasures that gradually destroy the city of life. The master of this city, the Self, is seated in the inner chamber of our being. Instead of having the profound consciousness of the master, the ego creates a false sense of individuality and ownership, and thus serious problems arise.

Because it indulges in sense gratification, the ego forgets the master and separates itself from the pure Self. This separation is actually the greatest of all pains for those who have already trodden the path and are conscious of the Self. The yogi is fully aware that the master of this city of life is the Self, not the ego. The yogi knows that it is the pleasures obtained from the nine gates that feed the ego, so he shuts all these gates with his power of discrimination and self-control. These nine gates then do not remain a source of distraction and misery. By being aware of the Reality and being free of the problems created by the ego, the yogi remains non-attached. His happiness is undisturbed.

In the city of life there are in fact ten portals. Nine are known by everyone, but the tenth is understood only by yogis. It is called *Brahma randhra* (the fontanel or soft spot on the crown of the head), and its function is only known by accomplished yogis. When the pranas (vital energies) depart or abandon their duties, the whole city of life crumbles, and a serious split or division is created. This is the separation that the ordinary man thinks of as death. Without the bridge that is formed by prana, the two units of life separate. One unit is the individual self and the unconscious mind; the other is the conscious mind, senses, and body. This is not actual death; it is only separation. Those who wait for death to release them from their circumstances are merely fantasizing about something that never occurs. They should instead devote their energies to accomplishing their task on this earth. When one's vision is limited, the horizon is not seen as it is. Death is a change and not annihilation. The wise who understand this are never affected by the horror of death created by ignorant minds. The wise person knows that he was never born and so he never dies. When a yogi leaves the body, he opens the tenth gate from which he can visualize the life hereafter. For a yogi there is no mystery concerning life here and hereafter. As a part of the eternal, he is never affected by any change, minor or major, even by death, but he remains in a state of calmness and tranquility. Ordinary minds are not aware of this tenth portal, for they are in the habit of enjoying the pleasures received from the other nine portals. They depart from the city of life without any knowledge of life hereafter. Because of their attachments and their pleasures they remain miserable here, and they carry their misery with them, remaining miserable in the hereafter.

न कर्तृत्वं न कर्माणि लोकस्य सृजति प्रभुः।
न कर्मफलसंयोगं स्वभावस्तु प्रवर्तते।। १४

नादत्ते कस्यचित्पापं न चैव सुकृतं विभुः।
अज्ञानेनावृतं ज्ञानं तेन मुह्यन्ति जन्तवः।। १५

ज्ञानेन तु तदज्ञानं येषां नाशितमात्मनः।
तेषामादित्यवज्ज्ञानं प्रकाशयति तत्परम्।। १६

तद्बुद्धयस्तदात्मानस्तन्निष्ठास्तत्परायणाः।
गच्छन्त्यपुनरावृत्तिं ज्ञाननिर्धूतकल्मषाः।। १७

14. *The Lord produces neither the agency for action nor the actions of people nor their union with the fruits of action; only nature is thus operative.*

15. *The all-pervading One neither takes anyone's sin nor anyone's merit. Knowledge is veiled by ignorance and thereby the creatures are deluded.*

16. *They who have destroyed that ignorance of theirs through knowledge, to them the knowledge illuminates that supreme One like the sun.*

17. *Their intellect dwelling in Him, the self absorbed in Him, intent upon Him, totally devoted to Him, their stains washed by knowledge, they no longer return by way of rebirth.*

In Verse 14 the word *prabhu* is used for the sovereign Self. One who has attained self-mastery is given this title. Such a master of yoga realizes that the pure Self has nothing to do with one's actions, wicked or good. And man is neither a doer nor is he responsible for anyone else's actions or for the fruits of their actions. It is the three qualities of nature—sattva, rajas, and tamas—joined together that cause action.

Man's knowledge remains clouded because of ignorance, so he remains in a state of delusion and confusion and acts from that confused state. Clouds can temporarily obscure the sun from human vision, but when the clouds are dispersed by the rays of the sun, the light is seen again. As the clouds temporarily obstruct the vision, so ignorance obstructs vision of the infinite. Ignorance is dispelled with the help of sadhana and knowledge.

The real Self has not created anything whatsoever; all manifestation is because of the gunas. The Self is a master, and the gunas are the subordinates. Nature functions under the will of the master, the real Self, but the Self remains aloof. The idea of the creation of the universe by God is dismissed by one who understands the philosophy of *ekoham bahu syam* (one manifested into many). There is no creation, for two cannot exist at the same time. There is nothing truly independent of the ultimate reality. Those who believe in duality cannot conceive of the profound truth of oneness without a second. Only one principle manifests and seems to become many, and that single splendid glory of one is not dependent upon any other principle.

Dualistic religions assert that one's sins, errors, and faults can be removed and purified by the Lord. They follow the system of self-centered prayer with the belief that their sins will be washed away by the Lord.

Religionists have developed a system of confession that may have a thera-peutic effect, but it does not remove the clouds of the mind. The belief in sin leads one to guilt feelings, and a guilty mind experiences depression and self-condemnation. All human beings suffer from guilt in various degrees. Guilt is a sort of repentance that occurs after one has already done something that he believes is bad. Becoming preoccupied with guilt and remorse merely compounds the problem, and asking for forgiveness may lead one to feel better, but what is really needed is a change in one's way of being so that he does not commit the same mistake again. Prayer that makes one aware of the source of strength within is helpful, but most of all one needs the will power to behave differently. When one has will power and is determined to apply all human endeavor to a new way of being, then the inner strength attained through prayer helps. A human being has free will but only fifty percent. The other fifty percent can be attained with the realization that the real source of strength lies in the depths of one's being. Mere confessions to priests or talking with friends does release one from the burden of guilt but does not keep one from repeating the action. Self-control and prayer that makes one aware of the source of strength within should both be applied at the same time. How can God possibly take responsibility for human errors and sins? That is a philosophy of the ignorant. People become irresponsible and do not pay attention to their duties and then claim that by visiting churches, temples, shrines, and sacred places their sins will be washed away. That is a conso-lation and a therapeutic solace but not a permanent remedy.

On the path of sadhana the yogi learns to understand that it is his past samskaras with their powerful motivations that force him to do that which he knows should not be done. Therefore, it is necessary to have self-control along with knowledge. Many students equate self-control with repression, but that is not correct. All repressions and suppressions—evident, hidden, or latent—are brought forward con-sciously and burned in the fire of knowledge. Self-control is a conscious act deliberately performed to free one from repression and suppression. Through sadhana alone the yogi is able to light the fire of knowledge and to burn all his samskaras. At that stage he realizes that it is not the

Self but the gunas that create delusion.

Those who find joy in practicing sadhana for the attainment of the Self become one with the Absolute. That is the highest state of sadhana. Those who are intellectuals but do not practice and experience directly never comprehend that state. The state of oneness is not at all the subject matter for debate and discussion; it is the profound experience of direct knowledge that can be comprehended only by those who are on the path of sadhana. Those who are following the path of sadhana with firm determination become free from samskaras. Their fetters are broken, and they attain that oneness and become free from the rounds of births and deaths.

Birth and death are two major changes experienced in human life, and one experiences these two events many times. A human being is born, he grows from infancy to childhood, childhood into adolescence, adolescence into adulthood, adulthood into middle age, and middle age into old age. Is it thus not true that we have died and been reborn many times in one lifetime? Then why does the horror of death mar the joys of the present? Only the ignorant are afraid and affected by what they imagine death to be. Death is essential in the process of growth. But the Self-realized are free, for all the mysteries of death and birth are already revealed to them. They are not only free from the fear of death but are free from the rounds of deaths and births.

विद्याविनयसंपन्ने ब्राह्मणे गवि हस्तिनि।
शुनि चैव श्वपाके च पण्डिता: समदर्शिन:।। १८
इहैव तैर्जित: सर्गो येषां साम्ये स्थितं मन:।
निर्दोषं हि समं ब्रह्म तस्माद्ब्रह्मणि ते स्थिता:।। १९

18. *Toward a philosopher endowed with knowledge and discipline, toward a cow, toward an elephant, and toward a dog as well as toward a cremation ground attendant, the wise are of a single eye.*
19. *They whose minds are established in equanimity have conquered the entire creation right here. Brahman is faultless and even; therefore they are established in Brahman.*

One who has attained the profound knowledge of Atman and sees the real Self as the Self of all is called a brahmana. A brahmana, enriched with the knowledge of Atman, is always modest and humble. Such a learned one who is devoted to acquiring knowledge of the Ultimate is also called a pandit, and he attains *samatvam* (evenness). He conquers the fear of death and is free from the bondage of birth and death. The real Self is free of attributes of all kinds. Those who realize the Self everywhere are absorbed in the Self. Just as the stream meets the ocean, becomes one with it, and can no longer be separated from it, the brahmana is no longer separated after becoming one with the Self of all.

The ordinary human being remains polluted by the sense of distinction. He thinks one person is good and another is bad; one attractive and another ugly; one rich and another poor. He reacts to such distinctions with either attraction or aversion. But the learned and realized one sees everyone alike. He is not affected by these distinctions, for he sees the Absolute smiling through all faces. Those learned ones behave with kindness and gentleness to all creatures. They love all and exclude none. The question might arise: how is it possible for anyone to treat a human being, dog, cow, rat, and ant equally? When one can easily discover differences in the characteristics of all creatures, how is it possible to treat all of them alike? A learned man knows the distinctions between creatures; he does not approach a dog for the sake of milk. But he acknowledges the real Self in both and admires each in its respective place. He knows that gold jewelry is fashioned into a variety of ornaments but that all of those ornaments are made of one and the same element: gold. He also has the knowledge to use the ornaments in the way that they should be used.

The ignorant do not have profound knowledge of birth and death. The secret of these two events is known only by the learned. They have already solved the riddles of these two occurrences, for past, present, and future are equally comprehended by them. They also have knowledge of the hereafter. For those who have attained Brahman, Brahman's knowledge is ever present.

न प्रहृष्येत्प्रियं प्राप्य नोद्विजेत्प्राप्य चाप्रियम्।
स्थिरबुद्धिरसंमूढो ब्रह्मविद् ब्रह्मणि स्थितः।। २०
बाह्यस्पर्शेष्वसक्तात्मा विन्दत्यात्मनि यत्सुखम्।
स ब्रह्मयोगयुक्तात्मा सुखमक्षयमश्नुते।। २१

20. *One should not be exhilarated upon attaining something pleasant nor should he tremble over attaining the unpleasant. A person of steady wisdom, entirely free of confusion, knowing Brahman, dwells in Brahman.*

21. *The happiness that he finds in the Self, whose self is unattached to external contacts, he with his self joined in the yoga of Brahman attains imperishable comfort.*

Those even-minded great men are neither excited by nor proud of their achievements, nor do they become disappointed or disgusted with that which is unpleasant. Their buddhi is firmly established in Brahman, and the knower of Brahman never becomes deluded. Those who are not attached to the objects of enjoyment experience everlasting happiness within themselves. Evenness leads such great ones to the attainment of perfection. They are revered by all.

This is an important lesson for all aspirants: one should not become overwhelmed by his attainments and should also not be affected by disagreeable situations. In all circumstances the great ones maintain their evenness. They do not lose their serenity, and they are not subject to the temptations and charms of the mundane world. Their tranquility comes with non-attachment; their peace and serenity remain undisturbed. Being one with Brahman, they remain in a state of joy everlasting yet ever changing.

Ordinarily people become imbalanced when they experience both success and failure. In success one becomes inflated with pride and thinks too much of himself, and in failure he becomes deflated and depressed. When one becomes inflated he sets himself for a fall, for he then creates a false impression of his worth, and the course of events established by his own unconscious is bound to bring him down. Similarly the depressed state is a deluded state in which one falsely identifies with his failure or supposed inadequacy. Although one may hold on to either state for some time, his own internal learning process will tend to eventually bring him to a state of balance. The wise man, however, avoids such swings of emotion; he has learned to balance his emotions and maintains that balance all the time. A tranquil mind is never deluded by these illusory events, whereas the mind of the ignorant is easily swayed by pain and pleasure.

Ordinary people find happiness only after obtaining the pleasurable objects of their desire, but those who are Self-realized experience the flow of perennial joy. The great yogis experience the happiness of perennial joy without interruption in the waking, dreaming, and sleeping states. The fountain of joy is within and can never be experienced if it is not realized within. As long as one finds delight in the temporary enjoyments of the world, perennial joy cannot be experienced. The desire to obtain joy through external experiences is always in vain.

Those who have intense thirst for knowledge cannot quench that thirst with the waters of streams and wells: only the knowledge of the Eternal quenches it. When in a systematic manner the aspirant practices inwardness, he learns to stop the outward flow, to experience the joy of the Eternal. He is constantly aware of that joy. Through yogic sadhana the yogi is able to reach a state of equilibrium, evenness, and tranquility. For him external pleasures do not have value, and he does not search for happiness in the external world. He knows that the source of happiness is within. He constantly remains aware of this truth, undisturbed and united with the Eternal.

ये हि संस्पर्शजा भोगा दुःखयोनय एव ते।
आद्यन्तवन्तः कौन्तेय न तेषु रमते बुधः।। २२
शक्नोतीहैव यः सोढुं प्राक्शरीरविमोक्षणात्।
कामक्रोधोद्भवं वेगं स युक्तः स सुखी नरः।। २३

22. *The pleasures that arise through contact are causes of sorrow alone; they have a beginning and an end, O Son of Kunti. A wise man is not delighted in them.*
23. *He who before leaving this body, rigid here, can learn to withstand the impetus rising from desire and action, he is joined in yoga. That man is happy.*

When an aspirant develops an awareness of and constantly feels the presence of Brahman, the state of uninterrupted happiness is experienced. Even when performing his duty, he maintains consciousness of the Eternal.

Contact with the objects of the world gives one only limited and momentary pleasure. The senses, trying to obtain boundless and imperishable pleasures, cannot succeed because the senses are limited, and the objects that give pleasure are not permanent. Pleasures last only for a short time. They are transitory in nature, and in between them one experiences many unpleasant states. The absence of the object of pleasure leads to anger, grief, depression, or anxiety. One becomes fearful of losing or not attaining the desired object and becomes envious or jealous of others' attainments. All of these unpleasant emotions arise from the search for sensory pleasure. Sensory pleasure is not capable of quenching one's thirst. The thirst of the human being can only be quenched by everlasting happiness.

Before his body stops functioning, a sadhaka attains a tranquil state of mind that prepares him for the transition that remains unknown to the ordinary human being. For ordinary people life hereafter is an unknown phenomenon, but it is not like that for the yogi or sadhaka. For the knowers of truth, existence on this earth is understood as preparation for the voyage to the unknown. They have already acquired the knowledge of that voyage in this lifetime, and they accomplish what is to be accomplished in this lifetime before the body falls apart. They do not postpone the real issue of life; rather they learn to postpone and even abandon the pleasures of the world for the highest happiness. They have the capacity to give up what is in the hand in order to attain that which is not experienced as yet but which will be fulfilling and satisfying. That is everyone's right: to attain the highest happiness, unalloyed knowledge, undisturbed peace, and tranquility.

The wise make all sincere efforts to attain happiness here and now. And many are successful in realizing the truth and in finding happiness before they leave their bodies. Such great men do not take off their garment, the physical body, in a helpless state as ordinary people do. They leave it consciously. They are free here and remain free wherever they go.

If one is not free from the desires of the mundane world and from the anger that results from unfulfilled desire, he is miserable here and will be miserable after leaving his body as well. Therefore, from the viewpoint of sadhana, it is the first and foremost duty of the sadhaka to strengthen his determination and devotion by building strong will power so that he does not allow his energy to be consumed by the trifles and pleasures of the mundane world. He knows that there is something higher that awaits him with all-embracing arms, with that rare love that gives one permanent happiness and everlasting joy. The great man does not postpone the task of attaining the state of nonattachment until the next life, but he accomplishes it in this lifetime. The so-called pangs of death that horrify and frighten the ordinary human being do not affect the great man because there is no attachment to the body.

अन्तः सुखोऽन्तरारामस्तथान्तर्ज्योतिरेव यः।
स योगी ब्रह्मनिर्वाणं ब्रह्मभूतोऽधिगच्छति।। २४

लभन्ते ब्रह्मनिर्वाणमृषयः क्षीणकल्मषाः।
छिन्नद्वैधा यतात्मानः सर्वभूतहिते रताः।। २५

कामक्रोधवियुक्तानां यतीनां यतचेतसाम्।
अभितो ब्रह्मनिर्वाणं वर्तते विदितात्मनाम्।। २६

24. He who finds comfort within himself, who finds zest and delight within himself, and whose light is within himself, such a yogi, having become Brahman, attains absorption into Brahman.

25. *The sages, with their stains dissolved, attain absorption into Brahman; their doubts sundered, their selves controlled, they delight in benefiting all beings.*

26. *Absorption into Brahman is close to those ascetics whose minds are controlled, who are devoid of desire and anger, and who have come to know the Self.*

Seeking happiness in the external world is like chasing a mirage: no matter how fast one may rush toward it, he never finds anything even when he reaches the place where he thought his goal lay. It is impossible to attain happiness in the external world, for happiness is only found deep in the innermost chamber of one's being. The Self is the center of happiness. Those who are realized are always filled with the happiness of the Self, and they alone find real peace in their hearts. With the light of knowledge, such illumined beings are able to remove all doubts from the mind. When the doubts are removed there is clarity of mind, and then one is able to see things as they are. This happens only when the knowledge of Atman is attained. That knowledge is all-encompassing, eternal, and everlasting. But those who become a victim of sense pleasures have no clarity of mind, are full of doubts, and are unable to see things in perspective. Their sufferings are countless, and they constantly create obstacles for themselves instead of removing them.

According to the message of the Bhagavad Gita, *Brahmanirvana* (absorption in Brahman) is a state of highest bliss. That blissful state is attained by those great ones who have sense control and whose doubts have been removed by the knowledge of discrimination. Such great ones live on the earth, serving all creatures selflessly. Those who have purified their hearts and minds, removing desire and anger, and who have perfect control over their minds find peace within and without.

Those who dedicate their lives to the service of mankind do not have selfish motivations and desires. It is easy for them to have control over their desires and anger, whereas selfish people have no self- control. They are uncontrolled, full of desire, and remain under the grip of anger. Anger is an outcome of unfulfilled desire. It is an evil that shatters the nervous system by imbalancing the body, breath, and mind. Those who are out to fulfill their selfish desires can never be happy, for such desire if fulfilled gives birth to many more desires and finally creates a whirlpool that makes one miserable. But those who are conscious of Brahman and find delight in having control over their minds are the great ones, enjoying peace within from the perennial source of peace and happiness, the Self.

स्पर्शान्कृत्वा बहिर्बाह्यांश्चक्षुश्चैवान्तरे भ्रुवोः।
प्राणापानौ समौ कृत्वा नासाभ्यन्तरचारिणौ।। २७
यतेन्द्रियमनोबुद्धिर्मुनिर्मोक्षपरायणः।
विगतेच्छाभयक्रोधो यः सदा मुक्त एव सः।। २८
भोक्तारं यज्ञतपसां सर्वलोकमहेश्वरम्।
सुहृदं सर्वभूतानां ज्ञात्वा मां शान्तिमृच्छति।। २९

27. *Keeping all external contacts out, and fixing the gaze between the brows, making prana and apana even-flowing between the nostrils,*

28. *The meditator (muni) whose senses, mind, and intellect are well controlled, who is intent upon liberation, who is devoid of desire, fear, and anger—he is indeed always free.*

29. *One attains peace upon knowing Me, the receiver of all sacrificial and ascetic observances, the great sovereign of all the world, and the friend of all beings.*

This passage explains a practical method of sadhana that helps one to attain a concentrated mind and then leads him to a higher step of one-pointedness. When the aspirant learns to be still, keeping his head, neck, and trunk straight in a comfortable and steady pose such as *sukhasana* (the easy pose) or *siddhasana* (the accomplished pose), and when he practices the same posture every day, the disturbances that arise from the body, such as tremors, twitches, shaking, and jerking, are tamed and brought under control.

Verse 27 states that the gaze should be fixed between the two eyebrows. This has two meanings. One is the practice of *trataka* (external gaze), which leads to some concentration of the mind but is primarily practiced to attain good eyesight. The other meaning is to concentrate the mind on the space between the eyebrows to gain control of the mind to the extent that is needed to achieve one-pointedness of mind and to turn it inward. There are numerous misunderstandings and misleading commentaries on this verse. Concentration on *ajna chakra*, a main center of focus during meditation, should be practiced internally and not externally. It is ludicrous for commentators to say that the eyeballs should be pushed upward and the gaze placed between the two eyebrows. If one does that, he will have a headache and will never want to do it again. Do not practice the gaze between the two eyebrows thinking that that is a form of meditation.

The second line of Verse 27 clarifies the practice but can be understood only by sadhakas, not by intellectuals. By focusing the mind on the space between the two nostrils, one increases the awareness of both breaths—inhalation and exhalation (prana and apana). Breath awareness and focusing the mind on the point between the two nostrils help the sadhaka to attain a state of *sushumna*, without which meditation on the ajna chakra between the two eyebrows is difficult. Other scriptures describe the two points—the tip of the nose and the space between the eyebrows—as practices of trataka (external gaze), but such practices of trataka are not related to the state of equilibrium between inhalation and exhalation. When both nostrils begin flowing freely instead of the breath flowing more predominantly through one nostril, and when prana and apana (the incoming and outgoing breaths) are equal, that is called the activation of sushumna. The two breaths are then in complete equilibrium with neither predominating. Without such equilibrium, sushumna cannot be active. Those who are on the path of sadhana and meditation should understand that without the application of sushumna, it is not possible to have control over the mind and its modifications. No matter how much one boasts about his methods of meditation, the practice is incomplete and the method is wrong if sushumna is not applied. The moment sushumna is applied, the mind experiences that state of joy that is quite different from the experience of any other joys in the world. During that time one has no desire to obtain the pleasures of the external world because the mind is in an elevated state of joy that is higher than any pleasure gained from the external world.

When concentration is strengthened and the mind is not allowed to use its usual channels (the senses), it spontaneously begins to attain one-pointed ness, which is a step beyond concentration. When one-pointedness of mind is attained and the mind is not allowed to go to the external world, it finds its way inward. That is the first step of meditation. When the sadhaka or yogi attains that state, he acquires direct control of the mind. Such a mind is free from fear and anger and finds liberation from the bondage arising from enslavement by sense pleasures. However, that liberation is not final liberation, for the one-pointed and inward mind has yet to light the fire of knowledge, in which all samskaras are burned. When that occurs a higher state of liberation is attained, but the final liberation is higher yet. That final liberation takes place when the jiva (individual self) unites itself with the pure Self, which is the Self of all, exactly as a drop of water unites with and becomes one with the ocean.

Verses 27 and 28 gave a brief account of the sadhana that brings freedom from the senses and sense pleasures and leads to control of the mind. Having control over the mind, one is able to control desire and anger. When meditation is deep and samadhi is experienced, liberation is finally attained. The liberated soul dedicates all of the fruits of his actions to the Lord alone, who is in everyone and who is everywhere. With this dedication he does not slip back to the consciousness of his own individuality.

Here ends the fifth chapter, in which Sri Krishna leads Arjuna on the path of action, which leads one to develop perfect control over his mind and to abandon all desires and anger, thus attaining liberation.

Chapter Six
The Path of Meditation

श्री भगवानुवाच
अनाश्रितः कर्मफलं कार्यं कर्म करोति यः।
स संन्यासी च योगी च न निरग्निर्न चाक्रियः।। १
यं संन्यासमिति प्राहुर्योगं तं विद्धि पाण्डव।
न ह्यसंन्यस्तसंकल्पो योगी भवति कश्चन।। २

The Blessed Lord said
1. *Without resorting to the fruit of action, he who performs the action that needs to be done, he is a renunciate and a yogi, and not one who has renounced ritual fires nor one who is actionless.*
2. *That which is called renunciation you should know that to be yoga, O Pandava. No one who has not renounced desires can become a yogi.*

The previous chapter teaches that renouncing desire for worldly pleasure and gain helps one to attain control over the mind. By giving up desires and gaining control over the mind, one can attain liberation. The highest liberation is attained only with Self-realization. In the first and second verses of this chapter, Sri Krishna says that *sannyasa* (renunciation) and karma yoga (the path of action) share certain requisites: performing one's own duty without any desire for the fruits, controlling the senses and the mind, and attaining a state of tranquility.

Now let us describe these two paths without considering one to be superior and one inferior and find out how they are distinct. In the path of renunciation, renouncing the fruits of actions comes later. First comes tyaga, literally abandoning all of one's personal possessions. Three main desires called three *eshanas* are renounced: the desire for a spouse and children, for wealth, and for name and fame. Along with this the practice of non-attachment (vairagya) is also strengthened, without which renunciation cannot be accomplished. It is said that a bird having two wings, tyaga and vairagya, is able to soar from this shore of life to the shore of eternity. The renunciate who is firmly established in the art of non-attachment and who has nothing of his own is a true renunciate. Such a renunciate is rare and is always revered because it is not easy to renounce the world of mine and thine. This path is for the fortunate few and not for the ordinary masses. It is called sannyasa yoga or jnana yoga.

The other path is the path of action. In that path one can have a wife, children, a home, and other means for living in the world, but non-attachment is strictly followed. In the path of action there is an important question to be considered: is it possible for the yogis who follow the path of action to perform actions in such a way that they do not create barriers and obstacles; can action become the means of liberation and lead one to Self-realization, the goal of human life? There are two main responses. First, good actions performed selflessly and with the fruits given as offerings to the Lord who is in everyone have no binding power. Selfless service is important. Second, good actions also bring good fruits, and those fruits can be utilized merely to enable one to live in the world so that he can discharge his duties effectively.

No matter which path one follows, he has to do actions; he cannot live without acting. Therefore, it is important to understand the nature of an action before one performs that action—whether he is doing sattvic action with self-mastery or is being controlled by rajasic or tamasic qualities and acting as a slave to those qualities. Sattvic actions alone lead one to the state of tranquility. Sattvic actions performed without the desire for fruits are considered to be liberating actions. All other actions bind the human being. Yogis who wish to attain the state of tranquility do their actions and duties selflessly and skillfully. They have all the necessary objects of the world but use them just for the sake of doing their duties.

Many students wonder how it is possible for anyone to realize the pure Self while doing his duties, for the renunciates say that without complete renunciation Self-realization is not possible. Renunciates also do their duties but only for Self-realization. They do not believe in doing actions for the people of the world. Renunciation is an inward journey, whereas the path of action is external, though the aim of both paths is one and the same. In the path of action there are allurements, charms, and temptations. In the path of renunciation, it is the samskaras (latent impressions) that are not yet dealt with that are the obstacles. Samskaras have a deep impact on human life. Because of their samskaras, yogis on the path of action are often led to do something that is not to be done. Therefore, purification of mind, action, and speech must be constantly practiced in both paths. These two paths have one and the same goal, though they seem to be distinct. Neither should be considered superior or inferior.

In practicality the real yogis and *sannyasins* are one and the same. On both the paths of action and renunciation, the key point is renouncing the fruits of actions. Those who have renounced the path of action but still lust for the fruits of action are not true renunciates. In the path of renunciation no external sacred fire is lit, and no sacrifice is offered to the fire. Rather, renunciates light the fire of knowledge and burn their samskaras. The path of renunciation is also referred to as yoga, for in the path of renunciation anything and everything is renounced but not the purpose, which is union of the individual self with the Self of all. That union is attained by the renunciate through meditation and contemplation. In the path of action one can attain that union by giving up all the fruits of actions and remaining completely non-attached.

आरुरुक्षोर्मुनेर्योगं कर्म कारणमुच्यते।
योगारूढस्य तस्यैव शमः कारणमुच्यते।। ३
यदा हि नेन्द्रियार्थेषु न कर्मस्वनुषज्जते।
सर्वसंकल्पसंन्यासी योगारूढस्तदोच्यते।। ४

3. *For a meditator (muni) desirous of ascending in yoga, action is
    said to be a supportive means. And when the same one has already
    risen in yoga, tranquility becomes his support.*
4. *When he is no longer drawn to the objects of senses nor to actions,
    having renounced all volitions of desire, he is then called 'one who
    has ascended to yoga.'*

One who wants to have perfect control over the mind and its modifications should master his internal states. It is only possible for one
to attain that control when he learns to practice in silence. A *muni* is
one who practices *mauna* (silence) in order to attain perfect silence.
When the muni makes efforts to achieve profound control over mind,
action, and speech and maintains perfect silence, he attains the state of
tranquility. Until one experiences perfect silence, he is not aware of the
profound difference between leading a life in the external world and
treading the path of the inward journey.

Silence is not understood by most people and is experienced by
only a few mendicants, for unless one fathoms the deepest state of
silence, silence is only a word, and one does not comprehend its meaning. Every human being wants to be in silence for some time. We often
hear a mother saying to her children, "Will you please be quiet?" She
asks the children to be quiet so that she is not disturbed, but her desire
is for more than external quietness: it is a desire to go to a deeper state
of silence. Consciously or unconsciously, everyone desires to go to the
deep state of silence, which is restful and refreshing and opens the gates
of new dimensions of life. Often silence answers the questions that are
not answered in any other way or by any other means.

The systematic method that leads one to the deepest state of silence
is called meditation. Sleep is very necessary for all creatures of the world
in order to have physical and mental rest, but the rest acquired through
meditation is far superior to the rest given by sleep. There is a difference between sleep and the deep state of silence. The ignorant person
sleeps every day and comes out of sleep no less ignorant because sleep
offers only rest. But if one learns to go to a deep state of meditation,

he is rested and at the same time his whole personality is transformed. That transformation cannot be attained without the inward method of meditation. Through meditation the mind attains a state of tranquility.

Meditation leads to mastery of the mind, and with that mastery, one attains quietude. Such a tranquil and equable mind, having no desire for sense pleasures, also has mastery in the performance of actions. Those who have gone beyond the jabberings of the mind, (sam-kalpa and vikalpa) attain the highest state of yoga.

Those who are not meditators experience only the known level of life. But with the help of meditation, one can have profound knowledge of all the subtle states within and ultimately attain the deep state of silence. Such an aspirant alone can experience both the known and unknown levels of life. The human being is a citizen of the inner world: he is an inner dweller first and a denizen of the external world afterwards. But ordinary people remain citizens of the external world and aliens to the internal world.

The yogi and sage remains aware that he is an inner dweller always. Once, for example, when our master was sitting quietly and calmly, a prince came to visit and said to him, "Sir, you seem to be lonesome." The master replied, "Because you have come! I have been enjoying in deep silence the conversation with my friend within. Now you have come and therefore I have become lonesome."

It is true that students, friends, and loved ones can make us lonesome. One should learn to establish friendship with the eternal friend within. Then he will never be lonely. Real meditators are never lonely, so those who do not want to be lonely should learn to meditate and go on doing meditation until they meet their beloved eternal friend who is seated in the silent chamber in everyone's being. Loneliness vanishes forever in that state of silence where the true friend resides. Loneliness and silence are two entirely different states of mind. In silence one has company, but in loneliness one is all alone. The yogis learn to attain that state of silence, and then they are able to realize directly the nature of both the external and internal worlds. Those yogis can observe both within and without from the height of tranquility.

The ancient yogis found that loneliness is the greatest of all diseases and that it has no remedy but to go to the deep state of silence where the eternal beloved is seated with long and tender arms to embrace one. That is the only therapy that removes loneliness. All company and associations in the external world eventually lead to separation and then to loneliness. But if one becomes aware of the eternal friend, he can efficiently play his role in the grand drama of life and will never become lonely. This knowledge is essential to remove the ignorance of loneliness. Then it does not matter which path one follows or to which end of the earth he travels. Going to the deepest state of silence with the help of a systematized and organized method of meditation is the highest of all therapies, but modern therapists have not yet understood the importance of meditative therapy. Modern therapy provides only one aspect of therapy: it allows the patient to let out his repressions and suppressions through speech and action. The patient receives a little solace, but he does not attain the control necessary to prevent him from becoming a victim of disturbances. Most therapists are afraid of introducing meditational therapy because of lack of practical knowledge and fear of the unknown. However, many beneficial results can be obtained by introducing preliminaries, such as stillness of the body and evenness of the breath, which have proven very helpful to those who are emotionally imbalanced. If such practices are introduced in a gentle and systematic manner, many psychosomatic illnesses can be eliminated.

What is the way for the people of the world who do not have much time for meditation and do not know the right method of meditation? The answer is to practice meditation in action as the Bhagavad Gita teaches. Be conscious of the Truth, the center of consciousness, and perform your actions selflessly with non-attachment. No matter where you are—in your office, in the kitchen, in the shopping center, or in the midst of a crowd—meditation in action can be practiced. Learn not to forget the center of consciousness within you. Do not allow your mind to be scattered, and whatever you do, do it with full attention. Beneath all your deeds there should be awareness of the center of consciousness within. If one thinks he is fit, he should practice meditation in silence.

Otherwise meditation in action is the message of the Bhagavad Gita, without which the path of action is difficult to tread.

उद्धरेदात्मनात्मानं नात्मानमवसादयेत्।
आत्मैव ह्यात्मनो बन्धुरात्मैव रिपुरात्मनः।। ५
बन्धुरात्मात्मनस्तस्य येनात्मैवात्मना जितः।
अनात्मनस्तु शत्रुत्वे वर्तेतात्मैव शत्रुवत्।। ६

5. *One should cause the deliverance of the self by the Self. One should not make the self sink. Self alone is the kinsman of the self; self alone is the enemy of the Self.*
6. *Self is the kinsman of his self by whom the self is conquered by the Self. In the apparent enmity from non-self, the Self alone is operating like an enemy.*

When the aspirant realizes that he is competent and resourceful, he gains confidence and begins following the inner path. Dependency on external resources cannot help him to tread that path. Having deep-rooted habits of depending on external resources leads the student again and again to search outside of himself. He thinks that visiting one shrine and then another and going from one teacher to another will help him, but the inner thirst remains unquenched. As long as one continues to seek the means and objects that give happiness in the external world, he does not find true happiness. So first of all a student should be led to realize that he already has all the means to tread the path of inner light and that external crutches cannot fulfill and satisfy his desire. Searching in the external world is in vain: seeking within is the only way. With firm determination one must use his will power to apply all the means that are at his disposal. One may strongly desire unfoldment and enlightenment, but as long as he does not find the right way and does not commit himself to a reliable and valid method of sadhana, he will be wasting his energy and might even meet disappointments that could kill his desire to continue seeking.

When one gets into his inner world, he gradually realizes that that which he was seeking outside is actually within. He comes to understand that he is fully equipped and has all the means at his disposal to attain Truth. Then he is on the path of inner light and knows that for attaining the Self, the Self alone is needed. Self is attained by the Self. And one's own resources are the only means for attainment. Treading the path of inner light is one of the greatest experiments that can be made by a human being.

Darkness prevails in the external world when the sun is obscured. But if someone is with the sun all the time, he will never encounter darkness. In the inner world the guiding light is always there, and one is never alone. But in the external world one has to depend on resources that are not always at his disposal and on the instructions of teachers and knowledge given by the scriptures. After one has examined the external resources and knows their limitations, he turns within. That is one of the brightest days in one's life. He is still a seeker, but he is no longer seeking in the external world. He has begun seeking within.

One encounters many inexplicable phenomena in the internal world. He may be bewildered and overwhelmed for some time, unable to accept and adjust to the subtle experiences. But when he pursues his sadhana he learns to differentiate between two types of experiences: some are negative and some positive, some are helpful and others unhelpful, some are misleading and others leading. One learns to reject those experiences that are not helpful and to accept those that are helpful in order to march toward deeper states of being. If he has patience, tolerance, and reliance on his inner strength, he pursues his sadhana with full determination and learns to discriminate and choose that which is helpful from that which is not. As one explores the inner world, there can be great confusion at times. But with the help of sadhana and the guiding light within, one attains clarity of mind and crosses safely over all obstacles. He follows the eternal light within, and that light leads him to its source: the pure Self. He, the seeker; light, the means—he is led to the kingdom of happiness, the pure Self. Thus a seeker elevates himself by the Self.

A seeker should never allow himself to slip back to the grooves of his past habits. The Self indeed is a real friend. If the seeker does not use his resources within but instead remains dependent on external resources, he becomes his own enemy. You are your own friend and your own enemy. He who has conquered his lower self through the guidance of his inner Self is a friend to himself; but one who has not been able to conquer his lower self is his own enemy. For conquering the lower self, self-control is needed. Self-control is indeed a friend, and without it the scattered forces of the mind create obstacles. A man of self-control and a man without self-control are like friend and foe respectively.

Students often project their incompetencies onto others and then blame them for their own inadequacies. That is an easy means of escape. No one wants to accept responsibility for his weaknesses and mistakes. But when the student becomes aware that he is his own friend and also his own enemy, then dawns the light of discriminative knowledge. That is another higher step attained in the path of Self-realization.

The student who does not have knowledge of the scriptures and has not been taught by a competent teacher is confused in discriminating between the real Self (Atman) and the lower self, which is a constituent of primordial nature, Prakriti. The lower self is called the mere self. The mere self is comprised of the body, senses, breath, conscious mind, and unconscious mind, which constantly undergo change. It is called the mere self or lower self because of its ever-changing nature. Behind the lower self shines the light of the Eternal. The pure Self is never born, so it never dies: it is everlasting and unchanging. One should learn to distinguish the lower self from the higher Self, for then one can learn to identify himself with the real Self instead of with the mere self.

जितात्मनः प्रशान्तस्य परमात्मा समाहितः ।
शीतोष्णसुखदुःखेषु तथा मानापमानयोः ।। ७
ज्ञानविज्ञानतृप्तात्मा कूटस्थो विजितेन्द्रियः ।
युक्त इत्युच्यते योगी समलोष्टाश्मकाञ्चनः ।। ८
सुहृन्मित्रार्युदासीनमध्यस्थद्वेष्यबन्धुषु ।
साधुष्वपि च पापेषु समबुद्धिर्विशिष्यते ।। ९

7. *The supreme Self of one pacified and self-conquered is harmo-nized in cold and heat, pleasure and pain, as well as in honor and dishonor.*
8. *His self satiated by knowledge and realization, absolute, having conquered the senses, joined in yoga, he is called a yogi, beholding a lump of clay, stone, or nugget of gold alike.*
9. *One is distinguished who holds the same view toward an affec-tionate friend, an enemy, a stranger, a neutral person, one hated, a kinsman, toward the saintly as well as the sinful.*

One who has successfully conquered this lower self with all its desires and appetites attains the highest state of uninterrupted peace, and he is above the influences of the pairs of opposites such as pain and pleasure, heat and cold. Such a great one is made fully content by the wisdom gained through yogic sadhana. One who is firmly established in the constant awareness of Atman (the pure Self) is aware of the lim-ited value of the mundane world, its objects and sense pleasures. He is no longer enticed by the pairs of opposites. For him a piece of rock and a heap of gold are alike. Such a yogi has attained perfection.

One who has conquered the appetites of the lower self is called *jitatma*. Such a yogi is free from all the charms and temptations of the external world and remains in Self delight. The joy that he finds within is not temporary and fleeting. By contrast, the pleasures that others seek outside are only temporary. The pleasures of the external world soon turn into pain, for in the absence of one, the other is experienced. But this is not the case with the joy of the yogi who is in the garden of delight all the time. It is not easy to recognize such a great yogi because ordinary people always remain busy protecting the image they have of themselves. They call that honor. And in want of honor and name and fame, one gets caught by the image he creates for himself, which is a false identity, a reflection of the lower ego. But those yogis who tread the inner path go beyond name and fame, honor and dishonor, and remain in a state of perpetual joy and delight. Those who know both the real Self and the mere self walk on the earth radiating their eternal delight through their behavior, and they are not concerned with name and fame, pain and pleasure. They care not who thinks what about them because they always feel that they are strangers in the world. The world is but a resting camp for them, and never their home. They are usually misunderstood, for only a few human beings have the capacity to understand them. Only other sages who have gained wisdom and knowledge through inner attainment can understand such great ones.

Previously, Sri Krishna taught Arjuna to be conscious of his honor, and that teaching does not contradict what is said here. Sri Krishna was reminding Arjuna of his duties by making him aware that he is a leader and a warrior, not a coward or ordinary person. Self-honor and self-respect remind one of his duties and the tasks he must fulfill. That kind of honor does not build a false image. But those who remain deluded by creating a false image because of their insecurities are not aware of their duties; they are selfish and egotistical and work only for sense gratification. Such people do not have self-respect because they know from within that they are not what they claim to be. They remain helpless because they are addicted to the pleasures of the senses, and they create defense mechanisms because of their fears and insecurities. These two kinds of people are quite distinct: one has true self-respect whereas the other merely creates a false image.

A teacher keenly observes the behavior of his students, and he finds that many students do not have respect for themselves. Instead they condemn themselves and try to hide the unwanted parts of their personalities by creating masks for themselves. The images they present to others are based on their insecurities. That is unhealthy and hinders the growth of the student. A good student is aware of and reveres his real Self, and he practices maintaining constant consciousness of the center within. That is real self-respect, and if one loses it he becomes the victim of vanity and creates defense mechanisms.

It does not matter to a sage whether anyone knows him or not, follows him or not. Only the prepared ones can understand the height of his realization and can be benefitted. But Arjuna is a leader and a warrior who is already followed by millions, and if he does not have profound knowledge of his dharma (duty), he will not be honored and followed by ordinary people. His position is different than that of the sage. He needs to perform his dharma skillfully, selflessly, and lovingly. The behavior of a leader becomes an example for the masses. He should therefore be cautious, vigilant, and conscious of his duties so that he does not create confusion for others. Ordinary people usually honor their leaders and guides, but a true leader and guide remains untouched, uninfluenced, and unaffected by the honors bestowed on him by others.

The great leaders and guides of humanity do not change their attitudes and lose their calm and balance because someone opposes them, someone misunderstands them, or someone does not follow them. For they are firm in the understanding that they are doing their dharma with full skill and confidence. Such great leaders treat saints and sinners alike. They do not judge others but accept them as they are. They neither hate nor uselessly praise. The attitude of the sage toward the saint and the evil doer remains even, and his faculty of judgment is never affected by extremes. He does not favor the saint and is not cruel to the person who does evil. He has attained evenness, tranquility, and peace, which are beyond a concern with virtue and vice. According to yoga sadhana, this state of mind is called the witnessing state; one learns to witness what is going on but does not involve himself in it.

योगी युञ्जीत सततमात्मानं रहसि स्थितः।
एकाकी यतचित्तात्मा निराशीरपरिग्रहः।। १०
शुचौ देशे प्रतिष्ठाप्य स्थिरमासनमात्मनः।
नात्युच्छ्रितं नातिनीचं चैलाजिनकुशोत्तरम्।। ११
तत्रैकाग्रं मनः कृत्वा यतचित्तेन्द्रियक्रियः।
उपविश्यासने युञ्ज्याद्योगमात्मविशुद्धये।। १२
समं कायशिरोग्रीवं धारयन्नचलं स्थिरः।
संप्रेक्ष्य नासिकाग्रं स्वं दिशश्चानवलोकयन्। १३

प्रशान्तात्मा विगतभीर्ब्रह्मचारिव्रते स्थितः।
मनः संयम्य मच्चित्तो युक्त आसीत मत्परः।। १४
युञ्जन्नेवं सदात्मानं योगी नियतमानसः।
शान्तिं निर्वाणपरमां मत्संस्थामधिगच्छति।। १५

10. *The yogi should incessantly place himself in yoga, dwelling in sol-itude, alone, his mind and self controlled, having no expectations, receiving no input into the senses.*
11. *Placing one's stable seat in a clean place neither too high nor too low, made of cloth, a black antelope skin, and kusha grass, one on top of the other,*
12. *There making the mind one-pointed, with the mind, self, and movement under control, sitting on the seat one should practice yoga for self-purification,*
13. *Holding the trunk, head, and neck straight, unmoving and still, observing the point in front of the nose, and not looking in various directions.*
14. *With a pacified self, with all fear banished, remaining in the vow of a celibate, controlling the mind, with the mind absorbed in Me, one should dwell joined in yoga and intent upon Me.*
15. *Thus uniting himself in yoga, the yogi with a well-directed mind reaches that peace the ultimate of which is absorption (nirvana), and the foundation of which is in Me.*

From the tenth verse onward a practical lesson is given that equally benefits ascetics and those living in the world. Knowledge received from sources other than the Self no doubt helps and inspires the sadhaka, but without direct knowledge and experience of the Self, the thirst for knowledge and attainment remains unquenched. When the sadhaka learns to light the Fire of knowledge, he begins treading the path of purification. He thereby attains a state in which all his samskaras are burned, and he is purified. When we say that everyone needs to be purified, it means that the mind ordinarily functions like a slave to one's samskaras and past habits. Then the mind is not functioning as an instrument of the Self. A profound, precise, and practical method of controlling the mind and its modifications is necessary. When one develops a strong desire to know truth and realizes his helplessness, he has no alternative but to follow the path of sadhana, the path of inner experience, the path of light and delight.

A yogi is he whose purpose of life is to unite himself with the absolute Truth. The term yogi is used for those who are making sincere efforts and practicing to attain a state of *samahita* (samadhi) and those who have already attained samahita. The path they follow is called *yoga sadhana.* If one really has a burning desire to practice, then he begins treading the path of sadhana. For that purpose a complete and practical method is expounded here. Deciding to go into solitude in order to follow the path of sadhana is the first dawning day of one's life. One needs a place where he can be free from all sorts of distractions such as noise and visitors coming and going. The place one chooses should not be damp or too warm or too cold. The hours before sunrise and after sunset are best for meditation. At other times one can practice yoga exercises. Both *asanas* and *pranayama* should be included in practice. Physical exercise keeps the body fit, and pranayama is important for regulating the motion of the lungs. Without fitness of the body and control of the breath, sadhana cannot be practiced. Food is another important factor. Nutritious food that is simple, fresh, and properly chewed should be eaten according to one's capacity. But one's time and energy should not be concentrated on food. Sadhana alone should be the center of one's activities.

Preparation for meditation is more important than the method of meditation. Without preparation of both the external environment and of oneself, meditation is not possible. The external environment should be kept neat and clean, undisturbed, and free from agitation. Anything that disturbs the mind creates an obstacle. The following conditions should be observed.

(1) In the beginning stage, meditation should be practiced in a quiet and peaceful room where external sounds do not disturb

the meditator. The room should be comfortable and not overly humid. Burning incense during meditation is injurious, but it can be burned before or after meditation if one wishes.

(2) There are two sets of yoga asanas (postures) that should be practiced. The postures for physical culture keep the body firm and are thus complementary to the postures practiced for meditation. The seat upon which one meditates should not be too high, for there is the possibility that the meditator may fall, and if the seat is too low insects may become a source of distraction. Another reason to keep oneself above the ground is to keep the body unaffected by the temperature and dampness. A wooden seat is preferred. It should be large enough so that one can sit comfortably. Wood is a poor conductor of heat and cold, and it is better than sitting on the ground or on metal or stone. *Kusha* is a grass that in ancient times was used as a base, and on top was a four-folded woolen blanket with a cotton spread over it. A tiger skin or deer skin was sometimes used instead of a blanket. Those were all used in order to have a cushion beneath and to insulate oneself from the ground because in ancient times the aspirant meditated in a cave or outside. Modern conveniences to control temperature, humidity, insects, and such were not available. Thus, the instructions given in the Bhagavad Gita may be modified to suit one's conditions and the material available.

(3) The meditator should sit in a posture that is comfortable and in which he can keep his body steady and his head, neck, and trunk straight. There are only a few postures that are used for meditation, and among these the accomplished pose (siddhasana) is preferable. One can also use the half lotus pose *(ardhapadmasana)* or the easy pose (sukhasana). The position one chooses is not so important. One can even choose to sit upright on a firm chair. That which is most important is to keep the head, neck, and trunk in a straight line and to arrange the upper and lower limbs in a definite way so that they do not create disturbance and discomfort for the body.

(4) Having seated himself firmly in siddhasana or in another posture, the meditator should gently close his eyes and focus the mind on the base of the bridge between the two nostrils. The word *nasagre* means in front of the two nostrils. It does not mean the tip of the nose, as some translators and commentators think, but the bridge between the two nostrils. By concentrating on that point the meditator becomes aware of the flow of both breaths. It is unfortunate that most commentators have only superficially commented on this verse, for students may practice on the basis of erroneous interpretations and injure themselves. How can one gaze on the tip of the nose and call that meditation? There is an exercise like that, but it is called trataka, gazing. It is a hatha yoga exercise for strengthening eyesight and concentration; it is not at all a part of meditation. The meditative method begins with the voluntary withdrawal of the senses and not with concentration of the mind through external gazes. The word *nasa* does not mean the tip of the nose but the nostrils, and *agra bhage* does not refer to the front of the tip of the nose. Rather it is the juncture at which the bridge that separates the two nostrils meets the top of the upper lip. Thus, the mind is fixed on the flow of both breaths so that sushumna is applied. Ordinarily one of the nostrils is predominant, but in sushumna both breaths flow equally.

(5) The mind and breath are interdependent; they react to one another. Breath is the barometer of the mind and the body, for it registers all the conditions of both. If something unusual happens in the mental world, the flow of the breath changes. And if the body is in pain or has a fever, the flow of the breath changes then as well. If one receives shocking news, the breath becomes more rapid, disturbing the motion of the lungs, the heart, the brain, and finally the mind. By focusing the mind on the flow of breath, the mind experiences a joy of concentration that purifies it. Many breathing exercises, especially when one is in an emotionally intense state, have been proven useful. The breath and mind are two inseparable friends.

(6) The purpose of meditation is threefold: first to apply sushumna; then to become conscious of the unknown and hidden levels of life, which is also known as awakening the primal force *kundalini;* and finally to experience a state beyond by attaining samadhi.

(7) In order to attain samadhi, the yogi takes a vow of celibacy. The word celibacy does not mean mere suppression of the sexual urge. *Brahmacharya* means walking in Brahman, being conscious of Brahman all the time. *Brahma* means shakti, and *charya* means how to direct. A brahmachari is able to master and direct his energies toward the attainment of the highest state of consciousness. Brahmacharya is not limited to the control of the sexual urge but also involves the control of mind, action, and speech. All one's energies should be directed toward Brahman consciousness so that the mind becomes one- pointed and turns inward. This inward flow of mental energy leads to the Self, the center of consciousness.

(8) Finally a yogi fathoms many levels of experience in his inner world. Those experiences are inexplicably delightful. Such a great man finally attains the state of oneness with the pure Self.

नात्यश्नतस्तु योगोऽस्ति न चैकान्तमनश्नतः।
न चातिस्वप्नशीलस्य जाग्रतो नैव चार्जुन।। १६
युक्ताहारविहारस्य युक्तचेष्टस्य कर्मसु।
युक्तस्वप्नावबोधस्य योगो भवति दुःखहा।। १७

16. *There is no yoga for one who eats much or who eats nothing at all or for one who is inclined to excessive sleep or one who awakes altogether, O Arjuna.*
17. *He whose food and enjoyment are balanced, whose movements in actions are balanced, whose sleeping and waking are balanced, his yoga becomes the eliminator of sorrows.*

Those who overeat and those who eat less than the body needs are not sensitive to the capacity of their bodies. They disturb their digestive systems and cannot regulate their bowels. Proper digestion is necessary for good health, and without good health, sadhana is not possible. When the yogi learns to regulate all the urges and refrains from overindulgence, he is able to attain profound control over his mind. But if one does not regulate his appetites by watching his capacity, perfection is never attained.

Many students fallaciously think that rigid austerities should be practiced on the path of yoga. Some inexperienced aspirants go on fasts for a long time because they think that physical mortification can help to purify both body and mind. It should be clear that except during a period of cleansing in which one practices *kriyas* such as the internal wash, the upper wash, the lower wash, and the complete wash, fasting is not recommended. Too much fasting affects one's resistance, and he may become a victim of disease. Yoga is a middle path. In yoga sadhana one should not touch the extremes: overeating or fasting, oversleeping or not sleeping enough.

In the modern world most people have not learned to regulate their appetites. They overindulge in sensual pleasures without taking heed of the harmful effects the indulgence has on their bodies and minds. Obesity, anorexia, and bulimia are three of the most frequent problems encountered by physicians and psychotherapists today. For most people food is symbolic of love and nurturance, so they either use food as a substitute for love and nurturance, or they reject food as they reject the insincere love of their parents. Bulimics do both. Many people also overeat because of sexual frustration.

Yogic practices lead one to become sensitive to the effects of overindulgence and austerities that are too severe. One is then able to find a natural balance in all areas of his life. Through sadhana one learns to regulate all aspects of his functioning and to gain mastery over the body, senses, and mind. He keeps the body free from disease and weakness, and he keeps the mind free from disturbance.

यदा विनियतं चित्तमात्मन्येवावतिष्ठते।
निःस्पृहः सर्वकामेभ्यो युक्त इत्युच्यते तदा।। १८
यथा दीपो निवातस्थो नेङ्गते सोपमा स्मृता।
योगिनो यतचित्तस्य युञ्जतो योगमात्मनः।। १९
यत्रोपरमते चित्तं निरुद्धं योगसेवया।
यत्र चैवात्मनात्मानं पश्यन्नात्मनि तुष्यति।। २०

18. *When a very well controlled mind remains stable in the Self alone, detached from all desires, then one is called joined in yoga.*
19. *As a lamp in a place without breeze does not tremble—this is the simile of a yogi whose mind is controlled practicing the yoga of the Self.*
20. *Where the mind ceases, withdrawn through the observance of yoga, where one sees the self in the Self, one is satiated in the Self.*

In yoga sadhana, samyama (self-discipline) is important. In fact, it is the very means for the renunciate to attain Brahman, for the yogi to attain samadhi, and for the man of action to perform his duty skillfully and selflessly. Non-attachment is part of that discipline. We have already explained that non-attachment and discipline should be properly understood. Discipline should not be seen as a punishment or as something imposed by teachers, and non-attachment should not be viewed as implying indifference, carelessness, or lack of love for others. Those who are not able to practice discipline cannot foresee its positive effects; they feel that discipline is not necessary. For fear of losing their little joys, they do not want to discipline themselves. So is the case with people who are attached to objects and human relationships because they use all these as crutches and as means to satisfy their sense gratifications. Such people misunderstand nonattachment. Non-attachment brings about the love divine, and it opens new horizons, which helps one understand that higher joys can be obtained in life.

No one in this world is satisfied. Everyone understands that and accepts it as a fact of life. But most people are afraid of the unknown and do not search for something higher. The ordinary person is not sure that the search for the unknown will give him something higher than what he has already. He is not happy as he is and yet is afraid of searching in the unknown. Dissatisfaction and fear are two great enemies of the human being; they create a great barrier in the process of unfoldment. The ordinary human being remains clinging to his dissatisfaction, not knowing anything better. But if he would begin to discipline himself and develop non-attachment, he would quickly begin to find something far better than what he leaves behind.

When the roving mind of the aspirant is brought back from its dissipated nature to a center of focus by meditative practices, when his mind becomes steady and one-pointed, and when he does not long for worldly desires, he is called a yogi. It is necessary to explain what is meant by the object or center of focus for the mind. Every person has his own mind that differs from the nature of other minds. The capacity for perceiving and conceptualizing differs in both degree and quality. The object that is recommended to the student as a point of focus during meditation is therefore a delicate matter. If the object is disagreeable to the student, he cannot practice. He begins fighting within himself instead of letting go. There are already innumerable objects in the mind, for the mind itself manufactures numerous objects and expresses them through symbols, ideas, fantasies, hallucinations, and dreams. The question rises: How will adding one more object to the mind be helpful? Verse 19 tells us that the object of meditation should not be anything but Atman, the pure Self. All of the objects created by the mind are partial and incomplete. But this object of meditation is all-encompassing and is the source of all other objects. That brings another question: how can one have as an object for his meditation something abstract, timeless, infinite, and eternal? To answer this question it is necessary to distinguish between concentration and meditation, which are two different states and experiences on the inner path.

There is no meditation in concentration, but there is already concentration in meditation. Many teachers these days think meditation can be attained without concentration. That ignorant idea is misleading. The mind as it is in its ordinary nature remains in a dissipated state. Without gathering together and concentrating the energy of the mind, the deeper state of meditation is not possible. The student who practices sitting in a quiet and calm place even for a short time can experience a bit of unusual joy, though he is not able to experience the deep joy of the meditative state. Why should one be afraid of concentration? Some say that concentration of mind can bring about strain and stress and thus should not be practiced. They even say that discipline is not needed, and they create simplified methods and call them meditation. Such teachings appear to make difficult sadhana easy, but these easy methods do not lead one to the higher dimensions of life.

For concentrating the mind, one needs something concrete: a form, image, or symbol that carries some meaning. Abstract thought can lead one to the contemplative state but not to a concentrated state of mind. Prescribing an object for the concentration of mind requires a skilled teacher. The best concentration is achieved when the student mentally centers his mind on the flow of the breath. It is easy for the mind to become concentrated if the breath is the focal point. That has many benefits. First the mind and breath, which are closely linked together, begin functioning in a coordinated way. When concentration is absent, the cooperation remains unconscious; it requires effort to establish coordination on a conscious level. Second, when the student concentrates on the breath, he is able to discover the defects in his breathing and becomes mentally aware of breathing patterns that need to be changed, such as jerky, noisy breathing or habits of inhaling shallowly or creating a pause between inhalation and exhalation. These bad habits are the sources of many physical imbalances and illnesses that cannot be treated with medicine.

In most great meditative traditions of the world, the breath is the center for focusing the mind. Only those teachers who do not have direct experience with the path of meditation and who have lost the sensitivity for the well being of their students prescribe a gross object as a focal point. With the breath as an object, the student is first led toward concentration, which gradually becomes more subtle. Following this fine thread of breath, he attains inwardness. The mind then acquires the capacity of subtlety, and one develops a penetrating sense of internal observation.

Concentration and meditation should ultimately lead one to Atman alone. One-pointedness of mind is an important requisite to help one accomplish that. When one learns to concentrate on the breath and removes all the defects that he finds in his breathing patterns, he tries to understand who it is that is inhaling and exhaling. There are traditions that believe in the coordination of *mantra* with the breath at this stage. Mantra is a Sanskrit word, sound, syllable, or set of words. It is a means to remove all the impurities of mind. There are a few mantras that are used while inhaling and exhaling that do not disturb the flow of the breath. The sadhaka reaches a point in his practice where he not only breathes the air but constantly remembers the mantra with each inhalation and exhalation. That leads the mind to constant awareness of the mantra. When the consciousness of the mantra is deepened, the mantra is able to guide the mind in the inner world.

The student is then taught to be aware of the inner light that already burns without flickering. When the mind experiences that light, it elevates itself to a state of joy that it did not experience before. That light which is within us is the finest and best form upon which to meditate. Without that light we would not be able to see, observe, verify, and discriminate anything in the external world. It is the light of consciousness that is experienced in a concentrated form. The mind then begins to see clearly; it is no longer clouded. Then the light of consciousness and mantra become one, because at that stage the mantra is not actually remembered, but its meaning and feeling are revealed. At first one remembers and repeats the mantra in a gross way, but gradually it is experienced in a more subtle way.

When one develops the feeling of constant awareness of the mantra, it unites with the mainstream of consciousness where light and sound are inseparably mingled. That is a perfect state of concentration. One has then attained profound control of the mind, and he experiences a constant closeness and union with the Self-illumined Atman. When the sadhaka has mastered the art of concentration, his mind is fixed on the Self only. The mind of an ordinary person is dissipated, disturbed, and fickle, but the mind of the sadhaka attains steadiness. Such a sadhaka has mastered and controlled the usual flow of mental energy that goes out to the external world. From the very beginning the object of concentration must be carefully chosen. At first it should be the breath and later breath with mantra well coordinated and united. In a higher stage sound and light are united, and in the highest state pure Consciousness alone exists.

Meditation is an inward process of therapy; it is able to remove all the impurities and weaknesses that are responsible for creating disorder and illness. Meditational therapy is quite different from hypnosis. In a hypnotic state, instead of having a direct experience of the unknown dimensions of life, one is influenced by suggestions from someone outside or by self-suggestion. Therapy based on hypnosis is an unguided method, for the therapist and client do not know what they will encounter next. They are being guided by their conscious and unconscious minds but not by the light of consciousness. Many times in such cases the therapist loses touch with the client, and the client with his consciousness. Many terrifying experiences may come from the unconscious of the client when the hypnotist is not able to maintain control over the hypnotic session. That form of therapy goes only so far. The great therapists of the past had to abandon that method, although lately hypnosis has been developed further and used successfully in certain cases. But those who practice hypnosis can never develop a profound training program that independently leads one to the source of knowledge and light. By contrast, on the path of meditation one is led to Self-realization.

सुखमात्यन्तिकं यत्तद् बुद्धिग्राह्यमतीन्द्रियम्।
वेत्ति यत्र न चैवायं स्थितश्चलति तत्त्वतः।। २१
यं लब्ध्वा चापरं लाभं मन्यते नाधिकं ततः।
यस्मिन्स्थितो न दुःखेन गुरुणापि विचाल्यते।। २२
तं विद्याद् दुःखसंयोगवियोगं योगसंज्ञितम्।
स निश्चयेन योक्तव्यो योगोऽनिर्विण्णचेतसा।। २३

21. *The ultimate happiness is that which is grasped by intelligence and is beyond the senses. When one knows this happiness, dwelling in it, he no longer moves from the knowledge of that reality,*

22. *Attaining which one no longer believes any other gain to be greater than that—staying in which, one is not shaken by even the greatest sorrow.*

23. *Now, that elimination of union with sorrows is to be known as yoga. That yoga should be practiced resolutely by one who has made his mind dispassionate.*

When the light of pure reason begins guiding the yogi, he is no longer victimized by the distress that is experienced by ordinary people. Then distraction and distress do not affect him in any way. That which is taken as a great calamity by the ordinary person is nothing serious for the yogi because he has attained the state of perfection by controlling the senses and mind and all its modifications. The word perfection is used in many situations. One can be considered to be perfect in many different things such as in writing, singing, gymnastics, and so on. But here perfection means that state of perfect control over the mind. The yogi attains that state only after his mind is fully concentrated and uninterruptedly flows toward the center of consciousness. This is a deep state of meditation, one of the stages of samadhi.

These verses explain that through the meditative method, buddhi becomes one-pointed, sharp, and able to fathom the subtler levels of life to which the sense organs have no access. The joy that is then experienced is unmeasurable and inexplicable, beyond the grasp of sense organs and mind. When one experiences this state, there is no chance that he may slip back to desiring the sense enjoyments, because he has already attained that joy which is infinitely superior to sensory pleasures. Verses 21, 22, and 23 explain the joyful experience of the yogi who has mastered his senses, mind, and buddhi. One who realizes this eternal joy experiences many benefits: (1) He is cheerful, calm, content, and undisturbed in all situations. (2) He does not depend on the senses to supply pleasure, for his joy is a million times higher than that attained from sensory pleasure. (3) He is not at all dependent on external experiences, for he has become self-reliant. (4) His is a joy that is experienced by the Self only. Self delights in Self. (5) His meditation is profound, and he is so established in meditation that he cannot do otherwise; he meditates all the time. (6) His happiness is of a supreme quality. It is infinite and words have no power to measure or explain it. (7) When that joy is attained, one is firm in knowing that there is no joy higher than that.

In the first chapters of the Bhagavad Gita, Arjuna identifies himself with his negative personality, so Sri Krishna leads him to remember his true Self. Arjuna then leaves his grief behind and commits himself to the yoga of perfection, mastery, and joy. That joy is unparalleled in its nature and is experienced directly from the fountain of joy itself. It does not depend on any object. It is a profound love without a beloved. It is love without an object, meditation without an object. Meditation is like falling in love. The difference is that ultimately it has no object, whereas love in the external world is held captive by the object.

संकल्पप्रभवान्कामांस्त्यक्त्वा सर्वानशेषतः।
मनसैवेन्द्रियग्रामं विनियम्य समन्ततः।। २४
शनैः शनैरुपरमेद् बुद्ध्या धृतिगृहीतया।
आत्मसंस्थं मनः कृत्वा न किञ्चिदपि चिन्तयेत्।। २५
यतो यतो निश्चरति मनश्चञ्चलमस्थिरम्।
ततस्ततो नियम्यैतदात्मन्येव वशं नयेत्।। २६

प्रशान्तमनसं ह्येनं योगिनं सुखमुत्तमम्।
उपैति शान्तरजसं ब्रह्मधूतमकल्मषम्।। २७
युञ्जन्नेवं सदात्मानं योगी विगतकल्मषः।
सुखेन ब्रह्मसंस्पर्शमत्यन्तं सुखमश्नुते।। २८

24. *Giving up all desires born of volition in their entirety, controlling the entire group of senses with the mind alone and from all sides—*

25. *Slowly, slowly, one should turn away with the help of intelligence, which is held in steadfastness, making the mind stable in the Self. Then one should think entirely of nothing.*

26. *In whatever direction the fickle and unstable mind wanders out, from that very direction one should pull it and bring it under the control of the Self alone.*

27. *The best happiness comes only to such a yogi whose mind is pacified, whose dust has settled, who has become identified with Brahman, and who is free of all stains.*

28. *Thus uniting the self in yoga, the yogi, free of all stains, easily enjoys the ultimate happiness, which is contact with Brahman.*

Verses 24 through 28 present a profound description of sadhana and inspire the aspirant. These verses also refer to the dark side of human nature and teach the student not to do that which is harmful to him. The pure Self should be the center of activity. From morning until evening and from evening until the next morning, all of the aspirant's activities should be directed only toward the attainment of Self. Because diversions are many, habits are strong, and attractions are immense, one needs a one-pointed mind, strong determination, and will power. Otherwise he will not be able to accomplish the purpose of life.

With the help of concentration, the sadhaka gathers together the dissipated forces of mind. With full strength he begins walking the path of the inward journey, One who is able to put his rajasic activities to rest consciously and voluntarily, whose mind has attained a state of quietness, finds his way in the world of inner experiences. Free from desire for pleasure and sense gratification, such a yogi identifies himself with his essential nature: the pure Self. This state of mind is not the result of sadhana practiced halfheartedly or sporadically. Rather it results from that sadhana which is given the highest priority. Then all the activities of life—thought, speech, and action—become auxiliary to sadhana. If the aspirant has patience and only one desire to fulfill—Self-realization—then alone is that state attained.

Modern students lack patience and determination; they want quick results without working hard. They are like children who sow the seed and pour water over it and the next morning dig up the seed to find out why it has not grown. Patience is a great virtue in sadhana. One who continues to follow the path of sadhana with firm determination and does not change his path no doubt attains the permanent abode of the Eternal. Suppose one's purpose is to travel to a distant city. One day he rushes forward on a road that leads to that city, but after a few hours of effort he turns back and the next day sets out on a different route. If he continues to do that, he will never reach his destination.

The following are essential) for an aspirant: (1) He should have profound knowledge of the path he is treading. (2) He should be fully equipped before he treads the path. That means he should discipline himself. (3) He should patiently and steadily tread his path. He should not forget his goal no matter what he does, whether he is studying, eating, or exercising. (4) The law of karma states that nothing is wasted and nothing is lost. One is bound to receive the fruits of his actions sooner or later. The student should have faith that his sadhana will not be wasted. (5) Before eating, sleeping, or practicing meditation and as many times as it is convenient and possible, one should dedicate his sadhana and surrender the fruits to the Lord of life. By following these principles, the sadhaka develops awareness of the Eternal and is no longer distracted by the temporal world. He experiences the greatest of all joys and happiness, which arises in the depths and heights of his inner Self.

सर्वभूतस्थमात्मानं सर्वभूतानि चात्मनि।
ईक्षते योगयुक्तात्मा सर्वत्र समदर्शनः।। २९
यो मां पश्यति सर्वत्र सर्वं च मयि पश्यति।
तस्याहं न प्रणश्यामि स च मे न प्रणश्यति।। ३०
सर्वभूतस्थितं यो मां भजत्येकत्वमास्थितः।
सर्वथा वर्तमानोऽपि स योगी मयि वर्तते।। ३१
आत्मौपम्येन सर्वत्र समं पश्यति योऽर्जुन।
सुखं वा यदि वा दुःखं स योगी परमो मतः।। ३२

29. *One whose self is joined in yoga, looking evenly at everything, sees the Self dwelling in all beings and all beings in the Self.*
30. *He who sees Me everywhere and sees everything in Me, for him I do not vanish nor does he vanish from Me.*
31. *He who, established in unity, devotes himself to Me, who am dwelling in all beings though operative in manifold ways, that yogi still remains in Me.*
32. *He who sees everything alike as similar to himself, O Arjuna, whether in comfort or discomfort, he is considered to be the highest yogi.*

The Self-realized yogi sees the eternal, omnipresent, omniscient, pure Self everywhere. He sees himself in all and all in himself. He realizes that the Self, the Lord of life, is in all beings and all are in the Lord. He knows that he cannot be separated from the universal consciousness, for he is one with it and is virtually that universal consciousness. Such a yogi's mind dwells in the state of evenness. For him pain and joy are the same, yet he remains sensitive to the pain and misery of others. He is aware of that which causes misery and also of that which brings worldly pleasure. His yoga practices and the attainment of a deep meditative state do not lead him to the black hole of nothingness but enable him to sympathize, love, help, and serve yet to remain in a state of tranquility. He is gifted with the special quality of knowledge through which he feels pain for those who suffer as though it were his own suffering. Such is the state of a yogi who is endowed with the great gift of sensitivity and yet is able to maintain evenness at the same time. He has the capacity to feel the misery of others but is not affected by it. He has learned the profound art of living and being; he lives in the world but is not of it.

The true meaning of the word samatvam (evenness) can only be realized by meditators and yogis. Others can merely intellectualize and speculate about its meaning. When the yogi touches the timeless and infinite knowledge in deep meditation, he is able to see the present, past, and future and can attain comprehensive knowledge of all three dimensions at a glance. Such a yogi has attained samatvam. He sees Atman everywhere. For him time, space, and causality do not create any limitations. With this limitless knowledge his mind becomes even, samatva. He loves all equally and hates none; he includes all and excludes none.

The yogi maintains his individuality yet is always fully conscious of Atman. Being one with the Eternal, he is free from destructibility even though the objects of the world are ever changing and subject to destruction. Such a yogi releases himself from the conditionings created by the three gunas and from the limitations of time, space, and causation. The entire chain of life from the unknown to the known and the known to the unknown, from birth to death and death to the hereafter is unveiled to him and reveals its secret. He is the knower of all events, yet he is free from the changes he experiences.

Such a great one is like a tank that is overflowing with water. The tank maintains its individuality even though the same water is both within and without and all around. The perennial flow of knowledge fills the yogi and keeps him overflowing. He is constantly aware of his eternal existence, but he still maintains his higher ego for the sake of serving others rather than for maintaining his individuality. He is firmly established in uninterrupted consciousness of the Absolute. The peace found in that state is a living peace, not like the peace one finds in a cemetery or in isolation. Such peace does not come to one who withdraws himself from his duty because he feels that he is not able to perform his duty skillfully. That peace comes only to one who stands at the edge that unites the human and divine. Such a yogi is considered to be a person of great wisdom and is adored by all.

अर्जुन उवाच

योऽयं योगस्त्वया प्रोक्तः साम्येन मधुसूदन।

एतस्याहं न पश्यामि चञ्चलत्वात्स्थितिं स्थिराम्।। ३३

चञ्चलं हि मनः कृष्ण प्रमाथि बलवद् दृढम्।

तस्याहं निग्रहं मन्ये वायोरिव सुदुष्करम्।। ३४

श्री भगवानुवाच

असंशयं महाबाहो मनो दुर्निग्रहं चलम्।

अभ्यासेन तु कौन्तेय वैराग्येण च गृह्यते।। ३५

असंयतात्मना योगो दुष्प्राप इति मे मतिः।

वश्यात्मना तु यतता शक्योऽवाप्तुमुपायतः।। ३६

Arjuna said

33. *I do not see the stability of this yoga through equanimity that you have taught, O Krishna, to be lasting because of the mind's fickleness.*

34. *The mind is indeed fickle, turbulent, very powerful, and strong. I believe its control to be as difficult as that of the wind*

The Blessed Lord said

35. *No doubt, O Arjuna, the mind is difficult to control and ever moving. But, O Son of Kunti, it can be held through practice and dispassion.*

36. *Yoga is difficult to be found by someone whose self is not in control—this is My view. But by someone who endeavors with a controlled self, it can be attained by appropriate methods.*

Arjuna accepts the validity of the teachings imparted to him, but like any student he wonders if it is really possible for him to attain the yoga of equanimity, for he recognizes that the mind is very restless, obstinate, and difficult to control. In the Vedas, Upanishads, and many other scriptures the mind is considered to be both an obstacle and at the same time a means of liberation. The conscious part of the mind is but a small part of the whole of the mind. Modern education makes an effort to cultivate only the conscious mind, which functions during the waking state. The rest of the mind remains unknown. That unknown part of the mind is called the unconscious. The functioning of the unconscious is difficult for the aspirant to comprehend and control. When the yogi talks of controlling the mind, it means the whole of the mind, not just the conscious part. Arjuna says that controlling the mind is comparable to controlling the wind, for it is impossible for anyone to have control over the wind.

The purpose of yoga sadhana is to understand the mind and its modifications (the way the mind functions in both the external and internal worlds) and to develop control over the mind. Self-control is that state in which one is not swayed by selfish desires or by the sense pleasures that are responsible for creating injurious ties of attachment. Attaining self-control is truly a difficult task. Hearing Arjuna's uncertainty Sri Krishna replies, "O Arjuna, no doubt the mind is dissipated and difficult to control. But when the sadhaka consistently makes sincere effort to isolate the mind from the objects of enjoyment and attachment, he can attain control of it." Vairagya (non-attachment) is an important means to attain control of the mind; it should be understood and practiced.

The human being's stay in the mundane world is very brief. On the path to eternity this world is just one of the camps. Therefore do not become attached to it. Always remember that this is not your permanent abode. Everyone is brought to that awareness many times in life, but again the strong desire for enjoying sensory pleasure distracts the mind. When someone very dear to us dies and we take that person's body to the cemetery, everyone there feels the presence of vairagya whispering its profound lesson. We are born to die; there is nothing in this world that is permanent and not subject to death. Death is an alarm that makes every human being realize that attachment to sense pleasures, to things of the world, and to relationships is painful.

Vairagya is the knowledge that dawns each time we go off the path and become attached to something of the world, for invariably that attachment causes pain and leads us to give up that attachment. That knowledge draws us, but strong habits and the desire to enjoy sensory pleasure do not allow us to pay heed to it. At the cemetery the knowledge of vairagya dawns for a short time. Everyone at the cemetery suddenly becomes a sage and begins realizing and talking about the impermanent nature of the temporal world. During that time everyone is attuned to one and the same reality, but after the body is buried and the mourners turn toward their homes, they forget the lesson that they received at the cemetery. Once more they become busy doing the same things as before.

Gain and loss are two experiences that the human being repeatedly encounters throughout life. When one gains something temporal, he becomes imbalanced and overjoyed. And when he loses it, he is plunged into sadness. Whatever is gained will sooner or later be lost. When one becomes aware that these two experiences always occur together, he realizes that attachment is unhealthy and the source of much misery. The yogi knows that sooner or later he will have to lose even the most well-loved things in the world. He constantly remembers that change is inevitable in the external world. He learns to maintain constant consciousness of the pure Self and adjusts himself to the changing situations of the mundane world.

To gain mastery over the mind, the development of nonattachment is essential. By practicing a well-designed sadhana and applying all the means one has, he can attain mastery. Creating one's own method of sadhana will not help in gaining control of mind, action, and speech. The proper means are those that have already been experienced by the great yogis in the past.

अर्जुन उवाच
अयतिः श्रद्धयोपेतो योगाच्चलितमानसः।
अप्राप्य योगसंसिद्धिं कां गतिं कृष्ण गच्छति।। ३७
कच्चिन्नोभयविभ्रष्टश्छिन्नाभ्रमिव नश्यति।
अप्रतिष्ठो महाबाहो विमूढो ब्रह्मणः पथि।। ३८
एतन्मे संशयं कृष्ण छेत्तुमर्हस्यशेषतः।
त्वदन्यः संशयस्यास्य छेत्ता न ह्युपपद्यते।। ३९

Arjuna said

37. *One who does not make full effort but maintains faith, his mind slipping away from yoga, thereby not attaining full accomplishment in yoga, what state does he come to, O Krishna?*
38. *Does he perchance, fallen from both, vanish like a broken up cloud established in nothing, O Krishna, lost on the path of Brahman?*
39. *Do indeed sunder this doubt in my mind, O Krishna, in its entirety. There is no other who can appropriately be considered a remover of this doubt.*

In these three verses Arjuna asks the same questions that are often asked by modern students. Even when a student tries his best, is faithful to his sadhana, and has firm faith in the path, he still encounters failures and may find himself on a plateau from whence he feels incapable of attaining his goal. With that concern Arjuna wants to know what happens to such people and if there is an alternative path to follow. Sometimes despite his sincere efforts, the aspirant docs not make progress on his inner path. That creates serious confusion in the mind of the aspirant, and he may find himself lost, not fit for either the path of spirituality or for the path of the world.

On the path to eternity and spirituality, one is like a pilgrim. Why should one be denied his right to complete his pilgrimage if he is sincere, truthful, and makes efforts with all his skill? Why is his path suddenly blocked? Why is he left in a state of limbo? These doubts not only affect Arjuna but all aspirants.

श्री भगवानुवाच
पार्थ नैवेह नामुत्र विनाशस्तस्य विद्यते।
न हि कल्याणकृत्कश्चिद् दुर्गतिं तात गच्छति।। ४०
प्राप्य पुण्यकृतां लोकानुषित्वा शाश्वतीः समाः।
शुचीनां श्रीमतां गेहे योगभ्रष्टोऽभिजायते।। ४१
अथवा योगिनामेव कुले भवति धीमताम्।
एतद्धि दुर्लभतरं लोके जन्म यदीदृशम्।। ४२

तत्र तं बुद्धिसंयोगं लभते पौर्वदेहिकम्।
यतते च ततो भूयः संसिद्धौ कुरुनन्दन।। ४३
पूर्वाभ्यासेन तेनैव ह्रियते ह्यवशोऽपि सः।
जिज्ञासुरपि योगस्य शब्दब्रह्मातिवर्तते।। ४४
प्रयत्नाद्यतमानस्तु योगी संशुद्धकिल्बिषः।
अनेकजन्मसंसिद्धस्ततो याति परां गतिम्।। ४५

The Blessed Lord said

40. *O Son of Pritha, neither here in this life nor there in the next is there any danger of his perishing. No one who performs blessed deeds at all goes to an evil state, O Beloved.*

41. *Attaining the worlds of performers of meritorious deeds, dwelling there for long periods, one who has fallen from yoga is born in the homes of pure and glorious people.*

42. *Or he is born in the family of wise yogis. A birth such as this is very difficult to come to in this world.*

43. *There he again gains union with the wisdom that came from his previous body. Then he undertakes further endeavor toward full accomplishment, O Prince of Kurus.*

44. *Because of that previous habit of practicing, he is carried even without his will. Desirous of knowing yoga, he transcends the verbal knowledge of God.*

45. *Purified of sins, endeavoring with effort, reaching accomplishment in more than one lifetime, then he attains the supreme state.*

In order to dispel the doubts of Arjuna, Sri Krishna explains that good deeds and good actions never vanish into nothingness. There is no evil power that can obstruct one from receiving the positive outcome of his sincere efforts. Arjuna thinks that there is no place for one who has failed to attain perfection in yoga either in the world or on the path of spirituality. That is not true. Only a few aspirants attain perfection in this birth, but others continue treading the path and are born again. Those who are not completely successful in treading their paths are born into families where they again have the opportunity to pursue their quest. Suppose one cannot complete his work today and that work is very important. Does he not try to complete the task the next day? After death the samskaras that are not fulfilled remain in the unconscious, and those desires and motivations compel the individual soul to assume a new garment called the body. Thus one does not begin afresh from the very beginning but continues from the point he last reached. Such a great task as Self-realization cannot possibly be accomplished in the small span of a single lifetime.

Birth does not happen by chance or by accident; it is not an event that occurs suddenly out of nowhere. If it were, one human being would not carry certain motivations, desires, and abilities that differ from those of another. Western thinkers are still bewildered by this philosophy. They are trying to find the answer to why one is born with certain characteristics in the world. Some great Western thinkers and philosophers believe in the philosophy of rebirth, but most psychologists do not accept the validity of reincarnation. Psychologists spend their time debating over whether heredity or learning is responsible for an individual's unique characteristics. They are trying to discover the answers by intellectualization and experiments conducted on superficial levels. Many cases of reincarnation and rebirth are documented every year in both the East and West. Those who have been following the spiritual path have access to the infinite library of their memories of the past and can recall them with full clarity. Without examining all the levels of consciousness of human life, how can anyone claim or prove that he did not exist before yet exists now? This very existence is proof that one has existed before.

Sri Krishna explains to Arjuna that the yogi who could not complete his task does not remain in limbo but starts again and completes his task in a future birth. He is born into a good family that offers him an environment conducive to the completion of his task. Such an aspirant sometimes feels that some unknown power is leading and guiding him to follow the path. It is actually his own powerful desire brought from the past that compels him to tread the path once again, but he is not conscious of that fact because his brain and the environment are new. On the path of spirituality if one is sincere and faithful but does not have the right means and environment, he cannot progress. The right means are a healthy body, a healthy environment, a sound and clear mind, determination, will power, self-confidence, and non-attachment. If any of these means is absent, progress is obstructed. But when the environment is conducive and the above mentioned means are strengthened, the difficulties one has encountered before are removed and the path becomes easy. One then attains perfection.

Typically students remain unaware of their potentials for many years. Sometimes a mental shock, a conversation with a sage, or visiting a familiar place reminds one of his past, and he can come in touch with that aspect of his personality that remained unknown until that point.

Most students want to know how many births are required to complete the journey to Self-realization. That is decided by the aspirant and not by Providence or by the teacher. If the aspirant learns to apply all his resources to make his mind one-pointed and inward, he can attain his goal in this lifetime. For those who have a wick, lamp, and oil and put them together, their lamp is ready to be lit. It is true that when the disciple is ready, the master appears. Lighting the lamp depends on both the disciple and the master. The aspirant's lamp is lit by the master, but one should not forget that that light is not the light of the master but was handed over to him in the same manner by the spiritual tradition.

तपस्विभ्योऽधिको योगी ज्ञानिभ्योऽपि मतोऽधिकः।
कर्मिभ्यश्चाधिको योगी तस्माद्योगी भवार्जुन।। ४६
योगिनामपि सर्वेषां मद्गतेनान्तरात्मना।
श्रद्धावान्भजते यो मां स मे युक्ततमो मतः।। ४७

46. *The yogi excels the ascetics. He is believed to be greater even than those endowed with knowledge. The yogi is greater than those who perform actions. Therefore, become a yogi, O Arjuna.*

47. *Among all the yogis, he who faithfully devotes himself to Me, with his inner self entered into Me, I consider him the one most united in yoga.*

Verse 47 refers to the 37th verse and answers Arjuna's question regarding an alternative path if one has not attained perfection on the path of yoga. As one jacket does not suit all, so one path does not suit all. Diverse are the paths, but the goal is one. The path of yoga is greater than the path of practicing austerities, for austerities are merely means to purify the mind. Austerities are external observances that are limited to physical cleanliness and to the control of the senses. They are practiced in many ways: by the ignorant in a rigid way and by the knowledgeable for the sake of purification of the body and senses. The yogi also practices austerities, but he goes further and practices higher sadhana in order to attain control over the mind and its modifications. He then directs all his mental energy toward the center of perfection. His goal is to attain samadhi, and he does not rest until he attains it.

There is another category of yogis whose minds are completely devoted, who have perfect faith, and who have completely surrendered themselves to the pure Self alone. They are considered to be special children of God. They are the chosen ones. Sri Krishna makes this comparison between different types of aspirants to help Arjuna understand that unwavering faith is a strong force that can lead the devotee to the highest perfection. The path of love in which one learns to give with reverence and dedication all that one has unhesitatingly and unquestioningly requires great strength. Therefore, commitment to that path is higher than commitment to the path of austerities. Here for the first time Sri Krishna mentions the path of devotion. The path of devotion is not the emotionalism that leads people toward chanting, dancing, shaking, and tears. It is complete giving until one has nothing further to give. The Lord says, "Empty thy vessel and I will fill thee." To be completely emptied, one must learn to be like the ocean, for the ocean continually evaporates itself yet is always full. By giving, the same is returned. The law of giving fulfills one. Love is giving and fulfillment.

Here ends the sixth chapter, in which the path of meditation and a glimpse of alternative paths are described.

Chapter Seven

Knowledge of the Absolute
in its Entirety

श्री भगवानुवाच
मय्यासक्तमनाः पार्थ योगं युञ्जन्मदाश्रयः।
असंशयं समग्रं मां यथा ज्ञास्यसि तच्छृणु।। १
ज्ञानं तेऽहं सविज्ञानमिदं वक्ष्याम्यशेषतः।
यज्ज्ञात्वा नेह भूयोऽन्यज्ज्ञातव्यमवशिष्यते।। २
मनुष्याणां सहस्रेषु कश्चिद्यतति सिद्धये।
यततामपि सिद्धानां कश्चिन्मां वेत्ति तत्त्वतः।। ३

The Blessed Lord said

1. *With your mind attached to Me, O Son of Pritha, uniting yourself in yoga, depending entirely on Me, listen to the way through which you will know Me in My entirety without doubt.*
2. *I shall teach you knowledge (jnana) together with realization (vijnana) in their entirety, knowing which thereafter nothing more remains to be known.*
3. *Among thousands of human beings only a few endeavor for perfection. Of those endeavoring accomplished ones, only a few know Me in reality.*

In the dialogue between Sri Krishna and Arjuna, Sri Krishna often uses the word "Me" for the real and pure Self. This might confuse and bewilder the modern student. One should not forget that Sri Krishna is a perfect enlightened incarnation and therefore is correct in using the words "I" and "Me" to refer to divinity rather than using the third person. That is a direct way of relating to the dearest disciples. Modern teachers become carried away and think that they too can talk in this way, but when they do, it is usually because of their egotism. In fact they have not attained a state of perfection but are trying to show off, which is very misleading to the student. It promotes only "gurudom" and not the Godhead. Many who claim to be men of God these days are indeed men, but they are hardly godlike. The student should be aware that a true teacher is completely selfless and loving. When a modern teacher asks his students to dedicate their time, money, and energy, and all that they have to him, his teaching is enveloped in egotism and selfishness. If the wants of a teacher are the same as those of his disciple, what is the difference between the two? How can such a teacher help a student? A good teacher is known for his selflessness. If that quality is absent, one should not follow him. It is better not to have a teacher than to be trapped by false teachings. A modern teacher cannot be compared with Sri Krishna and should not pretend to be. Sri Krishna was the greatest yogi that ever lived on the earth; he was unparalleled in knowledge in all respects.

Sri Krishna instructs his dear disciple, Arjuna, in the art and science of the knowledge that dispels ignorance and enables one to see truth clearly. He states that the aspirant should fix his heart on the highest alone and dedicate his whole life to the Lord, the Self of all. The aspirant should not allow his mind and emotions to travel in any other direction but should take refuge in the uninterrupted consciousness of Truth, through which flows the perennial knowledge of the Eternal in all its fullness. When that knowledge is attained, there remains nothing more to be attained. Among the thousands who travel on the path of spirituality, only a few individuals attain such perfection.

The sixth chapter explained attainment of the highest state through meditation. Having understood the method of meditation, Arjuna now wants to know the object of meditation and an alternative method for attaining the heights that are reached by yogis. This theme continues in chapters seven through eleven, and more explicit instructions are given to Arjuna.

Lessons imparted by an accomplished teacher directly to his beloved disciple have a more profound impact on the mind and heart of the student than reading and studying the scriptures. The questions that are not answered by the scriptures and teachings of the sages or by any other means are finally answered at the summit that one attains through direct experience. Without direct experience, doubts still lurk. Every aspirant longs to have direct knowledge. It is not that he does not believe in the teachings of the great sages and the scriptures; they do inspire and help him. But attainment of perfection is possible only through Self-realization. Therefore, a need arises for a perfectly devised method of preparing oneself to receive that knowledge.

The first instruction in this chapter is to maintain constant awareness that the Self alone exists. One should practice a method of sadhana to attain that insight, for without having knowledge of the goal and purpose of sadhana, nothing can be attained. Even if the sadhana is devised profoundly, if one does not have knowledge of his goal, he cannot progress, for he becomes a victim of allurements and is bound to stumble again and again. Many students begin practicing meditation without knowing why they are practicing. Practicing meditation without knowledge of the goal is like walking along a path without knowing one's destination. First the subject should be known in its entirety, and then one should pursue his practice.

Jnana and *vijnana* are two kinds of knowledge that we find in the scriptures. Jnana is knowledge of the Absolute; vijnana is the knowledge for devising the perfect method of sadhana. When one attains these two aspects of knowledge, he can tread the path and attain perfection. One among thousands reaches that perfection, and among those, only a fortunate few know the real Self in its entirety. Real knowledge is that knowledge after which nothing remains to be attained. The third verse explains that after attaining the state of samadhi or perfection, there still remains to be attained the highest state: Self-realization. In the state of perfection the aspirant attains the highest goal that an individual is capable of achieving. The last step is total expansion of the knowledge that he has attained: he becomes one with the Whole.

भूमिरापोऽनलो वायुः खं मनो बुद्धिरेव च।
अहंकार इतीयं मे भिन्ना प्रकृतिरष्टधा।। ४
अपरेयमितस्त्वन्यां प्रकृतिं विद्धि मे पराम्।
जीवभूतां महाबाहो ययेदं धार्यते जगत्।। ५
एतद्योनीनि भूतानि सर्वाणीत्युपधारय।
अहं कृत्स्नस्य जगतः प्रभवः प्रलयस्तथा।। ६
मत्तः परतरं नान्यत्किञ्चिदस्ति धनंजय।
मयि सर्वमिदं प्रोतं सूत्रे मणिगणा इव।। ७

4. *Earth, water, fire, air, space, mind, intelligence, and ego, this is My primordial nature, Prakriti, divided eightfold.*
5. *This is My immanent nature. Know My other transcendent nature, which has become the souls (jivas), O Long-armed One, by which this world is sustained.*
6. *All the beings have their origination in this; hold this to be true. I am the origin as well as the dissolution of the entire world.*
7. *There is nothing at all beyond Me, O Arjuna. Everything is woven in Me like gems on a thread to form a necklace.*

Every object in the world is gifted with a peculiar and unique quality. All that we see in the external world has some distinct quality that is not found in the same way elsewhere. Ultimately there is only one source from which all the innumerable aspects of phenomenal existence are manifest, but that source remains obscured from human vision.

In these verses Sri Krishna explains all the levels of manifestation from the gross to the subtlest. He addresses Arjuna as "long armed," meaning one who has the ability to grasp all-encompassing knowledge. That knowledge is imparted by the teacher only when the student has widened the horizon of his vision. Sri Krishna says that in the external world there are eight constituents: earth, water, fire, air, space, mind, intellect, and ego. He says to Arjuna, "These eight constituents make up my lowermost body, but within these there is another, highest essence. On this is sustained all beings. I am the originator, sustainer, and annihilator of this whole universe. Just as the beads are strung on a thread, everything is woven in me."

The aspirant should learn to identify himself with the source of manifestation. Then it will be easy for him to grasp the knowledge in the Bhagavad Gita. When the student is faithful, eager to receive that knowledge, and when he applies all his resources with full devotion, that knowledge is grasped. But one should not forget that for attaining that knowledge, he needs a profound method of sadhana devised by examining his own capacities and abilities.

रसोऽहमप्सु कौन्तेय प्रभास्मि शशिसूर्ययो:।
प्रणव: सर्ववेदेषु शब्द: खे पौरुषं नृषु।। ८
पुण्यो गन्ध: पृथिव्यां च तेजश्चास्मि विभावसौ।
जीवनं सर्वभूतेषु तपश्चास्मि तपस्विषु।। ९
बीजं मां सर्वभूतानां विद्धि पार्थ सनातनम्।
बुद्धिर्बुद्धिमतामस्मि तेजस्तेजस्विनामहम्।। १०
बलं बलवतामस्मि कामरागविवर्जितम्।
धर्माविरुद्धो भूतेषु कामोऽस्मि भरतर्षभ।। ११
ये चैव सात्त्विका भावा राजसास्तामसाश्च ये।
मत्त एवेति तान्विद्धि न त्वहं तेषु ते मयि।। १२

8. *I am the flavor in the waters, O Son of Kunti, and the radiance of the moon and the sun, I am pranava (OM) in all the Vedas, the sound in space, and manliness in men.*
9. *I am beautiful fragrance in the earth and brilliance in the sun, the living force in all beings, and I am asceticism in the ascetics.*

10. *Know Me to be the ancient seed of all beings, O Son of Pritha. I am the wisdom in the wise and the splendor in the splendid.*

11. *I am the strength in the strong, free of desire and attachment. I am that desire in beings which is not opposed to righteousness.*

12. *All the sattvic states, as well as the rajasic and the tamasic ones, originate from Me, know them to be thus. I am not in them, yet they are in Me.*

Sri Krishna further explains the nature of the elements of earth, water, fire, air, and space. He says to Arjuna that all the powers in the universe, "the fragrance of the earth, the taste of water, the luster of fire, the touch of the wind, the sound of space, the radiance of the sun, the light of the moon, the universal sound of OM, the life of the animate ones, the very essence of all beings, the desire to do one's duty, the valor of brave men, have risen from one source, and this I am." These verses do not explain the process of creation but that of manifestation. There is an important difference between these two words. The word creation is used in the philosophy of dualism. Dualists believe that apart from the existence of God, nature is also self-existent, and with the help of that nature, God created the world. There is another conception: God, the ultimate power of the universe, nature, and the individual soul are all self-existent. But these ideas are dismissed by the philosophy of *Advaita*, which holds that there is one and only one absolute Reality without a second and all that we see, the entire universe, is but a manifestation of the one Truth.

To help Arjuna understand this truth and to expand his consciousness, Sri Krishna explains that the fragrance of the earth, the taste of water, the luster of fire, the touch of the wind, and the sound in space are the manifestations of the absolute One. The aspirant should become aware that all these qualities of the different elements are but different faces of the same One.

Verse 8 refers to the sacred word OM (A-U-M), a universal sound that is the very theme of the Upanishads and Vedas. The three syllables, A, U, M, personify the waking, dreaming, and sleeping states. But the silent soundless sound is the fourth state called turiya. After attaining the state of turiya, the wise can visualize each state separately and yet all at once.* The Lord of life, though He manifested this universe, remains hidden beyond all the levels of consciousness, just as turiya, which contains waking, dreaming, and sleeping yet remains beyond them all. OM is called *pranava*. By constantly remembering this sound and understanding its meaning, one is led to the state of this soundless sound. When the aspirant uses this sound in both meditation and contemplation, he realizes its various aspects. The aspects of this sound from the gross to the subtlemost have been explained in Upanishadic literature and other scriptures on sadhana.

Before a student begins treading the path of bhakti yoga, jnana yoga, or the yoga of action, he should have sufficient knowledge of the nature of his body, senses, mind, intellect, and ego as well as of the source of this universe so that he can unhesitatingly begin practicing to attain that knowledge directly. When the student begins identifying himself with his essential nature and then expands his consciousness to the consciousness of the perfect state of being, he no longer identifies himself with the objects of the world. Such a state of perfection is considered to be the highest. Knowledge leads one from individual consciousness to universal consciousness. Sadhana leads the aspirant from his gross self to the subtlemost aspect of his being, and then he realizes that his real Self is the Self of the universe.

Three qualities function in the universe, and these qualities function in the same way in the human being. Sattva is the harmonious quality; rajas is the active and passionate quality; and tamas is slothful. All of the forms and means in the universe come out of these three gunas, and the gunas themselves come from the one single source of all, the Lord of life and the universe. The sun, moon, constellations, and the elements of earth come into existence from the Lord of life, the source of the universe. Because of these objects we become aware of the source behind all phenomena: the Lord of life. They exist because of the Lord, but He does not exist because of the existence of these objects. That is

* For more information, see *Enlightenment Without God*. Swami Rama, Honesdale, PA: Himalayan Institute, 1982.

why it is said, "All these objects are in Me, yet I am not in them." All things are in the Lord of life, but He is not in them.

त्रिभिर्गुणमयैर्भावैरेभिः सर्वमिदं जगत्‌।

मोहितं नाभिजानाति मामेभ्यः परमव्ययम्‌।। १३

दैवी ह्येषा गुणमयी मम माया दुरत्यया।

मामेवं ये प्रपद्यन्ते मायामेतां तरन्ति ते।। १४

न मां दुष्कृतिनो मूढाः प्रपद्यन्ते नराधमाः।

माययापहृतज्ञाना आसुरं भावमाश्रिताः।। १५

13. *This entire world, deluded by three states constituted of gunas, does not recognize Me as the immutable One beyond them.*
14. *This divine maya of Mine, consisting of gunas, is difficult to transcend. Only they who surrender themselves to Me go across this maya.*
15. *The basest among human beings, the deluded ones, evildoers, do not surrender to Me, their knowledge having been plundered away by maya as they have resorted to a demonic aspect.*

The whole world is deluded as a result of the illusory power of maya. Maya means that which exists and yet does not exist. The three gunas create an illusion for all human beings, and they are not able to see the power behind the illusion. All the activities of the human being—his mind, action, and speech—are controlled by the gunas, which motivate him to enjoy the objects but do not allow him to be aware of the self-existent Reality beyond all these phenomena. In the Isha Upanishad there is a prayer that says, "O Lord, remove this glittering disk which has hidden the truth." This means that the illusory power (maya) is full of temptations and charms that completely sway the human mind and senses, creating desire for the objects of the world. We all know that neither the objects nor the pleasures of the mundane world are permanent, yet our minds remain deluded in wanting to capture these pleasures. We suffer because of these delusions. The human mind and senses remain allured by the charms and temptations of the external world, by maya.

Maya has no existence of its own. It is not any particular being or object like the sun or moon but an illusion in the cosmos. Those who become aware of this fact and realize the truth that beyond all delusion lies the source of perennial light and life, which is self-existent, can cross the mire of delusion. Those alone who with sincere effort and the grace of God attain constant consciousness of the self-existent Lord of life cross the delusion of maya. They have made their minds one-pointed and inward and know the true nature of the Lord. But the mind that is dissipated and distracted and always goes out in search of the pleasures of the temporal world cannot comprehend that state. The mire of delusion created by maya is hard to cross. Maya veils the faculty of discrimination, judgment, and decision. One is then deluded, and in fact prefers to remain in that state. Those who have lost this faculty are called demonic or evil, for they create misery and suffering for themselves and others. Such people, having demonic attitudes and behavior, commit harmful acts and destroy knowledge because they are infatuated.

The question arises in every aspirant's mind: What is maya? The word *maya* signifies art, skill, or workmanship. As a potter creates a pitcher out of a lump of clay by using his skill, so maya with her three-fold gunas is able to create the illusion that is enjoyed by ordinary minds. The lump of clay, after being given a form by the skill of a potter, involves him in his own creation: he becomes attached to the pitcher he has created. He was not attached to the lump of clay but becomes attached after using his skill and fashioning the clay into a pitcher. Man thus models innumerable varieties of objects for his sense pleasure and becomes deluded, confused, and miserable. One who lives under that delusion does not perceive the truth that the pitcher is actually a lump of clay to which he has given a particular shape and to which he has become attached. The values that he projects onto the pitcher make him happy. But he becomes fearful that the pitcher might break, and if it should break, he becomes unhappy. Because of the virtues of the three gunas, one has the skill to fashion a lump of clay into a pitcher, but from the attachment that results come all the emotional problems that consume our energy and time. When we study this entire process, we find that the three gunas create a vicious cycle that is difficult to break.

Now let us examine the threefold quality of maya. The human being goes to the state of sleep because of the predominance of tamas. The moment he wakes up, rajas is predominant and leads him to activity. Then he likes to enjoy the sense objects. But when sattva is predominant, one remains in a state of joy and peace. The aspirant can become aware of the influence of the gunas in all human activities, mental and physical. He can measure the progress of his sadhana by observing which guna becomes predominant in his daily life. When he is sad, disappointed, and distressed, it is the influence of tamas; when he is active, busy in doing and in wanting to do, it is rajas; when he is calm and joyous and feels delighted from within, the sattva quality is predominant. Yogis consciously attain the state of sattva by applying sushumna with a particular exercise involving the combined effort of concentration and breathing. During that state one spontaneously lifts his body consciousness to the higher dimensions of life. Calmness and quietness reflect a tranquil state in which sattva is predominant.

The threefold quality of maya arises from the source of the life stream, the Lord of life. But the highest of all, the Lord of all, remains beyond them. Maya is called divine. It is a power of the Lord and cannot be dispelled by ordinary austerities and mortifications. Special effort and profound sadhana alone help to cut the fetters of the bondage created by that delusion. When human endeavor fails, the sadhaka remembers the Lord in the same way that the infant cries for his mother's help. That powerful one-pointed devotion brings the grace of the Lord to the aid of the sadhaka. When the yogi makes sincere effort to attain the state of sattva and devotes his sattvic effort to the Lord, he becomes free from the delusion of maya. The tamasic attitudes of those who remain in the deluded state, always desiring to enjoy the pleasures of the senses, create misery for them. Because of their infatuation, they create darkness for themselves. Such ignorant people actually destroy the great gift given to human beings by Providence.

चतुर्विधा भजन्ते मां जनाः सुकृतिनोऽर्जुन।
आर्तो जिज्ञासुरर्थार्थी ज्ञानी च भरतर्षभ।। १६
तेषां ज्ञानी नित्ययुक्त एकभक्तिर्विशिष्यते।
प्रियो हि ज्ञानिनोऽत्यर्थमहं स च मम प्रियः।। १७
उदाराः सर्व एवैते ज्ञानी त्वात्मैव मे मतम्।
आस्थितः स हि युक्तात्मा मामेवानुत्तमां गतिम्।। १८
बहूनां जन्मनामन्ते ज्ञानवान्मां प्रपद्यते।
वासुदेवः सर्वमिति स महात्मा सुदुर्लभः।। १९

16. *Four kinds of people, performers of good deeds, devote themselves to Me, O Arjuna: the distressed, the seeker of knowledge, the seeker of fulfillment of a wish, and the one who knows, O Bull Among the Bharatas.*

17. *Of these, the one endowed with knowledge, ever united in yoga with single-pointed devotion is distinguished. I am most beloved of the one endowed with wisdom, and he is also My beloved.*

18. *All these others are excellent, but one endowed with knowledge is My own self—this is My view. Such a one whose self is joined in yoga is stablished in Me, consequently in a state higher than which there is none.*

19. *At the end of many lifetimes one endowed with knowledge attains Me, knowing 'the Indweller is All.' Such a great-souled one (mahatma) is very difficult to find.*

There are four categories of people who are devoted to the Lord. In the first category are those who are needy and in distress, who suffer mentally and physically. They are not successful in attaining wealth in the temporal world, and they are miserable and suffer from all kinds of diseases. That type of person worships God to fulfill his mundane desires and has no knowledge of the nature of the Self. He prays to the Lord to fulfill his desires and does not pray when his desires are met. That kind of devotee is the most petty one, yet compared to those who do not pray to God and do not have any consciousness of higher dimensions of life, those who pray longing to fulfill their worldly desires are superior because they at least believe in the existence of God, Their search eventually leads them to realize the importance of selfless prayer and finally leads them to the realization of the Self, the highest goal of human life. To believe in God for whatever reason is far better than non-belief. How unfortunate are those who do not make efforts to believe in the reality of the Self. They deny their own existence.

The next category of worshipers seeks knowledge with the desire to know the mystery of human relationships, of life, and of the universe. That person's devotion to the Lord does not arise out of misery or failure experienced in the external world but out of the desire to know the highest truth. His desire to know is predominant. To satisfy his intellectual curiosity, he pursues the path of enlightenment. If he pursues it for a long time and learns to unfold himself to a point where pure reason begins functioning, he becomes able to discriminate between the mundane and the Absolute. That class of seekers is definitely superior to the first category of devotees who pray to God merely because they are distressed, miserable, and unable to fulfill their desires. Desiring to know the highest truth is superior to longing to have worldly needs and desires fulfilled.

In the third category are those aspirants who have sharpened their faculty of discrimination and know the difference between the pure Self and the not-self, the imperishable and the perishable. Such an aspirant makes sincere efforts to realize the highest truth. He searches for a competent teacher and follows the path to enlightenment that is imparted to him. With the help of meditation, he directs his energies only toward realizing the Self. He proves to be the highest of all seekers. His devotion does not arise out of worldly distress, anxiety, or intellectual curiosity. In his search for truth there lies a purity of heart and mind. Those who have been practicing the path of light and life in the past start treading the same path again and continue pursuing their path until they reach the end.

The fourth class is composed of those fortunate ones who have already attained wisdom. Such an aspirant has realized the real Self, so for him nothing remains to be attained. He has already attained the state of tranquility and is superior to those in the other classes that have been described. Such a jnana yogi is the finest of all. He is dear to the Lord, and the Lord is dear to him. The man of wisdom is called *mahatma*. Such high souls are rare and become torch bearers and examples for all aspirants. Because of these great mahatmas, the spiritual knowledge flows uninterruptedly.

Though all four classes pray and are devoted to one and the same Lord, the highest is the realized one who has attained the state of equanimity and equilibrium. Those in the highest class do not have any desire at all, whereas the seekers in the other three classes still have desires. Such a great man is firmly established in his conviction because he already knows the truth. He knows that this entire universe has come out of the truth. The man of wisdom can never slip from the heights of attainment. He is steadfast and has attained oneness with the divine. Therefore he is divine.

When one seriously thinks about life and its purpose, it becomes clear that one lifetime is not sufficient to attain the ultimate goal. Self-realization is attained through the effort of many lifetimes. If that effort is uninterrupted, one is sure to attain his goal.

कामैस्तैस्तैर्हृतज्ञानाः प्रपद्यन्तेऽन्यदेवताः।
तं तं नियममास्थाय प्रकृत्या नियताः स्वया।। २०
यो यो यां यां तनुं भक्तः श्रद्धयार्चितुमिच्छति।
तस्य तस्याचलां श्रद्धां तामेव विदधाम्यहम्।। २१
स तया श्रद्धया युक्तस्तस्याराधनमीहते।
लभते च ततः कामान्मयैव विहितान्हि तान्।। २२
अन्तवत्तु फलं तेषां तद्भवत्यल्पमेधसाम्।
देवान्देवयजो यान्ति मद्भक्ता यान्ति मामपि।। २३

20. *Many, their knowledge plundered away by so many desires, resort to other deities, undertaking this and that observance, impelled thereto by their own nature.*

21. *Whatever form or aspect of mind a devotee wishes to worship with faith, toward that very form or aspect of Mine I establish his unshaken devotion.*
22. *Endowed with that faith, he endeavors to practice the worship of the same; thereby he gains the fulfillment of those very wishes provided by Me.*
23. *But the fruit of theirs, whose wisdom is thus limited, comes to an end. Those who sacrifice to the deities go to the deities. Those who are devoted to Me come even to Me.*

Though the paths are various, the goal is one and the same. Even they who do not have profound knowledge of human existence and the universe around them, whose mental horizons have not expanded, and who worship various gods are benefited because of the ultimate source of light and life, the only one self-existent truth. This one truth is manifest in millions of ways. When one devotes his time and prays to one aspect of the truth, he indeed gains solace and is helped, but the ultimate truth still remains beyond his vision. Only those who know truth directly become liberated.

The aspirant who has a longing to enjoy the objects of the senses destroys his knowledge because his longing creates barriers and obstacles for him. Such an aspirant remains under the control of the three gunas, which delude his mind. He worships all sorts of objects, experiences, and achievements in the mundane world.

These verses do not merely refer to gods as we usually think of them. When one has a strong desire for an object or an achievement, that desire is inevitably fulfilled. If a desire is powerful enough, it fulfills itself. When one is devoted to fulfilling a desire, he makes that desire the object of his devotion, his god. And his devotion toward that God satisfies him, for he attains what he is seeking. In the Old Testament the first commandment is "Thou shalt have no other gods before Me." This means that one should not worship or become devoted to money, possessions, power, fame, or other mundane attainments. Sri Krishna takes a different perspective and says that if one worships or devotes himself to mundane objects he is bound to attain them through God's grace, but the reward received is only temporary and mundane. One who is devoted to the material gets only the material; one who is devoted to wealth gets only wealth. If one does not seek that which is more abundant and fulfilling and which is equally available, he does not gain the ultimate reward.

The ordinary person with limited knowledge chooses a symbol, begins worshipping that symbol, and makes it the object of his devotion. He performs many rites because the human mind has the tendency to be dependent on the form and is not able to comprehend the knowledge and vision of the formless. One who functions from his lower mind cannot have a vision of the attributeless and formless. Even today many religions believe that God is a being who fulfills the desires of those who beseech him. No doubt that helps one to some extent, but still he is not able to break the fetters and the bondages created by his limited conceptions. The ordinary person worships gods or believes in the existence of God, but he is not aware that there exists only one Reality without a second.

Sri Krishna explains to Arjuna that humanity can be divided into four groups. Some people believe in fulfilling their sense pleasures, others out of curiosity try to know and believe, and a small number attain truth by following the path of yoga. But only a fortunate few are Self-realized and are capable of leading others.

Ordinary men and women think, act, and worship according to the guna that is predominant in them. Sri Krishna says that one who has no knowledge of the real Self indulges in a mockery of worship because of his ignorance. Those who have no knowledge of the eternal presence of the infinite are infatuated and worship gods without realizing the one truth. But those who do not worship any image and whose minds have attained a state of tranquility are truly free.

अव्यक्तं व्यक्तिमापन्नं मन्यन्ते मामबुद्धयः।
परं भावमजानन्तो ममाव्ययमनुत्तमम्।। २४
नाहं प्रकाशः सर्वस्य योगमायासमावृतः।
मूढोऽयं नाभिजानाति लोको मामजमव्ययम्।। २५

वेदाहं समतीतानि वर्तमानानि चाऽर्जुन।
भविष्याणि च भूतानि मां तु वेद न कश्चन।। २६
इच्छाद्वेषसमुत्थेन द्वन्द्वमोहेन भारत।
सर्वभूतानि संमोहं सर्गे यान्ति परंतप।। २७

24. *The unwise believe Me, though unmanifest, as having come to manifestation, not knowing My supreme, immutable, and unexcelled aspect.*
25. *I am not vivid to all, veiled by the yoga-maya. This deluded world does not know Me, who am unborn and immutable.*
26. *I know all the past and all the present ones, O Arjuna, and all the future beings. No one, however, knows Me.*
27. *Through the delusion of the dual opposites which arises through desire and enmity, O Descendant of Bharata, all beings enter delusion at the time of birth, O Scorcher of Enemies.*

The absolute Truth is not subject to destruction. It is the supreme of all. The Lord knows all beings in all three times—past, present and future—but no one knows the Lord. The Lord is hidden behind His own power, and it is not easy to realize Him. The ignorant do not know this truth because they are infatuated with the pleasures of the mundane world. They do not understand that which has the power to manifest Itself as an incarnation. The ignorant are not capable of understanding the unborn, never-dying One. From desire springs the pairs of opposites such as misery and joy. Almost everyone is infatuated by the pairs of opposites and is deluded by them. Those who are under the influence of the pairs of opposites have no conception of the truth and therefore are not capable of comprehending the glory of the Lord. Their minds and senses remain engrossed with sense pleasures, and they do not even think of improving or unfolding themselves. But those fortunate ones who are not infatuated and who are free from the pairs of opposites are liberated. Their whole being remains devoted to the Lord alone.

Contemplation of and meditation on external pleasure leads one to further delusion, but the aspirant who is conscious of the ultimate reality meditates and contemplates only on the highest of truth. With the help of self-discipline, such an aspirant acquires extraordinary power: the power of supreme knowledge, which is the source of all knowledge. Many aspirants do not understand the distinction between the manifest and the unmanifest One. The word *avyakta* means unknown, unseen, imperceivable. *Vyakta,* however, may be perceived with the help of the sense organs. The sadhaka attempts to go beyond vyakta to attain knowledge of avyakta, but the ignorant have no power to go beyond the mire of delusion created by the senses. They do not know if there is anything that exists beyond sense perception. Their minds remain engrossed in sense pleasures, and they have no comprehension of the unknown phenomena of life, of the supreme power that is eternal and infinite. The ignorant think that the ultimate truth is a particular being or has a particular form; they do not comprehend the whole. To know the whole is real knowledge, but to think of the whole as being limited or as an individual being is sheer ignorance.

To regard the infinite as just part of itself is a gross error. As a wave in the ocean is not the whole ocean, so all the creatures are but fragments of the one whole. To consider the supreme One as having a form means that one is thinking of the undivided as being divided. Sun, moon, stars, space, fire, water, and earth are but mere aspects of the whole; they are only small parts of the infinite. Instead of meditation on one individual aspect of the universe, the wise meditate on the supreme fountainhead of life and light from which proceeds the whole universe. But because of their limited knowledge, the ignorant ones engage in the worship of gods in various forms. Those whose minds are dissipated and who lack control and concentration can focus their minds on forms in the beginning and can eventually be led to the formless.

There are two schools of meditation. One believes in meditation on the forms, the other on the formless. But since ordinary minds cannot comprehend meditation of the formless, a form is useful for them in the primary stage of meditation to help them attain concentration of mind. Ultimately meditation should go to a deeper level that is beyond forms and names.

येषां त्वन्तगतं पापं जनानां पुण्यकर्मणाम्।
ते द्वन्द्वमोहनिर्मुक्ता भजन्ते मां दृढव्रताः।। २८
जरामरणमोक्षाय मामाश्रित्य यतन्ति ये।
ते ब्रह्म तद्विदुः कृत्स्नमध्यात्मं कर्म चाखिलम्।। २९
साधिभूताधिदैवं मां साधियज्ञं च ये विदुः।
प्रयाणकालेऽपि च मां ते विदुर्युक्तचेतसः।। ३०

28. *But those people of meritorious deeds whose past sin is reaching an end, they, freed of delusion with regard to the pairs of opposites, devote themselves to Me with very firm vows of observance.*

29. *They who, resorting to Me, endeavor for freedom from old age and death, come to know the entire Brahman, the complete spiritual affairs, and the entire range of action.*

30. *They who know Me with reference to the beings, with reference to the deities, as well as with reference to sacrificial observances, even at the time of their departure their minds are united in yoga and they know Me.*

Perfection can be attained by performing actions skillfully and with full devotion. When a one-pointed mind has been achieved and all the energies are directed toward Self-realization, all action becomes a form of worship. Then the aspirant identifies himself with his essential nature which is truth, happiness, and bliss. He knows that the worshiped one and the worshiper are one and the same. All the qualities of the ocean are found in a single drop of water. Qualitatively they are one and the same. Realizing that truth, the aspirant fulfills the purpose of his life and becomes perfect. He is no longer affected by the pairs of opposites.

Those who have made sincere efforts and have completed all endeavors attain freedom from old age and death. Ordinarily in old age the mind remains preoccupied; it goes to the old habit grooves that have been created in one's past. But when one makes full effort to meditate and contemplate on the innermost center of his being, he does not suffer from his old patterns. Death reveals its mystery to him. Thus he knows that one lives after death, that the Self remains eternal and unchanged, and that it is only the body that dies. He is not afraid of dying; he remains fearless both here and hereafter. Truth alone makes one fearless. Many devotees and aspirants make efforts to remember and maintain awareness of the center of consciousness at the time of death but are unable to do so because their meditation has not been strengthened and their minds still flow toward the grooves of their past habits. But those who have remained constantly aware of the center of consciousness are, at their hour of departure from this world, fearless, free, and happy.

Here ends the seventh chapter, in which the mystery of the unknown and the known is revealed

Chapter Eight
Knowledge of the Eternal

अर्जुन उवाच

किं तद्ब्रह्म किमध्यात्मं किं कर्म पुरुषोत्तम।

अधिभूतं च किं प्रोक्तमधिदैवं किमुच्यते।। १

अधियज्ञ: कथं कोऽत्र देहेऽस्मिन्मधुसूदन।

प्रयाणकाले च कथं ज्ञेयोऽसि नियतात्मभिः।। २

श्री भगवानुवाच

अक्षरं ब्रह्म परमं स्वभावोऽध्यात्ममुच्यते।

भूतभावोद्भवकरो विसर्गः कर्मसंज्ञितः।। ३

अधिभूतं क्षरो भावः पुरुषश्चाधिदैवतम्।

अधियज्ञोऽहमेवात्र देहे देहभृतां वर।। ४

Arjuna said

1. *What is Brahman with reference to the spiritual Self (adhyat-man)? What is karma, O Highest of Persons? What is it with reference to beings (adhibhuta), and what with reference to the deities (adhidaivata) is it said to be?*

2. *What is it with reference to sacrificial observances within this body (adhiyajna), O Madhu-sudana, and how are You to be known at the hour of departure by those of controlled selves?*

The Blessed Lord said

3. *The indestructible syllable, the supreme Brahman, the very transcendental nature is the inward spiritual Self. The emission, which*

> *is the cause of the production of the aspects of beings, is called*
> *karma.*
> 4. *The perishable aspect is the one referred to concerning the being,*
> *and the conscious principle Purusha is of the deities. As sacrificial*
> *observances it is I in this body, O Best of the Body-bearers.*

At the end of chapter seven, Sri Krishna tells Arjuna that one should know Brahman, *adhyatma*, karma, *adhibhuta*, *adhidaivata*, and *adhi-yajna*, and that at the final hour of departure one should contemplate and meditate on the highest Lord alone. Arjuna does not comprehend the meaning of these words and wants to understand their profundity.

In the eighth chapter Sri Krishna answers all of Arjuna's questions. First he explains that Brahman is the highest of all principles. The supreme Brahman alone exists and is the source of manifestation. Brahman is eternal and immutable. It is not subject to change, death, or destruction. Brahman is not different from the innermost Self of every individual. Brahman is the liberated state of consciousness. It is the state in which Sri Krishna abides, and that state of consciousness can also be attained by the aspirant. Those who have attained a state of tranquility and equanimity have the knowledge of Brahman.

The word adhyatma is used for the supreme Brahman as it exists in every individual soul. There are two aspects of Brahman: the unmanifest and the manifest. As Brahman begins the process of manifestation. It divides itself into the transcendent subject (adhyatma) and the unmanifest source of all objects (*mula-prakriti*). Adhyatma refers to Brahman as the transcendent subject in every being.

Whatever is done that results in beings coming into existence is called karma. Karma is the power that brings about the origination of all beings. It is the creative fire by which life is developed, elevated, and evolved. The existence of all living beings comes about because of the law of karma. The transcendent subject (adhyatma), the basis of all objectification (mula-prakriti), and the creative principle (karma) are all aspects of Brahman.

Sri Krishna says that he should be known in each of his aspects.

All the objects that come into being are called bhuta. All the names and forms of the universe are perishable and subject to destruction. Whatever objects appear to exist in the material world are only forms of Prakriti, and the term adhibhuta refers to their perishable nature. In contrast to this, adhidaivata is the principle of pure consciousness, *Purusha*, which is everywhere and which is above all divinities. The term adhiyajna means "myself as sacrifice." Sri Krishna as the supreme Lord, the pure consciousness, rules over all sacrifice and is the recipient of all sacrifice. All sacrifices are directed toward the Self, and that is called adhiyajna. The sacrifice that is continually taking place in the body is also directed toward the Self. The Upanishads say that human life is a long series of sacrifices that should last for at least one hundred years.

अन्तकाले च मामेव स्मरन्मुक्त्वा कलेवरम्।
यः प्रयाति स मद्भावं याति नास्त्यत्र संशयः।। ५
यं यं वापि स्मरन्भावं त्यजत्यन्ते कलेवरम्।
तं तमेवैति कौन्तेय सदा तद्भावभावितः।। ६
तस्मात्सर्वेषु कालेषु मामनुस्मर युध्य च।
मय्यर्पितमनोबुद्धिर्मामेवैष्यस्यसंशयम्।। ७
अभ्यासयोगयुक्तेन चेतसा नान्यगामिना।
परमं पुरुषं दिव्यं याति पार्थानुचिन्तयन्।। ८

5. *He who departs remembering Me at the last moment, after leaving the body, he comes to identify with Me; there is no doubt in this.*
6. *Remembering whichever aspect of mine as he leaves the body at the end, he reaches that very aspect, O Son of Kunti, identified and always nurtured by that aspect.*
7. *Therefore remember Me at all times, and fight. With your mind and intelligence surrendered to Me, you will come to Me alone, without doubt.*
8. *With a mind joined in the yoga of practice, and wandering nowhere else, contemplating the supreme, divine Person, one goes to Him, O Son of Pritha.*

Verses 5 through 8 explain how the aspirant should prepare himself for life hereafter. He should not be haunted by thoughts, desires, and attachments to the mundane world. At the last hour of one's departure from this world, he should remember the Lord of life, for one's last desire determines the course of his rebirth. If during that time the aspirant thinks only of the Lord, nothing of the world influences the course of his transition. How can one remember the Lord at that time? Every great tradition teaches a way to remember the Lord, either by remembering a mantra, a word, a syllable, or a set of words. When the pranas (inhalation and exhalation)—which create a bridge between the conscious and unconscious life, the mortal and immortal parts of life— abandon their duties, the conscious mind, breath, senses, and body separate from the unconscious part of life. All the desires, merits, and demerits remain in the unconscious. One's prominent desires prompt him to assume a new garment. That is called rebirth.

During that transition period, remembering a mantra is useful; it enables the voyage to be comfortable. At the time of death ordinary people remember their worldly attachments and pleasures. That magnifies the pain and leads the mind to sorrow. But the aspirant who has clarity of mind remembers the name of the Lord and thus does not have unpleasant experiences at the time of departure. When the mantra is remembered consciously, it is recorded by the unconscious. During the time of departure when the conscious mind fails, any thought or desire that is prominent in the unconscious leads the individual according to its nature. It is very important to repeatedly remember the name of the Lord during one's lifetime so that the impression created by repeated remembrance is the strongest impression in the unconscious, for it is the strongest motivation that becomes the leader. Many aspirants are not aware of the profound effects of remembering the mantra, but they should understand that no action remains unrecorded in the unconscious. The student should not be concerned about consciously noticing a result but should continue remembering the mantra so that it becomes embedded in the unconscious. There is no doubt that the aspirant who constantly remembers the Lord at the time of departure attains liberation.

Many students wonder about life hereafter. After death one does not go to any hell or heaven but remains in his own habit patterns. Hell and heaven are merely the creations of one's own mind and habits. Those who understand the meaning of life know that the final hour is the deciding factor for whether one's voyage to the unknown will be pleasant or unpleasant. They prepare themselves for that hour. They depart from this world with a free mind and conscience, enjoying the eternal joy of the infinite. Whatever state an aspirant habitually remembers, the same he attains after leaving his body. One who has an auspicious state as his goal will reach it after death, and he who remembers worldly pleasures will continue to long for those pleasures after leaving his body. His desires, however, cannot be fulfilled in the state between death and birth, for then he has no senses and no objects with which to fulfill his desires. Thus he suffers. Those who are meditators, however, attain the deep state of tranquility and are never affected by the desire for worldly pleasure. They attain the state of perfection by identifying themselves with the Lord, and they finally become one with the Lord.

कविं पुराणमनुशासितारमणोरणीयांसमनुस्मरेद्यः।
सर्वस्य धातारमचिन्त्यरूपमादित्यवर्णं तमसः परस्तात्।। ९

प्रयाणकाले मनसाऽचलेन भक्त्या युक्तो योगबलेन चैव।
भ्रुवोर्मध्ये प्राणमावेश्य सम्यक् स तं परं पुरुषमुपैति दिव्यम्।। १०

यदक्षरं वेदविदो वदन्ति विशन्ति यद्यतयो वीतरागाः।
यदिच्छन्तो ब्रह्मचर्यं चरन्ति तत्ते पदं संग्रहेण प्रवक्ष्ये।। ११

सर्वद्वाराणि संयम्य मनो हृदि निरुध्य च।
मूर्ध्याधायात्मनः प्राणमास्थितो योगधारणाम्। १२

ओमित्येकाक्षरं ब्रह्म व्याहरन्मामनुस्मरन्।
यः प्रयाति त्यजन्देहं स याति परमां गतिम्।। १३

9. *He who contemplates Him who is the master of intuition, the ancient One, the giver of all commandments, more minute than the minute, sustainer of all, whose form is beyond thought, having*

the solar hue, beyond darkness,

10. *At the hour of departure, with an unmoving mind, endowed with devotion and with the power of yoga, making the prana enter between the eyebrows properly, he reaches the supreme, divine Person.*

11. *The indestructible syllable that the knowers of Veda know, that which the ascetics, free of attachments, enter, seeking which they practice celibacy, I shall teach you that word briefly.*

12. *Closing all the doors of the body and retaining the mind in the heart, placing the prana in the crown of the head, established in the concentration of yoga—*

13. *OM, this is Brahman consisting of a single, indestructible syllable. He who, enunciating it and contemplating it, goes forth abandoning his body, he reaches the supreme state.*

The Lord is omniscient, omnipresent, and omnipotent. He is the most ancient seer, and there is nothing that He does not know. He is the controller and ruler of all. He is extremely subtle and is not visible through the eyes of ordinary human minds. To meditate on Him is difficult. He is full of light without any tinge of darkness. At the time of departure one should remain in deep meditation on the Lord with full devotion and one-pointedness.

Sri Krishna gives a brief explanation of the practice of meditation that incorporates a subtle breathing method. When the aspirant learns to be still in a steady posture, he finds that the incoming and outgoing breaths draw the attention of his mind. Meditation can only be profound if sushumna is applied. Sushumna is a joyous state of mind in which the meditator spontaneously attains an unusual calmness without any external distraction. One of the signs and symptoms of this state of mind is that the breath flows freely and equally through both nostrils. In the ordinary state, one of the nostrils remains predominant.

Breath and mind are interdependent and are in the habit of reacting simultaneously. When the breath is calm and serene, the mind attains a state of joy. The aspirant should focus his mind at the space between the two eyebrows and should learn to visualize the light of life, through which one sees, senses, and knows. When his meditation is strengthened the light becomes more and more clear, and he finally reaches the source of light and life. The yogi who regularly practices meditation for a long time without interruptions in his practice attains that state. With the desire to attain the center of consciousness within, he observes complete celibacy. Here celibacy does not refer to practice only on a physical level but should be performed with mind, action, and speech.

The yogi who learns to meditate by applying sushumna and incorporating the sacred syllable OM can attain a state of equilibrium. It is interesting to note that all mantras cannot be adjusted to the inhalation and exhalation process. OM is a smooth sound and does not create jerks or irregular rhythms in the breath. Yogis remember that sound all the time; it has been praised by the Vedas, the most ancient scriptures in the library of man.

Those who cast off their mortal bodies remembering the Lord definitely reach the highest state. But one should not wait for the last hour of departure and learn to meditate only during the last days of his life. The wise person knows that in reality one experiences death every moment. We die millions of times in one lifetime, and millions of times we are born. Every moment that passes by is like a moment of death. One moment dies and another moment is born; one experience dies and another comes into being. Death precedes birth and birth precedes death, yet we experience a continuity of consciousness through these deaths and births. In a similar way the pure consciousness remains through the deaths and births of the physical body.

The human being is on a pilgrimage. His goal is the eternal abode, where he finds perfect happiness, peace, and bliss. The ignorant ones who consider this earth their permanent abode are deluded. Every moment of life until one reaches his eternal abode is precious. Therefore one should remember the Lord in every moment. That practice is called *ajapa japa*. Those who remember the name of the Lord in every breath of their lives are the fortunate few. When a student learns to remember the name of God in silence with a one-pointed mind and strengthens that habit, he can continue practicing anywhere and everywhere he goes. Thus ajapa japa leads one to constant awareness of the Self, which helps him during the period of departure.

अनन्यचेताः सततं यो मां स्मरति नित्यशः।
तस्याहं सुलभः पार्थ नित्ययुक्तस्य योगिनः।। १४
मामुपेत्य पुनर्जन्म दुःखालयमशाश्वतम्।
नाप्नुवन्ति महात्मानः संसिद्धिं परमां गताः।। १५
आब्रह्मभुवनाल्लोकाः पुनरावर्तिनोऽर्जुन।
मामुपेत्य तु कौन्तेय पुनर्जन्म न विद्यते।। १६

14. *He who, without turning his mind to any other, remembers Me incessantly—to that yogi, who is ever united in yoga, I am easily available, 0 Son of Pritha.*
15. *Upon reaching me, the great-souled one, having attained the supreme fulfillment, no longer comes to rebirth, which is an impermanent abode of sorrows.*
16. *All the way to the realm of Brahman, all the worlds revolve again and again, O Arjuna. Upon reaching Me, however, O Son of Kunti, there is no more rebirth.*

When the aspirant analyzes his existence in this world, he realizes that there is nothing permanent here. He focuses his mind on the Lord alone and remembers Him all the time. That constant awareness gives him freedom from the dissipation of the mind, and then he establishes himself in the consciousness of the eternal Self. Such a yogi is not born again and again; he is not subject to the rounds of deaths and births. The accomplished yogi is not required to come back again, for he has already attained liberation. The law of death and rebirth is not applicable to him.

सहस्रयुगपर्यन्तमहर्यद्ब्रह्मणो विदु:।
रात्रिं युगसहस्रान्तां तेऽहोरात्रविदो जना:।। १७
अव्यक्ताद्व्यक्तय: सर्वा: प्रभवन्त्यहरागमे।
रात्र्यागमे प्रलीयन्ते तत्रैवाव्यक्तसंज्ञके।। १८
भूतग्राम: स एवायं भूत्वा भूत्वा प्रलीयते।
रात्र्यागमेऽवश: पार्थ प्रभवत्यहरागमे।। १९

17. *People who know day and night know that the day of Brahma extends to a thousand aeons, and the night extends to a thousand aeons also.*

18. *All the manifest entities arise from the unmanifest upon the coming of the day, and upon the coming of the night they dissolve into that very thing called the unmanifest.*

19. *This aggregate of beings and elements, born again and again, is then dissolved at the coming of the night, quite helplessly, O Son of Pritha, and it is produced again upon the arrival of the day.*

There are four *yugas* or ages: Krita, Treta, Dvapara, and Kali. The four together are called a *mahayuga*, a great age. One mahayuga consists of 4,326,000, years. One thousand mahayugas make one day of Brahma, and the night of Brahma is of the same duration. The day and night together are called a *kalpa*.* Three hundred and sixty such units of day and night make one year of Brahma, and one hundred such years is the life of Brahma. With each day of Brahma the universe comes into being, and at the close of that day all beings merge into the unmanifest Prakriti. That process goes on eternally.

These verses explain that which physics and astronomy are trying to discover through external means: when the universe began, how it evolved, and if and when it will be annihilated. According to this view

---

* The cosmology presented here explains that a universe exists for four billion three hundred and twenty six million years before its annihilation. Estimates of the age of our universe given by modern astronomers and geologists have ranged from 1.8 to 20 billion years.

the universe goes through an endless cycle of creation and annihilation. Each cycle takes a vast length of time as measured by the human frame of reference but a much shorter time from the perspective of a more comprehensive state of consciousness. Physics has introduced to the modern world the concept that time is relative, but now we see that such a conception existed long ago in the cosmology of the ancient Vedic scriptures.

In these verses Sri Krishna makes Arjuna aware of the grand scale of the universe and the relative insignificance of all that Arjuna is attached to in his small world. These verses also give an inkling of the vastness of the universe over which Sri Krishna presides.

परस्तस्मात्तु भावोऽन्योऽव्यक्तोऽव्यक्तात्सनातनः।
यः स सर्वेषु भूतेषु नश्यत्सु न विनश्यति।। २०
अव्यक्तोऽक्षर इत्युक्तस्तमाहुः परमां गतिम्।
यं प्राप्य न निवर्तन्ते तद्धाम परमं मम।। २१
पुरुषः स परः पार्थ भक्त्या लभ्यस्त्वनन्यया।
यस्यान्तःस्थानि भूतानि येन सर्वमिदं ततम्।। २२

20. *But beyond that primordial unmanifest Prakriti is another eternal unmanifest Entity who does not perish when all the beings perish.*
21. *The unmanifest is called the indestructible syllable that is said to be the supreme status, upon attaining which they no longer return to the world. That is My supreme abode.*
22. *He is the transcendent Self (Purusha) to be attained through devotion distracted toward none other, inside whom dwell all the beings and by whom is all this spanned and pervaded.*

The time comes when the entire universe is annihilated by the great design of the Absolute. When everything that is manifest is destroyed, one unchanging principle remains that is never destroyed. That principle is called *Akshara* (immutable). It is the highest abode of the Absolute. The aspirant who has secured the knowledge of and attained that abode is no longer subject to birth and death. That eternal, unchanging, and everlasting principle is the highest goal of the aspirant. In that dwell all beings. It is the unmanifested pure Consciousness that is eternal and changeless, whereas all else goes through a process of birth and death. That unmanifest Reality is beyond the process of Prakriti and does not perish when the universe perishes. It is never changing and is everlasting, eternal, and infinite.

यत्र काले त्वनावृत्तिमावृत्तिं चैव योगिनः।
प्रयाता यान्ति तं कालं वक्ष्यामि भरतर्षभ।। २३
अग्निज्योतिरहः शुक्लः षण्मासा उत्तरायणम्।
तत्र प्रयाता गच्छन्ति ब्रह्म ब्रह्मविदो जनाः।। २४
धूमो रात्रिस्तथा कृष्णः षण्मासा दक्षिणायनम्।
तत्र चान्द्रमसं ज्योतिर्योगी प्राप्य निवर्तते।। २५
शुक्लकृष्णे गती ह्येते जगतः शाश्वते मते।
एकया यात्यनावृत्तिमन्ययावर्तते पुनः।। २६

23. *The time, departing in which the yogis return or do not return, I shall tell you of that time division, O Bull among the Bharatas.*
24. *Fire, light, the day, the moonlit fortnight, the six months of the northern solstice—departing in that time, the people who know Brahman go to Brahman.*
25. *Smoke, night, the dark lunar fortnight, the six months of the southern solstice—there the yogi attaining the lunar light returns.*
26. *These white and dark directions of the world are said to be perennial. By one he no longer returns, by the other he returns again.*

Sri Krishna teaches Arjuna the knowledge of the two paths that deal with the art and science of death and dying. What is the right time to depart from this mortal world? Those who are Self-realized cast off their bodies in the daytime during the bright half of the month while the sun is in its northern course. They then attain Brahman. Those who follow the path of action drop their bodies at a nocturnal hour during the dark half of the month while the sun is in its southern course, and they are reborn again. The path of those who are Self-realized is called the path of light, whereas the path of those who die during the six months when the sun is in the southern course is called the path of smoke. Both paths exist eternally, but one leads to emancipation and the other to rebirth. The words *agni, jyoti, shukla* are applied to the bright half of a month and indicate the light that shows the path. The words *dhuma, ratri, krishna* are applied to the dark half of the month and indicate darkness or ignorance. These verses do not just refer to the external universe but to the internal processes occurring within each person.

There are two paths: the path of good (selfless service) and the path of evil (selfishness). By following the path of good and dedicating all the fruits of one's actions, one remains liberated in the midst of performing his duty. But following the path of pleasure and living a selfish life leads to sorrow and pain. The path of good is the path of freedom, whereas the path of selfishness causes births and deaths.

According to yoga there are three paths. The path of *pingala* (the right breath) is the path of the sun, light, and day; the path of *ida* (the left breath) is that of night and darkness. The yogi who knows how to change from ida to pingala and from pingala to ida has complete control over the course of these two breaths. Such a yogi knows how to apply sushumna and thus attains a state of tranquility, of samadhi. That is the third path. Only two of these paths are mentioned in the Bhagavad Gita: the path of light and the path of darkness. The yogi who follows the path of the sun or light does not have to stumble through the dark path of ignorance. But one who does not have knowledge and does not practice yoga must go through the dark path. In his desire for the mundane objects of the world, his vision is obscured and his eyes remain blindfolded. His life is controlled by the gunas, for he does not practice the path of self-control. But the great yogi has self-control, and following the path of light, he reaches the highest abode of Brahman. The ignorant man, however, is subject to rebirth and suffers as a result of his selfishness.

The ordinary person does not have control over the time he departs. He is swayed by Prakriti (the three gunas), which determines the course of his life. But the yogi has profound control over his senses and mind. He can choose to cast off his body according to his wish, for he already understands life and its values thoroughly. For the yogi, dropping the body is just like taking off a garment. He does not remain attached to his body or to any other relationship related to the body. When the body is no longer a fit instrument, he decides to cast it off according to his will. The ordinary person does not have such a dynamic will or knowledge of the relationship of the body with the Self. The path of light, knowledge, and sun is the path the great ones tread.

नैते सृती पार्थ जानन् योगी मुह्यति कश्चन।
तस्मात्सर्वेषु कालेषु योगयुक्तो भवार्जुन।। २७
वेदेषु यज्ञेषु तप:सु चैव दानेषु यत्पुण्यफलं प्रदिष्टम्।
अत्येति तत्सर्वमिदं विदित्वा योगी परं स्थानमुपैति चाद्यम्।। २८

27. *Knowing these two paths, no yogi is ever confused. Therefore, O Arjuna, be united in yoga in all times.*
28. *The fruit of merit that has been stated with regard to the Vedas, the sacrifices, ascetic endeavors, and charities—the yogi surpasses it all, knowing this, and attains the primal and supreme peace.*

One who has knowledge of both paths—the path of light and the path of darkness—is never deluded by the darkness, by ignorance, for he knows the consequences of both paths. Such a yogi is never trapped by the charms, temptations, and allurements of the external world. Every moment of his life is devoted to the path of yoga. He never abandons the practices of yoga, so there is no chance of his downfall. He follows the path of yoga with full faith and a one-pointed mind. Yoga is an art and science that means skill in action, equanimity with regard to plea-sure and pain, and freedom from attachment to mundane enjoyments.

One who follows yoga is never deluded.

Scriptural knowledge is helpful only to a certain extent, but the true yogi attains direct knowledge, which helps him to go beyond to the heart of the teachings of the Vedas. He is definitely superior to one who follows the scriptures and performs sacrifices according to the instructions given in the scriptures. Direct knowledge alone leads to salvation. Two categories of yogis have been explained here. Those fortunate ones who have no attachments and who have attained the knowledge of skillful action are definitely superior to those who do their duties by performing daily rites and living in the world. The yogi of the first category attains the highest state of tranquility and equanimity and remains unaffected by the influences of the external world. He is never disturbed. Sri Krishna leads Arjuna to this path of skillful, selfless action and non-attachment.

Thus ends the eighth chapter, in which the knowledge of the eternal is explained.

Chapter Nine

Knowledge of the Royal and Secret Path

श्री भगवानुवाच

इदं तु ते गुह्यतमं प्रवक्ष्याम्यनसूयवे।

ज्ञानं विज्ञानसहितं यज्ज्ञात्वा मोक्ष्यसेऽशुभात्।। १

राजविद्या राजगुह्यं पवित्रमिदमुत्तमम्।

प्रत्यक्षावगमं धर्म्यं सुसुखं कर्तुमव्ययम्।। २

अश्रद्दधानाः पुरुषा धर्मस्यास्य परंतप।

अप्राप्य मां निवर्तन्ते मृत्युसंसारवर्त्मनि।। ३

The Blessed Lord said

1. *To you who are free of all intolerance I shall tell this secret-most knowledge together with its realization, knowing which, you will be freed from all that is impure.*

2. *The royal science, the royal secret, this is the unexcelled purifier, the attainment of which is evident, meritorious, immutable, and very easy to accomplish.*

3. *The persons not having faith in this law (dharma), O Scorcher of Enemies, not finding Me, keep returning on the path of death and the worldly cycles.*

Real knowledge and higher knowledge are described separately here. Knowledge relating to the factual world is considered to be real knowledge, yet there is another, higher state of knowledge in which one attains complete freedom from all pain and misery. Before one attains the highest state of knowledge, he should have knowledge of the real. Real here means that which is subject to sense perception. When one comprehends the nature of the temporal and evident reality, he discovers that all the objects of the external world are ever changing. Then he wants to understand the law underlying all those changes, for he knows that there must be something permanent beyond those changes. He distinguishes between two phenomena: one is subject to change and the other is eternal.

Sri Krishna imparts the secret knowledge of the eternal to Arjuna, but this does not imply that he is being prejudiced in favor of Arjuna. The word *guhya,* used in the first verse, means hidden, unrevealed, and not comprehended by ordinary minds. But actually there is no secret in the path of knowledge. Anyone who desires that knowledge can attain it, but one who is engrossed in worldly pleasures and whose mind is dissipated and distracted does not have the power to understand and assimilate the higher knowledge. Thus it remains a secret to him. These verses say that the higher knowledge, the secrets of the royal path, are imparted only to those whose minds are one- pointed, who follow the path of yoga, and who have firmly decided to dedicate their lives to attaining the highest knowledge. A competent teacher instructs his student according to the ability of the student's mind. When the student advances on the path, the teacher goes on revealing further secrets to him that he cannot impart to beginners.

The knowledge that is expounded in this chapter is called *raja vidya* (royal knowledge). There is a difference between royal knowledge and other paths. The road that leads one to the royal house is clean and clear and guides the aspirant. The milestones and road markers help him understand how far he has travelled on the path and how far and in which direction he has yet to tread. Modern students tend to follow this path, for it is a highly systematic approach. If one continues to faithfully follow this path, he finally reaches the royal palace where the king resides in his splendid eternal glory.

There is another meaning that can be derived from this verse. Raja vidya is the vidya (knowledge) that helps one to know the secrets of governing a kingdom. How should a raja (king) conduct himself and govern the kingdom? How can an individual govern the kingdom of life within and without? In both situations the state of equanimity should be attained first, for without it establishing self-government within or ruling the masses outside is impossible. Leaders should have profound knowledge of life within and without before they assume the duty of leading the masses. One who has not established control and mastery over himself is not capable of leading others. He cannot do justice to his task if he has not yet attained the state of equanimity.

With direct experience the yogi learns to understand all the laws that govern the city of life. He also knows the eternal principle that remains deep seated in the inner chamber of his being. The yogi learns to govern the city of life and becomes a master, whereas the ordinary person has no knowledge and skill to do so. He is governed and controlled by the forces of nature, and he always wants to enjoy the pleasures of the world. He is enslaved by his desires. One who does not follow the path of yoga but instead seeks to enjoy the fruits of his actions is subject to birth and death. It is as though he is born and dies without any purpose.

In this chapter Sri Krishna expounds the profound knowledge that will help Arjuna understand his internal organization so that he can be free from delusion. Sri Krishna first imparts the knowledge of the temporal and real world and then leads Arjuna to the higher knowledge that can only be attained directly and not through any other source. Knowledge of the scriptures and teachings of the sages do inspire us, but direct knowledge alone enables one to attain the highest wisdom.

मया ततमिदं सर्वं जगदव्यक्तमूर्तिना।
मत्स्थानि सर्वभूतानि न चाहं तेष्ववस्थितः।। ४
न च मत्स्थानि भूतानि पश्य मे योगमैश्वरम्।
भूतभृन्न च भूतस्थो ममात्मा भूतभावनः।। ५
यथाकाशस्थितो नित्यं वायुः सर्वत्रगो महान्।
तथा सर्वाणि भूतानि मत्स्थानीत्युपधारय।। ६

4. *All this is pervaded by Me whose form is unmanifest. All beings are dwelling in Me; I am not dwelling in them.*
5. *Nor are the beings dwelling within Me. See My yoga of sovereignty. My Self is the bearer of beings, nurturing the beings, yet not dwelling in the beings.*
6. *As the great wind dwelling in the sky reaches everywhere, so all the beings are dwelling within Me—be certain of this.*

That which is self-existent, complete, and full in itself does not need any support. The whole universe has arisen from the unmanifested power of the Lord. The entire administration of this universe is governed efficiently by the Lord. All beings rely on that one power, but that power does not rely on any being, for it is independent in and of itself. It nourishes and protects all beings yet is not bound up in them. Atman is the very cause and source of the activities of all beings. As the air exists in space and moves about in space, so all things have their existence and movement within the Lord.

In an organization there are many administrative officers, but above all these governing authorities there is one who has supreme authority to govern the entire organization. Similarly in the city of life there are many governing powers, but over all is *Ishvara*. In both the individual and the universe, the highest Self is the presiding divinity that directs and protects the universe and the individual life. The same governing principle is in the individual as is in the universe.

सर्वभूतानि कौन्तेय प्रकृतिं यान्ति मामिकाम्।
कल्पक्षये पुनस्तानि कल्पादौ विसृजाम्यहम्।। ७
प्रकृतिं स्वामवष्टभ्य विसृजामि पुनः पुनः।
भूतग्राममिमं कृत्स्नमवशं प्रकृतेर्वशात्। ८
न च मां तानि कर्माणि निबध्नन्ति धनंजय।
उदासीनवदासीनमसक्तं तेषु कर्मसु।। ९
मयाध्यक्षेण प्रकृतिः सूयते सचराचरम्।
हेतुनानेन कौन्तेय जगद्विपरिवर्तते।। १०

7. *All beings, O Son of Kunti, come to My own primordial nature, Prakriti, at the end of a cycle (kalpa); and again at the beginning of the next I release them in various forms.*
8. *Controlling My primordial nature, Prakriti, I emit again and again this entire aggregate of beings and elements, which is help-less because of the control of Prakriti.*
9. *Nor do these acts bind Me, O Arjuna, as I remain neutral, above them, unattached to those karmas.*
10. *With Me as supervisor, primordial nature brings forth the animate and the inanimate world. Through this process as the cause, O Son of Kunti, the world keeps changing and revolving.*

According to the Vedic scriptures, half a kalpa (day of Brahma) lasts for 4,326,000,000 human years. That is the time period from the manifestation to the dissolution of the universe. When the universe is dissolved, all beings return to the primordial nature for aeons, and man-ifestation then begins again with the next half kalpa. This cycle goes on endlessly. The pure Self presides over the manifestation of Prakriti, of the universe with all its forms and names.

At the time of both dissolution and manifestation, the pure Self remains unaffected by actions performed by its primordial nature, Prakriti. The pure Self uses Prakriti to manifest the universe. The pri-mordial nature manifests both the animate and inanimate. During the manifestation and dissolution, all beings are helplessly swept up into the grand process. Ultimately the power over all beings rests with the Self. The process of manifestation occurs so that the beings that are manifest may elevate their consciousness and ultimately realize their identity with the universal Self. In Verse 10 the word *suyate* is used. It comes from the root "su" meaning to bring forth or to bring about pros-perity. Thus, the Self brings about the prosperity of all that is manifest.

अवजानन्ति मां मूढा मानुषीं तनुमाश्रितम् ।
परं भावमजानन्तो मम भूतमहेश्वरम् ।। ११

मोघाशा मोघकर्माणो मोघज्ञाना विचेतसः।
राक्षसीमासुरीं चैव प्रकृतिं मोहिनीं श्रिताः।। १२

11. *Only the foolish attribute to Me a lesser station when I assume human bodies—not knowing My supreme aspect, which is the great Lord of all beings.*
12. *Of vain expectations, with vain actions, their knowledge in vain, devoid of wisdom, they have resorted to the enticing, demonic, and evil nature.*

When there is a great need the Lord assumes a human form to help human beings attain awareness of the Supreme. In his human disguise the Lord seems to act like a human being, and ordinary people take Him as such. They are unable to appreciate His divine qualities that express themselves in His human form. Those who are confused and deluded do not understand and accept the presence of the Lord in a human body. Even for the wise it is difficult to comprehend how the finite vessel carries the infinite within, how the Lord can resort to a human body that moves about in this world. Many people disregard Him, and some even despise Him. What He stands for threatens deluded people who are infatuated with the objects and pleasures of the mundane world. They wish to cling to their values and attachments, so they react venomously to any kind of teaching that puts forth a contrary way of living. Thus, many of the great teachers of the world who advocated non-attachment and love were assassinated by those who frantically clung to the world. The worldly person stands for everything that is opposed to the bringers of light, and the bringers of light stand in opposition to the values of the worldly person.

The royal power that resides in every human being is very subtle and invisible and cannot be grasped by sense perception. That power is superior to all other powers. It dwells in every living creature from the minutest to the largest. The ignorant do not recognize and acknowledge that power of powers. In their deluded condition they despise the Lord by despising other human beings. But truth is always victorious. Their longings and actions eventually prove to be in vain because they are attached and resort to evil. They continue to act foolishly and wrongly, and thus create sorrow and misery for themselves. They are finally brought down by their own actions.

It is a law of Providence that the ignorant eventually suffer because their actions are motivated by the desire to fulfill their selfish ends. Selfishness contracts the human personality; it does not allow it to expand. But the law of life is expansion, and one who learns to expand his individual consciousness to the universal consciousness by being selfless and non-attached finds enjoyment in establishing himself in his true nature, which is peace, happiness, and bliss.

महात्मानस्तु मां पार्थ दैवीं प्रकृतिमाश्रिताः।
भजन्त्यनन्यमनसो ज्ञात्वा भूतादिमव्ययम्।। १३
सततं कीर्तयन्तो मां यतन्तश्च दृढव्रताः।
नमस्यन्तश्च मां भक्त्या नित्ययुक्ता उपासते।। १४
ज्ञानयज्ञेन चाप्यन्ये यजन्तो मामुपासते।
एकत्वेन पृथक्त्वेन बहुधा विश्वतोमुखम्।। १५

13. *The great-souled ones, however, resorting to the divine nature, devote themselves to Me with their minds on no other, knowing Me as the immutable origin of all beings and elements.*
14. *Always glorifying Me and endeavoring with firmness of observances and vows, always bowing with devotion, ever joined in yoga, they worship Me.*
15. *Others through the sacrificial observances in knowledge, in unity and multiplicity, worship Me in various ways, who am facing in all directions.*

Great men meditate and contemplate on the divine and thus attain a state of wisdom in which they identify themselves with divinity, and their nature becomes divine. Their minds remain one-pointed in the knowledge that the Lord is the first cause of all beings and is imperishable. With one-pointed devotion they dedicate their minds, actions, and speech to the Lord alone, and they serve the Lord through their pure devotion. They have a single desire to attain the goal of human life. All of their energies are thus directed toward the Lord. They are resolute in their disciplined way of living, and they practice discipline in all aspects of life. They see the Lord everywhere and in everyone. And they salute everyone because they know that the Lord dwells in every being.

There are others who perform sacrifices in the form of knowledge. Such a yogi surrenders all that he knows with his limited mind; he empties himself and opens himself to divine wisdom. Knowledge is a means to attain the goal of life. The wealth of a yogi is his knowledge; he has nothing but knowledge. He has no desires, wants, or attachments. In the path of self surrender, one surrenders all that he has, and the yogi has only his knowledge to surrender. Thus, the yogi sacrifices his knowledge and becomes one with the Absolute. He realizes the absolute one without a second. He does not go to a state of unconsciousness but remains fully conscious, identifying himself with the center of pure consciousness. That is the most profound state of wisdom and not a state of unconsciousness, as some modern psychologists assume.

There are others who serve the Lord in various ways. Some perform their duties skillfully with full devotion and with an attitude of selfless service. They follow the spiritual path with great determination. Such great people always work for the prosperity of all beings. Great men and mahatmas know the power of the Absolute to be the means by which society can prosper. Maintaining harmonious attitudes, they perform selfless actions for the well being of all people, and they are always enthusiastic in the spirit of selfless service. These great people are always modest, saintly, and generous. They always work for the welfare of both the individual and society.

अहं क्रतुरहं यज्ञः स्वधाहमहमौषधम्।
मन्त्रोऽहमहमेवाज्यमहमग्निरहं हुतम्।। १६

पिताहमस्य जगतो माता धाता पितामहः।

वेद्यं पवित्रमोंकार ऋक्साम यजुरेव च।। १७

गतिर्भर्ता प्रभुः साक्षी निवासः शरणं सुहृत्।

प्रभवः प्रलयः स्थानं निधानं बीजमव्ययम्।। १८

तपाम्यहमहं वर्षं निगृह्णाम्युत्सृजामि च।

अमृतं चैव मृत्युश्च सदसच्चाहमर्जुन।। १९

16. *I am the sacrificial act, I am the sacrifice, I am the offering given to the saintly ancestors, I am the herb of oblation, I am the mantra, I am the clarified butter, I am the fire, and I am the act of burning the offering.*

17. *I am the father of this world, mother, sustainer, grandfather, the one to be known, the purifier, OM, Rig-Veda, Sama-Veda, as well as Vajur-Veda.*

18. *I am the goal, nurturer, master, witness, dwelling, refuge, friend, origin, dissolution, place, pledge, the imperishable seed.*

19. *I scorch; I release the rain and hold it back also. I am the principle of immortality as well as death, existence as well as non-existence, O Arjuna.*

The Lord is the self-existent reality. He is never born and therefore is not subject to change, death, or decay. He remains the same in the past, present, and future. The origin and dissolution of the universe is all within Him. He is both immortal and mortal. He exists and yet does not exist. Nothing exists without His existence. Therefore, He is everything.

When a ritual is performed and a sacrifice is offered, the collection of herbs used for the offering, the mantras, the clarified butter to be offered to the fire, and the act of offering are all different forms of the same principle: Brahman. The dedication, the offering, the fire, the oblation offered, and the one who offers are all Brahman. The giver, the enjoyer, the food, and the eater are nothing else but Brahman. Although objects in the world seem to be different from one another, they are in fact various aspects of the same Reality. As various kinds of ornaments are made out of the same gold metal, so the underlying principle of different forms, names, and objects of the world is one and the same.

The Lord is the father and mother of this universe. The universe arises from Him, it is sustained by Him, and it is finally absorbed into Him alone. The highest Lord is OM; the syllable OM is the designator of the Lord. The phrase *avati iti* OM means "one who protects is called OM." Only the Lord protects, and no one else. All four Vedas—Rig, Sama, Yajur, and Atharva—praise the same supreme Lord. They are also aspects of the Lord. The fire, sun, moon, stars, wind, water, and earth are but forms that have come from one absolute reality. The aspirant should be constantly aware of only one reality though he experiences that Reality in various names and forms. When one becomes aware of the unity in diversity, he realizes the pure Self, the Self of all.

त्रैविद्या मां सोमपाः पूतपापा
    यज्ञैरिष्ट्वा स्वर्गतिं प्रार्थयन्ते।
ते पुण्यमासाद्य सुरेन्द्रलोकमश्नन्ति
    दिव्यान्दिवि देवभोगान्।। २०
ते तं भुक्त्वा स्वर्गलोकं विशालं क्षीणे पुण्ये मर्त्यलोकं विशन्ति।
एवं त्रयीधर्ममनुप्रपन्ना गतागतं कामकामा लभन्ते।। २१
अनन्याश्चिन्तयन्तो मां ये जनाः पर्युपासते।
तेषां नित्याभियुक्तानां योगक्षेमं वहाम्यहम्।। २२

20. *The master of three sciences (vidyas) who drink soma and whose sin is purified, having performed sacrifices, seek to reach heaven. They, reaching the meritorious world of the king of gods, enjoy the celestial pleasures of gods in heaven.*

21. *They, having enjoyed that vast, celestial world, upon the exhaustion of merit, enter the world of mortals, thus resorting to the law of threefold existence! Desiring desires, they remain in the cycles of coming and going.*

22. *Those people, however, who having no other, worship contemplating Me, I bear their prosperity in this world and the next as they are ever joined to Me in yoga.*

Those who enjoy the objects of the world and desire to have the same enjoyment in heaven perform good deeds. Good deeds like charity, sacrifice, and austerities are no doubt superior to selfish deeds. But reaping the fruits of one's actions, even if the actions are good, brings only momentary happiness. One who performs good deeds enjoys the fruits of his actions in the yonder world, but even heavenly enjoyments do not bring everlasting happiness. After experiencing joys in the yonder world, one is reborn again and returns to the mortal world. But the aspirant who is fully committed to Self-realization devotes his whole life to the Lord alone, desiring neither worldly pleasures nor heavenly joys. And the Lord looks after and protects those who are totally absorbed in Him. Their happiness never diminishes; it is everlasting.

The Vedas expound three different vidyas: sukta vidya (knowledge of good utterances and thoughts), yajur vidya (knowledge of sacrificial acts), and sama vidya (knowledge of meditation and devotion). The aspirant who wishes to obtain the objects of his enjoyment makes efforts with good thoughts, good actions, meditation, and devotion to increase those pleasures. Such an aspirant is called a sakama (desiring) worshipper. The vast majority of aspirants worship and perform devotional practices and various types of rituals and sacrifices in order to secure specific desires. In today's world most people pray to God to fulfill their wants. They worship God to secure the fruit that will give them enjoyment. Whatever good they do in the world is to secure objects that bring pleasure, and they aspire to have pleasure in heaven as well. That is called sakama upasana, devotion with a motive.

In ancient times aspirants performed various kinds of sacrifices for the sake of prosperity, for the sake of the common good, or to fulfill desires for earthly enjoyments. Some aspirants performed a special kind of ritual called soma sacrifice. Those who used to drink soma wanted their mundane desires fulfilled. In ancient times soma sacrifice was performed as a ritual, and the preparations were done with austerities. From the very beginning the ritual was performed with a single motive in mind, which helped the participants to concentrate on the specific motive for which the ritual was performed. Much has been written in the Vedic scriptures about soma: the way it was obtained, prepared, and used while performing sacrifice. It is said that soma is a creeper found in the higher mountains and that when its juice is extracted, it creates a delightful intoxication and stimulation in the mind. The ancients knew a profound way to extract the juice of the soma creeper and often used it in their rituals. It has been said that soma has the capacity to help the aspirant make his mind concentrated by bringing about a supersensual joy.

The yogic method of drinking soma is entirely different and unique, and only a fortunate few yogis know how to derive soma from within and thus remain elevated in their spiritual endeavors. When the yogi applies *khechari mudra* by inserting his tongue upward behind the roof of the palate, from there he tastes the soma or nectar that is everflowing from Brahma randhra, a cavity in the crown of the head. With the help of that nectar, the yogi prolongs the span of his life. Those who do not know how to take that nectar remain brutish because that ever-flowing nectar is then taken by the kundalini. That is why the primal force in the human body, kundalini, remains intoxicated and asleep. Depriving kundalini of that nectar, the yogi consciously drinks it himself. When the primal force, kundalini, does not receive the nectar, she wakes up and ascends through all the *chakras* to the final abode at *sahasrara* chakra. Then all that has been unconscious and unknown comes forward, and one attains the knowledge of unity. This is one of the rarest practices experienced by yogis. It requires an accomplished yogic pose and bandhas (locks) along with khechari mudra. This method of taking soma leads the yogi to a state of divine intoxication in which he is aware of the Self only. The external way of extracting soma from herbs is far inferior to this method.

The ancient soma has been compared to the natural and synthetic hallucinogenics used today such as mescaline, peyote, and LSD. Though these are different from soma, they may well be in the same family of hallucinogens and may produce similar results. People today take such drugs for various purposes, and their experiences match their purposes as well as vividly bringing forth latent impressions from the unconscious. If one is preoccupied with sensory pleasure, such pleasure is greatly heightened by hallucinogens. And if one is inclined toward spiritual experiences, it is those experiences that are heightened. Except for the use of peyote by American Indians, today there is no systematic ritual to direct the hallucinogenic experience along beneficial lines, though modern experimenters have attempted to develop ritualized and guided hallucinogenic sessions with that purpose in mind.

There is considerable controversy today about whether hallucinogens are beneficial or harmful. Arguments have been put forth for both the positive and negative effects of their use. It is true that psychoactive drugs can lead one to intense concentration on a single object, and that concentration can lead one to a vivid exploration of the unconscious, to altered states of consciousness, to a sense of transcending time, and to the awareness of the illusory nature of one's ordinary mode of experiencing. One then sees that his ordinary reality is insubstantial and only a relative reality. Yet one may ask, as vivid as these experiences might be, are they genuine or merely hallucinations? Are they the same as those experiences of the yogis who develop concentration and a one-pointed mind through their own efforts? It seems that hallucinogens merely bring forth that which is already in one's unconscious mind. They give one a glimpse of supersensual realms and of the powers and forces that underlie the material world experienced by the senses. But such drugs cannot lead one beyond his already developed capacities to know, comprehend, and enjoy the subtle realms and underlying truths. And they cannot lead one beyond manifestation to experience the unmanifest Brahman.

While hallucinogens may help one to become less identified with the waking reality and to become aware of alternate realities, one who uses them may pay a great price for ingesting them. The experience itself gives a shock to the nervous system, and if one is not prepared for such experiences, he can become emotionally disturbed. The intense energy released through such experiences drains one and subsequently leads him toward a tamasic state, from which it takes one some time to recover his energy. Repeated use may lead one to become "burned out," depressed, and unable to perform his actions in the world. Thus, he does not accomplish the purpose of his life. He becomes passive and dependent on such experiences and in between slips back to a state of inertia and lethargy.

There is no shortcut to Self-realization. The path must be followed with determination. Through self-discipline one must attain non-attached action, meditation, and contemplation. Actions performed with motives or desires do not lead to everlasting happiness. Yogis therefore devote their whole lives to performing actions without any desire to reap the fruits of their actions. Such great yogis lead society and live for the welfare of others, for they do not have any selfish desires.

येऽप्यन्यदेवता भक्ता यजन्ते श्रद्धयाऽन्विताः।
तेऽपि मामेव कौन्तेय यजन्त्यविधिपूर्वकम्।। २३
अहं हि सर्वयज्ञानां भोक्ता च प्रभुरेव च।
न तु मामभिजानन्ति तत्त्वेनातश्च्यवन्ति ते।। २४
यान्ति देवव्रता देवान्पितृन्यान्ति पितृव्रताः।
भूतानि यान्ति भूतेज्या यान्ति मद्याजिनोऽपि माम्।। २५

23. *Even those devotees of other deities who sacrifice endowed with faith, they too, O Son of Kunti, sacrifice to Me alone, even though in an inappropriate manner.*
24. *I alone am the receiver of the offerings of all sacrifices, and I alone am their master. However, they do not recognize Me as such and therefore they slip from Reality.*
25. *Those whose vows are directed toward gods go to the gods. Those whose vows are addressed to the ancestors go to the ancestors. Those who sacrifice to spirits go to those spirits. Those who sacrifice to Me come to Me.*

In any way one worships, whether it be to any god, deity, or other aspect of Brahman, he in fact worships Brahman alone. All worship, ritual, and prayer are offered to the one Brahman only, for Brahman alone exists without a second. All the reverence and respect shown by the worshipper is actually shown to Brahman. But the ignorant who do not recognize Brahman fall back to the world because of their ignorance. A worshipper identifies himself with the worshipped one. Those who worship spirits identify themselves with the nature of spirits, whereas those who worship Brahman identify with the nature of the Lord.

When a student starts seeking, he wants to try all the methods of sadhana mentioned in the scriptures. He does not have the patience to steadily practice one path but changes his path every now and then. Some of the ignorant ones even worship spirits because they do not have knowledge of the absolute Truth. These verses contain a warning to all seekers that they should carefully understand the various paths and select the pure and clear path that leads to Brahman alone. It is important for aspirants to select a valid and profound path so that they reach the highest Brahman. A competent teacher or yogi can help the student select the best path for him to follow.

पत्रं पुष्पं फलं तोयं यो मे भक्त्या प्रयच्छति।
तदहं भक्त्युपहृतमश्नामि प्रयतात्मनः।। २६
यत्करोषि यदश्नासि यज्जुहोषि ददासि यत्।
यत्तपस्यसि कौन्तेय तत्कुरुष्व मदर्पणम्।। २७
शुभाशुभफलैरेवं मोक्ष्यसे कर्मबन्धनैः।
संन्यासयोगयुक्तात्मा विमुक्तो मामुपैष्यसि।। २८

**26. Whoever offers Me a leaf, flower, fruit, or water, with devotion—
that gift of a person of controlled self, offered with devotion, I accept.**

27. Whatever you do, sacrifice, or give, whatever austerities you per-
form, O Son of Kunti, surrender that as an offering unto Me.
28. Thus, you will be freed from the bondages of actions whose fruits
are beautiful or ugly; your self, united in the yoga of renunciation,
liberated, will reach Me.

The Lord accepts any offerings no matter how insignificant- even a leaf, flower, fruit, or a small amount of water—if it is given with full devotion. This does not mean that aspirants should use only these objects for worship. It means that which is important is the feeling of devotion. The Lord does not need anything, for everything already belongs to Him. Offerings are only expressions of devotion.

Those who offer the fruits of their actions to others without any selfish motivation, no matter how big or small the fruits, are making offerings to the Lord. Learning to give is a great virtue. It is as good for oneself as it is for others. By offering fruits, one learns giving and is benefited in two ways: he practices non-attachment and acknowledges the presence of the Lord in others. Thus, giving is a step toward non-attachment and at the same time acknowledges the presence of God in all beings.

Verse 26 teaches the aspirant to give or offer whatever he can according to his capacity. Those who acquire this habit cannot stop giving, and finally they give all that they have as an offering to the Lord. Giving and giving up bring one and the same result. These two virtues are the highest of all and help the aspirant in self-unfoldment. Any self-less action performed is a devotion to the Lord.

When the aspirant dedicates everything to the Lord and directs all his energy with mind, action, and speech to the Lord alone, his actions and the fruits of his actions no longer bind him. Actions performed as worship to the Lord do not create bondage. Great men solely dedicate their lives and perform all their actions for the selfless service of mankind. They do not ever experience bad or good fruits of their actions because they live for the service of the Lord performed through service to mankind.

समोऽहं सर्वभूतेषु न मे द्वेष्योऽस्ति न प्रियः।
ये भजन्ति तु मां भक्त्या मयि ते तेषु चाप्यहम्।। २९
अपि चेत्सुदुराचारो भजते मामनन्यभाक्।
साधुरेव स मन्तव्यः सम्यग्व्यवसितो हि सः।। ३०
क्षिप्रं भवति धर्मात्मा शश्वच्छान्तिं निगच्छति।
कौन्तेय प्रतिजानीहि न मे भक्तः प्रणश्यति।। ३१
मां हि पार्थ व्यपाश्रित्य येऽपि स्युः पापयोनयः।
स्त्रियो वैश्यास्तथा शूद्रास्तेऽपि यान्ति परां गतिम्।। ३२
किं पुनर्ब्राह्मणाः पुण्या भक्ता राजर्षयस्तथा।
अनित्यमसुखं लोकमिमं प्राप्य भजस्व माम्।। ३३

29. *I am alike to all beings; no one is hated or beloved of Me. However, those who devote themselves to Me with devotion, they are in Me; I am also in them.*
30. *Even if a person of very bad conduct devotes himself to Me following no other, he should be considered only saintly; he is embarked on right determination.*
31. *Very quickly he becomes a person whose self is virtuous and attains eternal peace. O Son of Kunti, do know for certain! My devotee does not perish.*
32. *Making themselves depend on Me, even the lowly born as well as women, traders, and servants reach the supreme status—*
33. *How much more so the meritorious brahmanas, devotees, and royal sages. Having come to this transient, unhappy world, do devote yourself to Me.*

Sri Krishna continues teaching Arjuna that the real Self maintains an attitude of evenness toward all beings. The supreme Brahman is never partial in any way. It has neither hatred nor favor for anyone. The aspirant who devotes his life to Brahman alone remains in Brahman consciousness, and Brahman dwells in him. When the yogi attains the height of tranquility beyond body, breath, senses, and mental consciousness and maintains constant consciousness of Brahman within himself, he realizes that there is none who is a friend to him and none whom he can hate. For he has gone beyond the pairs of opposites and has attained the state of evenness. His life is completely transformed because he realizes the omnipresence of Brahman within himself and himself in Brahman. It is just like a river meeting the ocean. When a river meets the ocean, it becomes the ocean. Constant consciousness of Brahman leads the yogi to attain such a state.

History reveals that many people of ill conduct were able to liberate themselves by becoming solely devoted to the Lord. Many such people after complete self-transformation became well known and respected sages. Having resolved all of their conflicts, even ill-behaved men can attain the height of equilibrium. Therefore, everyone has the opportunity to reform, improve, and unfold himself. That is possible when one turns his mind inward and with full concentration and meditation attains a state of tranquility. Tranquil-minded people neither hate nor lust. When the human mind wanders in the grooves of hatred and lust, it becomes blinded by the pairs of opposites. But one who has attained the summit of equanimity behaves with evenness. He then performs his duty righteously, impartially, and in a non-attached way. Such a sage attains everlasting peace and is not lost in the jungle of confusion. A true devotee of the Lord is in peace always.

Verse 32 states that even the lowly born and people without much intelligence can attain enlightenment if they devote their lives to the Lord alone. The words "lowly born" refer to those who do not get much opportunity to study and learn and who do not have means and amenities by birth. Those who do not have the opportunity to have a good upbringing can also attain the highest state.

Those who have already trodden the path in their past lives are born with certain virtues and samskaras that lead them again on the path of enlightenment. Then it is easy for them to accomplish or complete that which they could not in their previous lives. This lesson teaches all aspirants not to waste their time and energy in worldly plea-sures. It is best for them to devote all their time to God in this mortal world of ours. A life devoted to the Lord is the best of all lives. That is the purpose of human birth.

मन्मना भव मद्भक्तो मद्याजी मां नमस्कुरु।
मामेवैष्यसि युक्त्वैवमात्मानं मत्परायणः।। ३४

34. *Let your mind be fixed on Me. My devotee, sacrifice unto Me, bow unto Me. Intent on Me, thus joining yourself in yoga, you will come only to Me.*

The last verse in this chapter instructs the earnest aspirant to sys-tematically attain the highest state of perfection. The mind should be wholly applied and devoted to the real Self alone. The Lord of life seated in the deepest chamber of our being should be the sole object of med-itation. When the mind is not allowed to roam around but is focused on the Lord only, it is purified and becomes one-pointed and inward. When a meditative mind flows uninterruptedly to its object, it attains a state of tranquility, peace, and happiness.

A consistent method of meditation, contemplation, and prayer along with devotion to none else but the Lord helps one to attain this state. Such an aspirant sacrifices all the fruits of his actions to the Lord alone. His mind, action, and speech are fully dedicated to the Lord. His aim of life is the attainment of the Lord. Such yogis are liberated. They attain the highest perfection and become one with the highest.

Here ends the eighth chapter, in which the secret knowledge of the royal path, called raja vidya, is imparted.

Chapter Ten

The Glorious Manifestations
of the Lord

श्री भगवानुवाच

भूय एव महाबाहो शृणु मे परमं वचः।
यत्तेऽहं प्रीयमाणाय वक्ष्यामि हितकाम्यया।। १

न मे विदुः सुरगणाः प्रभवं न महर्षयः।
अहमादिर्हि देवानां महर्षीणां च सर्वशः।। २

यो मामजमनादिं च वेत्ति लोकमहेश्वरम्।
असंमूढः स मर्त्येषु सर्वपापैः प्रमुच्यते।। ३

The Blessed Lord said

1. *Furthermore, O Mighty-armed One, hear my supreme words, which I will tell you, with the wish to benefit you, loving one that you are.*

2. *The groups of gods do not know my origin nor do the great sages. I am indeed the origin of the gods and of the sages, one and all.*

3. *He who knows Me as unborn and beginningless, great sovereign of the worlds, not confused from among human beings, he is freed from all sins.*

The profound teachings imparted by Sri Krishna gradually dispel Arjuna's doubts. The heart of the divine teacher is like that of a mother who always wishes for the well being of her child. Teaching an important truth, Sri Krishna says that even the gods do not know the mighty Lord, and the sages also cannot comprehend His majesty. The gods and sages are born from the highest Lord; the Lord, being father of all, is the father of the gods and sages. They are his children. The Lord existed with all his glory and majesty long before the gods and sages. They are not able to understand the highest Lord in his profundity. One who knows the Truth realizes that the highest Lord of the universe was never born, that He is without beginning and end, that He is eternal and infinite. True knowledge is knowing the Lord who is without beginning and end. He is eternal and perfect. He does everything selflessly for the spiritual unfoldment of all beings, and it is for that purpose that He manifests the universe. He is kind and merciful in looking after the welfare of even the smallest of creatures. Realizing that truth, the aspirant also leads a selfless life and serves those who are weaker than himself. One who practices selflessness becomes free from all sin and bondage. He becomes pure and liberated.

बुद्धिर्ज्ञानमसंमोहः क्षमा सत्यं दमः शमः।
सुखं दुःखं भवोऽभावो भयं चाभयमेव च।। ४

अहिंसा समता तुष्टिस्तपो दानं यशोऽयशः।
भवन्ति भावा भूतानां मत्त एव पृथग्विधाः।। ५

महर्षयः सप्त पूर्वे चत्वारो मनवस्तथा।
मद्भावा मानसा जाता येषां लोक इमाः प्रजाः।। ६

एतां विभूतिं योगं च मम यो वेत्ति तत्त्वतः।
सोऽविकम्पेन योगेन युज्यते नात्र संशयः।। ७

4. *The discriminating faculty, knowledge, freedom from confusion, forgiveness, truth, control, pacification, comfort, discomfort, being, non-being, fear as well as reassurance;*

5. *Non-violence, equanimity, satiety, asceticism, charity, reputation, disrepute—all of these various kinds of situations of beings happen only from Me.*

6. *The seven ancient great sages and the four Manus, My aspects, were born of My mind, whose progeny are all these worlds and people.*
7. *He who knows this magnificence (vibhuti) and yoga in its reality here becomes united with unshakable yoga.*

All of the innumerable qualities such as intelligence and knowledge that exist in human beings arise from the ocean of infinity, the Lord Himself, as do the seven seers and the four *Manus* (law givers) who in turn give rise to all the creatures. The qualities are called bhavas (mental creations) of the Lord; they are the manifestations of the glory of the Lord, and the power that creates or manifests is the Lord's power. From the all-pervading mind of the Lord arise the mental entities. Intelligence and knowledge are ever-flowing streams from the ocean of infinity. The majesty of the Lord is displayed in the manifestation of the virtues mentioned in these verses. The aspirant who knows and is fully conscious that all manifestations arise from the Lord attains perfection.

The yogi is he who is in union with the Lord. When the yogi knows that happiness and misery, success and failure, fame and infamy are the bhavas of the Lord and that all creatures possessed of these bhavas have arisen out of the Lord, then in all situations he maintains a tranquil mind. For such a yogi every aspect of the universe is but an aspect of the mighty Lord Himself. One who remains in union with the Lord remains fearless.

अहं सर्वस्य प्रभवो मत्त: सर्वं प्रवर्तते।

इति मत्वा भजन्ते मां बुधा भावसमन्विता:।। ८

मच्चित्ता मद्गतप्राणा बोधयन्त: परस्परम्।

कथयन्तश्च मां नित्यं तुष्यन्ति च रमन्ति च।। ९

तेषां सततयुक्तानां भजतां प्रीतिपूर्वकम्।

ददामि बुद्धियोगं तं येन मामुपयान्ति ते।। १०

तेषामेवानुकम्पार्थमहमज्ञानजं तम:।

नाशयाम्यात्मभावस्थो ज्ञानदीपेन भास्वता।। ११

8. *I am the origin of all; everything proceeds from Me. Thinking thus, the wise, filled with the sentiment of devotion, devote themselves to Me.*
9. *Their minds absorbed in Me, their pranas entering into Me, enlightening each other, narrating about Me, they are ever satisfied and ever delighted.*
10. *To them who are ever joined in yoga and who devote themselves with pleasure and love, I confer that yoga of wisdom whereby they come close to Me.*
11. *Dwelling in their inner Self, to favor them, out of compassion I destroy their darkness born of ignorance with the brilliant lamp of knowledge.*

The Lord is the source of all manifestation. In the whole of the universe there is not a single object that is not dependent on the Lord. The fundamental cause of all is the highest Lord. Knowing that truth, the aspirant fixes his mind solely on the Lord and dedicates his life to Him. That dedication brings knowledge of the Lord to him, and he then imparts that knowledge to other aspirants. Such a devotee sings the praises of the Lord and always remains joyful. The aspirant who practices yoga without interruption secures that knowledge. He always remains in union with the Lord. The pure knowledge received from that union removes all ignorance and enables the aspirant to achieve anything and everything that is to be achieved.

One who has firm faith, full confidence, and devotion to the Lord alone remains fearless and carries out the sacred mission of the Lord. He has lifelong dedication to the Lord and gladly courts death while carrying out the divine mission. He walks on the earth fearlessly and gives the message of fearlessness to others. To impart that knowledge becomes his prime duty; he teaches the knowledge of the divine in a simple and lucid manner wherever he goes. He always sings the song of divine joy, which gives him the highest of happiness. One whose life is fully dedicated with mind, speech, and action to the Lord alone remains ever filled with divinity. Such a great one is called a perennial yogi. In all situations of life, his sadhana is never interrupted. His love of life is service to the Lord, and with his heart and mind full of love for God, he always remains in sadhana. Sadhana becomes his life. One who has attained this buddhi yoga, the yoga of pure reason, always remains in union with the Lord. He perennially enjoys the love divine. In the mind and heart of such a yogi remains the presence of the Lord all the time. Because of pure knowledge, ignorance does not exist at all.

अर्जुन उवाच

परं ब्रह्म परं धाम पवित्रं परमं भवान्।
पुरुषं शाश्वतं दिव्यमादिदेवमजं विभुम्।। १२

आहुस्त्वामृषयः सर्वे देवर्षिर्नारदस्तथा।
असितो देवलो व्यासः स्वयं चैव ब्रवीषि मे।। १३

सर्वमेतदृतं मन्ये यन्मां वदसि केशव।
न हि ते भगवन्व्यक्तिं विदुर्देवा न दानवाः।। १४

स्वयमेवात्मनात्मानं वेत्थ त्वं पुरुषोत्तम।
भूतभावन भूतेश देवदेव जगत्पते।। १५

वक्तुमर्हस्यशेषेण दिव्या ह्यात्मविभूतयः।
याभिर्विभूतिभिर्लोकानिमांस्त्वं व्याप्य तिष्ठसि।। १६

कथं विद्यामहं योगिंस्त्वां सदा परिचिन्तयन्।
केषु केषु च भावेषु चिन्त्योऽसि भगवन्मया।। १७

विस्तरेणात्मनो योगं विभूतिं च जनार्दन।
भूयः कथय तृप्तिर्हि शृण्वतो नास्ति मेऽमृतम्।। १८

Arjuna said

12. *The supreme Brahman, the supreme abode, the supreme purifier are You, the eternal Spirit (Purusha), the divine first God, unborn and all-pervading.*

13. *So say all the sages and the celestial sages—Narada, Asita, Devala, and Vyasa—and You Yourself are also telling me so.*

14. *I believe all that You are telling me to be true, O Keshava. Neither*

gods nor demons know Your origin, O Blessed Lord.

15. *By yourself alone You know Yourself, O Unexcelled Spirit, O Nurturer of Beings, Lord of Beings, God of Gods, Master of the World.*

16. *It behooves You to tell me all Your celestial magnificences (vibhuti) by which magnificences You dwell pervading all of these worlds.*

17. *Ever contemplating You, how may I know You, O Yogi; in what aspects are You to be contemplated by me?*

18. *Tell me more in detail Your yoga and magnificence, O Krishna. Hearing this nectar-like speech, I am not satiated.*

Having received the knowledge directly, Arjuna realizes that the Lord is present everywhere. In these verses he praises the profound teachings of Sri Krishna with eagerness to know more about the Lord of life and of His glory. The supreme Brahman, the highest and holiest abode, is the final destination of all aspirants. The sages who have already trodden the path of light and have attained the purest knowledge have described the Lord as eternal, birthless, and infinite, the all pervading center of omnipresence. He is the Purusha found in the deep recesses of the city of life and throughout the universe. Sages like Narada, Asita, Devala, Vyasa, and many others who have attained Self-realization describe the Lord in one and the same way; their descriptions do not differ in any way.

The 14th verse explains that neither those who are godlike nor those who are demonic have any knowledge of the Lord. The words godlike and demonic are used respectively for students of good and bad character. In ancient times all kinds of students possessing various qualities used to study together in the *gurukulas, ashrams,* or places of learning where spiritual knowledge was imparted. Here the student would sit at the feet of his guru in order to learn the paths of spirituality and receive teachings on divine knowledge. It is said that *Indra,* the king of gods, and Virochana, the king of demons, stayed at the gurukula of Prajapati for many years to master the science and knowledge of the Self. But neither of the two could grasp that profound knowledge. The god's aim was the attainment of Self-realization, whereas the goal of the demon was the enjoyment of sense pleasures. Indra, being of a divine nature, stayed in the gurukula for one hundred years to accomplish his goal of Self-realization, but Virochana, the demonic king, abandoned his studies and went back to the world to enjoy its pleasures.

The highest Lord is sovereign among all gods; He is the master of the universe. It is He alone who knows Himself thoroughly. Though He is omnipresent and omnipotent. His manifestation differs from one place to another. Ordinary people do not know that the Lord is everywhere, that the presence of the Lord is in everything, even in the smallest molecule. Although Arjuna understands that the Lord is all pervading, he is eager to know the mystery of manifestation in diversity.

Aspirants like Arjuna who desire to meditate on the highest Lord fail to understand the idea of meditation on the imperceptible omnipresent. They wonder: If there is nothing concrete to meditate upon, how can one meditate? The Lord is formless. How is one able to meditate on the formless? How is it possible for one to meditate on something that has no shape, form, or size? That is Arjuna's question in Verse 17. All aspirants have one and the same question when they are made aware of the formless Lord of all. In the 18th verse Arjuna, realizing that in meditation he will have to concentrate his mind on some form, asks a specific question: he wants to know what is the special and significant manifestation (*vibhuti*) of the supreme Lord upon which he can focus his mind during meditation. Sri Krishna answers that question in the following verses.

श्री भगवानुवाच
हन्त ते कथयिष्यामि दिव्या ह्यात्मविभूतयः।
प्राधान्यतः कुरुश्रेष्ठ नास्त्यन्तो विस्तरस्य मे।। १९

अहमात्मा गुडाकेश सर्वभूताशयस्थितः।
अहमादिश्च मध्यं च भूतानामन्त एव च।। २०

आदित्यानामहं विष्णुर्ज्योतिषां रविरंशुमान्।
मरीचिर्मरुतामस्मि नक्षत्राणामहं शशी।। २१

वेदानां सामवेदोऽस्मि देवानामस्मि वासवः।
इन्द्रियाणां मनश्चास्मि भूतानामस्मि चेतना।। २२

रुद्राणां शंकरश्चास्मि वित्तेशो यक्षरक्षसाम् ।
वसूनां पावकश्चास्मि मेरुः शिखरिणामहम् ।। २३

पुरोधसां च मुख्यं मां विद्धि पार्थ बृहस्पतिम् ।
सेनानीनामहं स्कन्दः सरसामस्मि सागरः ।। २४

महर्षीणां भृगुरहं गिरामस्म्येकमक्षरम् ।
यज्ञानां जपयज्ञोऽस्मि स्थावराणां हिमालयः ।। २५

अश्वत्थः सर्ववृक्षाणां देवर्षीणां च नारदः ।
गन्धर्वाणां चित्ररथः सिद्धानां कपिलो मुनिः ।। २६

उच्चैःश्रवसमश्वानां विद्धि माममृतोद्भवम् ।
ऐरावतं गजेन्द्राणां नराणां च नराधिपम् ।। २७

आयुधानामहं वज्रं धेनूनामस्मि कामधुक् ।
प्रजनश्चास्मि कन्दर्पः सर्पाणामस्मि वासुकिः ।। २८

अनन्तश्चास्मि नागानां वरुणो यादसामहम् ।
पितृणामर्यमा चास्मि यमः संयमतामहम् ।। २९

प्रह्लादश्चास्मि दैत्यानां कालः कलयतामहम् ।
मृगाणां च मृगेन्द्रोऽहं वैनतेयश्च पक्षिणाम् ।। ३०

पवनः पवतामस्मि रामः शस्त्रभृतामहम् ।
झषाणां मकरश्चास्मि स्रोतसामस्मि जाह्नवी ।। ३१

सर्गाणामादिरन्तश्च मध्यं चैवाहमर्जुन ।
अध्यात्मविद्या विद्यानां वादः प्रवदतामहम् ।। ३२

अक्षराणामकारोऽस्मि द्वन्द्वः सामासिकस्य च ।
अहमेवाक्षयः कालो धाताहं विश्वतोमुखः ।। ३३

मृत्युः सर्वहरश्चाहं उद्भवश्च भविष्यताम् ।
कीर्तिः श्रीर्वाक्च नारीणां स्मृतिर्मेधा धृतिः क्षमा ।। ३४

बृहत्साम तथा साम्नां गायत्री छन्दसामहम् ।
मासानां मार्गशीर्षोऽहं ऋतूनां कुसुमाकरः ।। ३५

द्यूतं छलयतामस्मि तेजस्तेजस्विनामहम् ।
जयोऽस्मि व्यवसायोऽस्मि सत्त्वं सत्त्ववतामहम् ।। ३६

वृष्णीनां वासुदेवोऽस्मि पाण्डवानां धनंजयः।
मुनीनामप्यहं व्यासः कवीनामुशना कविः।। ३७
दण्डो दमयतामस्मि नीतिरस्मि जिगीषताम्।
मौनं चैवास्मि गुह्यानां ज्ञानं ज्ञानवतामहम्।। ३८
यच्चापि सर्वभूतानां बीजं तदहमर्जुन।
न तदस्ति विना यत्स्यान्मया भूतं चराचरम्।। ३९
नान्तोऽस्ति मम दिव्यानां विभूतीनां परंतप।
एष तूद्देशतः प्रोक्तो विभूतेर्विस्तरो मया।। ४०

The Blessed Lord said

19. *Indeed I shall tell you of My celestial magnificences, but only the main ones, O Best of the Kurus. There is no end to my details.*

20. *I am the Self, O Master of Sleep, dwelling in the heart of all beings, and the beginning, the middle, as well as the end of all beings.*

21. *Of Adityas I am Vishnu; of luminosities I am the sun with rays; of Maruts I am Marichi; of heavenly bodies I am the moon.*

22. *Of Vedas I am Sama-Veda; of deities I am Indra; of senses I am the mind; of beings I am awareness.*

23. *Of the Rudras I am Shiva; of the Yakshas and Rakshasas I am Kuvera, the ruling deity of wealth; of the Vasus I am fire; of the high-peaked ones I am Meru.*

24. *Know Me, O Son of Pritha, the chief of the priests, Brihaspati. Of commanders I am Skanda; of the lakes I am ocean.*

25. *Among great sages I am Bhrigu; of speeches I am the one indestructible syllable OM; of sacrifices I am the sacrifice called japa; of immovable ones I am the Himalaya.*

26. *Of all the trees I am the holy fig; of celestial sages I am Narada; of Gandharvas 1 am Chitrartha; of adepts I am the sage Kapila.*

27. *Among horses know Me to be Uchchaihshravas born of the nectar of immortality; of the chiefs of elephants Airavata; and among human beings the king.*

28. *Of weapons I am the thunderbolt; of cows I am the celestial wish-fulfilling cow; of progenitors I am passion; of snakes I am Vasuki.*

29. *Among Nagas I am Ananta; of sea creatures I am Varuna; among ancestors I am Aryaman; of controlling ones I am Varna, the god of death.*

30. *Among Daityas I am Prahlada; among calculators I am time; among beasts I am the lion; among birds I am Garuda.*

31. *Among blowing ones I am wind; among weapon-bearers I am Rama; of fish I am the crocodile; among the streams I am the Ganges.*

32. *I am the beginning, the end, as well as the middle of creation. Of sciences I am the spiritual science; and of the discussants I am debate.*

33. *Of letters I am the letter A; of compounds I am the compound of duality (dvandva); I am the imperishable time, I am the ordainer facing in all directions.*

34. *I am the death that plunders all, and I am also the origin of those who will come in the future. Among feminine forces I am glory, affluence, speech, memory, intuitive wisdom, steadfastness, and forgiveness.*

35. *Of hymns I am Brhat-saman; of meters I am Gayatri; of months I am Margasirsha; of seasons I am the flowery spring.*

36. *Of deceiving ones I am gambling; of the brilliant I am brilliance; I am the victory, the initiator of determination, as well as the inner strength of those endowed with power.*

37. *Of Vrishnis I am Krishna; of Pandavas I am Arjuna; also among Munis I am Vyasa; and among those endowed with intuition I am Ushanas.*

38. *Of controlling ones I am the staff; of those desiring victory I am the essence of polity; of secrets I am silence; and of the knowing ones I am knowledge.*

39. *Whatever is the seed of all beings I am that, O Arjuna. There is no moving or unmoving entity that may exist without Me.*

40. *There is no end to My celestial magnificences, O Scorcher of Enemies; I have told this detail of My magnificences only by way of illustration.*

In these verses the vibhutas, the extraordinary powers and manifestations of the Lord, are enumerated. The word *bhuti* means victory, happiness, and strength, and the word *vibhuti* means having special power and great strength. The self-existent Reality is in the sun and in the smallest particle; it is in all that exists. But the ordinary person perceives the manifestation of the Lord in only a small number of things. He recognizes the presence of the supreme Lord only in such things as religious symbols, but in fact the Lord exists everywhere with one and the same equanimity. The ordinary person finds it difficult to realize that truth.

In this universe of ours, there are innumerable objects. Therefore, the manifestations of the Lord are endless. The supreme Self is the dweller in the heart of every being. He is the beginning, the middle, and the end of this universe. He is the Self of every being. There is not even the smallest unit of matter or energy over which He does not have governing authority. The entire universe is His divine expansion. For those who are not able to grasp this grand idea of the all-pervading nature of the Lord, seventy manifestations are mentioned in these verses. These verses explain only the prominent manifestations of the Lord. They are examples of the Lord's power to manifest rather than an all-inclusive list. These glorious and majestic manifestations of the Lord are mentioned in response to Arjuna's questions as to what the object of meditation should be. But for contemplators it is not necessary to choose such objects for the concentration of the mind because they are already aware of the omnipresent and omnipotent power in all objects of the universe, from the most minute to the most enormous.

Initially the meditator finds it difficult to control his dissipated mind. To aid those who are unable to meditate without a concrete object, the teacher recommends either a symbol, a light, or a sound that helps the student gather together the dissipated condition of the mind. In our long, unbroken lineage of meditation, it is recommended that the beginning meditator focus his mind on the flow of his breath. That makes one aware that all creatures of this universe are sustained by one and the same vital force, prana, the only one life giver for all creatures. Concentrating on the flow of the breath has two definite benefits. First, because mind and breath are closely linked, concentration on the breath makes the breath become smooth, even, and calm, and the mind also becomes stilled. Second, the aspirant becomes aware that there is only one force that sustains the entire universe and all creatures. The realization that there is one absolute Truth has immense philosophical value, for when one becomes aware that there is only one life force in all creatures, he learns to love all as he loves himself.

Sri Krishna gives many alternatives for aspirants who are prepared to meditate but do not know how to choose the objects of their meditation. He mentions the sun as one of these. Some manuals recommend gazing at the sun, but that can be injurious to the optic nerve and can lead one to lose his eyesight, so aspirants should not use gazing at the sun as the object of meditation. The scriptures offer a glimpse of how one should practice, but the meditational methods should be learned only under the guidance of a competent teacher. No yoga exercise— whether it be *hatha yoga,* pranayama, or *raja yoga*— should ever be practiced on one's own.

Having received the profound teachings of Sri Krishna, Arjuna is now eager to know the practical way of meditation. The experience of the ancients and those great ones who have already trodden the path of meditation guides students in their advancement. The scriptures say that the aspirant should first have profound knowledge of the universe and all its forms, and of Brahman from which this universe arises and by which it is sustained and returns to its primal source. Without having profound knowledge of the universe, the human being, the other creatures, and their relationship to one another, it is not of much use to abruptly begin the practice of meditation. Without building a profound philosophy, practice or sadhana remains incomplete.

The supreme Self is the Lord of all from whom arise all beings in the beginning, who sustains them in the middle, and to whom they return in the end. He is the origin of all. Nothing in the universe is excluded from this power of powers. Anything that is considered to be a special manifestation such as the sun, moon, stars, and oceans actually has the same presence of the Lord that exists in all things— animate and inanimate, large and small. The sun among objects that shine, the moon among the bodies of the solar system, the mind among the instruments of knowledge, OM among the sacred sounds, the king among men, the lion among the animals, Garuda among the birds, Rama among the brave, and Vyasa among the sages are some of the special manifestations of the Lord, although His manifestations are endless. After one becomes aware of the Lord's manifestations, he finally meditates on the highest Lord who is the source of light, life, knowledge, and the whole of the universe.

यद्यद्विभूतिमत्सत्त्वं श्रीमदूर्जितमेव वा।
तत्तदेवावगच्छ त्वं मम तेजोंशसंभवम्।। ४१
अथवा बहुनैतेन किं ज्ञातेन तवार्जुन।
विष्टभ्याहमिदं कृत्स्नं एकांशेन स्थितो जगत्।। ४२

41. *Whatever aspect there may be filled with magnificence, glory, or energy, know each and every one to be born of a particle of My brilliance.*
42. *Of what use is it for you to know much more? Only with a particle of Mine I dwell holding this entire world.*

Poets and sages vainly praise the grandeur, beauty, and loftiness of different aspects of the Lord's manifestation. But manifestations are only fragments of the beauty of the whole. There is only one pervading power, and this universe is just a fraction of its manifestation. Of what use is it to grasp a partial view? That is only a glimpse of the part and not the knowledge of the whole. To know partial truth is not to attain the knowledge of the infinite. "Therefore, Arjuna, attain the knowledge of the whole, the supreme Lord." Wherever grandeur, extraordinary beauty, or unusual loftiness exists, it is solely because of the Lord's manifestation. Whether that beauty is in human beings, animals, or any other aspect of manifestation in the universe, it is the Lord alone that smiles through all these faces.

Thus ends the tenth chapter, in which the teachings of Sri Krishna on the glorious manifestations of the Lord are explained.

Chapter Eleven
Yogic Vision

अर्जुन उवाच
मदनुग्रहाय परमं गुह्यमध्यात्मसंज्ञितम्।
यत्त्वयोक्तं वचस्तेन मोहोऽयं विगतो मम।। १
भवाप्ययौ हि भूतानां श्रुतौ विस्तरशो मया।
त्वत्तः कमलपत्राक्ष माहात्म्यमपि चाव्ययम्।। २
एवमेतद्यथात्थ त्वमात्मानं परमेश्वर।
द्रष्टुमिच्छामि ते रूपमैश्वरं पुरुषोत्तम।। ३
मन्यसे यदि तच्छक्यं मया द्रष्टुमिति प्रभो।
योगेश्वर ततो मे त्वं दर्शयात्मानमव्ययम्।। ४

Arjuna said

1. *Through the words of the supreme secret called spiritual knowledge, which You have taught out of Your grace and kindness to me, thereby this delusion of mine has vanished.*

2. *I have heard from You in detail of the creation and dissolution of beings as well as Your imperishable greatness, O You having eyes like lotus petals.*

3. *As You have spoken of Yourself thus, O Supreme Sovereign, I wish to see Your lordly form, O Unexcelled Spirit.*

4. *If you believe that it can be seen by me, O Lord, then show me Your immutable Self, O Lord of Yoga.*

This chapter is more important than the previous chapters, for it explains both aspects of the Lord: formless and with form. It also describes the goal of mankind. Arjuna understands that the highest secret of adhyatma (spiritual knowledge) has been imparted to him as a special grace. He also admits that the knowledge expounded by Sri Krishna has dispelled delusion from his mind. He has attained the profound knowledge of the origin of all manifestation and of the universe, for Sri Krishna has imparted the knowledge of the greatness of the supreme Brahman to him.

A great master of yoga, Sri Krishna now leads Arjuna further on the path of Self-awareness. Arjuna still has two desires. One is to have profound knowledge of the indescribable and ineffable power of Brahman. Brahman is formless and unmodifiable. It cannot be perceived by the sense organs nor known by the mind. Arjuna's other desire is to see the formless Brahman manifest into forms. He wants to experience both the abstract and concrete manifestations of Brahman. Arjuna requests Sri Krishna to lead him to direct experience of the self-existent power of the Lord.

श्री भगवानुवाच
पश्य मे पार्थ रूपाणि शतशोऽथ सहस्रशः।
नानाविधानि दिव्यानि नानावर्णाकृतीनि च।। ५
पश्यादित्यान्वसून्रुद्रानश्विनौ मरुतस्तथा।
बहून्यदृष्टपूर्वाणि पश्याश्चर्याणि भारत।। ६
इहैकस्थं जगत्कृत्स्नं पश्याद्य सचराचरम्।
मम देहे गुडाकेश यच्चान्यद्द्रष्टुमिच्छसि।। ७
न तु मां शक्यसे द्रष्टुमनेनैव स्वचक्षुषा।
दिव्यं ददामि ते चक्षुः पश्य मे योगमैश्वरम्।। ८

The Blessed Lord said

5. *See My multifarious, divine forms of many hues and configurations, by hundreds and by thousands.*

6. *See the Adityas, Vasus, Rudras, Ashvins, as well as Maruts; see many wonders that have not been seen before, O Descendant of Bharata.*

7. *Today see the entire world with everything animate and inani-*
   mate, here dwelling in one, in My body, O Master of Sleep, and
   whatever else you wish to see.
8. *However, you cannot see Me merely with this eye of your own. I*
   give you a divine eye. See My lordly yoga.

Sri Krishna says, "O Arjuna, I have innumerable forms of diverse colors and shapes. There are many miraculous things that you have not seen before. The whole universe, both animate and inanimate, exists in one part of My divine body. You are not able to see the whole of My form with your sense perception. Therefore, I will give you a *divya chakshu* (divine eye) through which you can see the form of the Lord as a whole."

According to yogic scriptures the yogi, who with the help of meditation uses his whole being for seeing, has a divine eye that gives him profound vision of the entire universe in a single glance. When the mind is led beyond the concepts and conditionings of time, space, and causation, it can fathom the unfathomable and attain a state of timelessness and infinity. A teacher who is a perfect master of yoga has the capacity to expand the consciousness of his beloved student, to open his divine eye. Sri Krishna performs *shaktipata:* he bestows that power and grace on Arjuna, enabling him to see the magnanimous form of the Lord. When the student has practiced meditation and when he is exhausted and all his efforts have failed, the yogi gives a profound touch to such a student, enabling him to open his divine eye. Sri Krishna, a great teacher and the greatest of yogis, opens Arjuna's divine eye so that he can have a vision of the power of the supreme Lord at one glance.

The yogi can open his own divine eye when he is able to bring his consciousness to the summit of the here and now. Mind is in the habit of either brooding on the past or imagining the future; it has no experience of the present. During meditation the mind is focused on the now and thus is capable of having a vision of past, present, and future simultaneously. That is called the timeless state of mind. One who has practiced meditation for a long time understands that it is possible for the meditator to know things happening in the future long before they occur in the external world. These experiences are not accidental or prophetic but are the outcome of a one-pointed mind, which has the capacity to go beyond the conditionings of time.

Ordinarily human beings can see the diverse forms of the Lord such as the sun, moon, stars, and other aspects of manifestation with the help of their eyes. But they do not have the capacity to see the entire universe. Therefore, it is necessary for Sri Krishna to bless Arjuna and open his divine eye. To see the whole universe, the form of the Lord, one needs divya chak-shu. Without a divine eye, the divine yoga cannot be experienced.

संजय उवाच

एवमुक्त्वा ततो राजन्महायोगेश्वरो हरिः।
दर्शयामास पार्थाय परमं रूपमैश्वरम्।। ९

अनेकवक्त्रनयनमनेकाद्भुतदर्शनम्।
अनेकदिव्याभरणं दिव्यानेकोद्यतायुधम्।। १०

दिव्यमाल्याम्बरधरं दिव्यगन्धानुलेपनम्।
सर्वाश्चर्यमयं देवं अनन्तं विश्वतोमुखम्।। ११

दिवि सूर्यसहस्रस्य भवेद्युगपदुत्थिता।
यदि भाः सदृशी सा स्याद्भासस्तस्य महात्मनः।। १२

तत्रैकस्थं जगत्कृत्स्नं प्रविभक्तमनेकधा।
अपश्यद्देवदेवस्य शरीरे पाण्डवस्तदा।। १३

ततः स विस्मयाविष्टो हृष्टरोमा धनंजयः।
प्रणम्य शिरसा देवं कृतांजलिरभाषत।। १४

Sanjaya said

9. *Having stated thus, O King, Krishna the Sovereign of great yoga showed to the son of Pritha his supreme, Lordly form—*

10. *Having many faces and eyes, with many wondrous views, wearing many divine ornaments, bearing many divine weapons held ready;*

11. *Wearing divine garlands and vestments, anointed with divine perfumes, comprising all wonders, the endless God facing in all directions.*

**12. *If there were to rise the brilliance of a thousand suns in heaven,
that would be similar to the brilliance of that great-souled One.***

**13. *Then the Pandava saw there in the body of the God of gods the
entire universe, divided multifariously, dwelling in One.***

**14. *Then possessed by amazement, that Dhananjaya, with his hairs
standing on end, with his hands clasped and bowing with his head,
addressed God.***

Let the reader remember that Sanjaya also had divya chaksu,
a divine eye. He was appointed to observe the entire battlefield, and
he submitted first-hand reports to the sage *Vyasa*. Vyasa recorded all
the teachings of the Bhagavad Gita that were imparted by the yogi Sri
Krishna to his beloved friend and disciple, Arjuna. Dhritarashtra, the
blind king, also requested Sanjaya to explain to him what was taking
place on the battlefield. Sanjaya told Dhritarashtra that Sri Krishna,
the great Lord of yoga, has opened Arjuna's divine eye and is showing
him the form of the highest Lord. That form has innumerable faces,
countless eyes, is endowed with all sorts of glistening ornaments, holds
countless weapons in His innumerable hands, wears many glistening
garlands and garments, and is full of divine fragrance. It is more lustrous than the light that thousands of suns could radiate.

Arjuna has this profound vision of the whole universe in the body
of the God of gods. Astonished, his hair stands on end; he bows with
praying hands and stands before the Lord. Bowing indicates submis-
sion and self-surrender; praying hands means that one is conscious that
the individual soul and the universal soul should unite. That union is
the purpose of human life. Praying hands is a gesture that the student
makes to his revered teacher. It is also the way of greeting someone in
Indian culture and means, "I bow to the divinity in you."

Sanjaya is able to see the universal form of the Lord because he
has the same divine eye as Arjuna. There are, in fact, other heroes in
the battlefield who are able to see the divine form of the Lord. They are
equally gifted by the grace of God and the grace of their yoga teachers. Although we often hear and use the word grace, it has never been

satisfactorily explained by philosophy and psychology. Grace comes to one who deserves it. It does not come out of desire. When the aspirant has attained a height of spiritual knowledge and when he has exhausted all human efforts, then dawns the knowledge to that deserving one who has honestly, sincerely, and truthfully followed the path of yoga. No doubt it is a gift received by the aspirant, a reward he receives to enable him to accomplish the task he has assumed. Many students without making sincere efforts pray to God for His grace. In their hearts and minds, they are fully aware that they do not deserve grace, yet they desire it. Desire not, but deserve, and you will have it.

अर्जुन उवाच

पश्यामि देवांस्तव देव देहे
    सर्वांस्तथा भूतविशेषसंघान्।
ब्रह्माणमीशं कमलासनस्थ
    मृषींश्च सर्वानुरगांश्च दिव्यान्।। १५

अनेकबाहूदरवक्त्रनेत्रं
    पश्यामि त्वां सर्वतोऽनन्तरूपम्।
नान्तं न मध्यं न पुनस्तवादिं
    पश्यामि विश्वेश्वर विश्वरूप।। १६

किरीटिनं गदिनं चक्रिणं च
    तेजोराशिं सर्वतो दीप्तिमन्तम्।
पश्यामि त्वां दुर्निरीक्ष्यं समन्ताद्
    दीप्तानलार्कद्युतिमप्रमेयम्।। १७

त्वमक्षरं परमं वेदितव्यं
    त्वमस्य विश्वस्य परं निधानम्।
त्वमव्ययः शाश्वतधर्मगोप्ता
    सनातनस्त्वं पुरुषो मतो मे।। १८

अनादिमध्यान्तमनन्तवीर्य-
    मनन्तबाहुं शशिसूर्यनेत्रम्।
पश्यामि त्वां दीप्तहुताशवक्त्रं

स्वतेजसा विश्वमिदं तपन्तम्।। १९

द्यावापृथिव्योरिदमन्तरं हि

व्याप्तं त्वयैकेन दिशश्च सर्वाः।

दृष्ट्वाद्भुतं रूपमुग्रं तवेदं

लोकत्रयं प्रव्यथितं महात्मन्।। २०

अमी हि त्वां सुरसंघा विशन्ति

केचिद् भीताः प्राञ्जलयो गृणन्ति।

स्वस्तीत्युक्त्वा महर्षिसिद्धसंघाः

स्तुवन्ति त्वां स्तुतिभिः पुष्कलाभिः।। २१

रुद्रादित्या वसवो ये च साध्या

विश्वेऽश्विनौ मरुतश्चोष्मपाश्च।

गन्धर्वयक्षासुरसिद्धसंघा

वीक्षन्ते त्वां विस्मिताश्चैव सर्वे।। २२

रूपं महत्ते बहुवक्त्रनेत्रं

महाबाहो बहुबाहूरुपादम्।

बहूदरं बहुदंष्ट्राकरालं

दृष्ट्वा लोकाः प्रव्यथितास्तथाहम्। २३

नभः स्पृशं दीप्तमनेकवर्णं

व्यात्ताननं दीप्तविशालनेत्रम्।

दृष्ट्वा हि त्वां प्रव्यथितान्तरात्मा

धृतिं न विन्दामि शमं च विष्णो।। २४

दंष्ट्राकरालानि च ते मुखानि

दृष्ट्वैव कालानलसन्निभानि।

दिशो न जाने न लभे च शर्म

प्रसीद देवेश जगन्निवास।। २५

अमी च त्वां धृतराष्ट्रस्य पुत्राः

सर्वे सहैवावनिपालसंघैः।

भीष्मो द्रोणः सूतपुत्रस्तथासौ

सहास्मदीयैरपि योधमुख्यैः।। २६
वक्त्राणि ते त्वरमाणा विशन्ति
दंष्ट्राकरालानि भयानकानि।
केचिद्विलग्ना दशनान्तरेषु
संदृश्यन्ते चूर्णितैरुत्तमांगैः।। २७
यथा नदीनां बहवोऽम्बुवेगाः
समुद्रमेवाभिमुखा द्रवन्ति।
तथा तवामी नरलोकवीरा
विशन्ति वक्त्राण्यभिविज्वलन्ति।। २८
यथा प्रदीप्तं ज्वलनं पतंगा
विशन्ति नाशाय समृद्धवेगाः।
तथैव नाशाय विशन्ति लोका-
स्तवापि वक्त्राणि समृद्धवेगाः।। २९
लेलिह्यसे ग्रसमानः समन्ता-
ल्लोकान्समग्रान्वदनैर्ज्वलद्भिः।
तेजोभिरापूर्य जगत् समग्रं
भासस्तवोग्राः प्रतपन्ति विष्णो।। ३०
आख्याहि मे को भवानुग्ररूपो
नमोऽस्तु ते देववर प्रसीद।
विज्ञातुमिच्छामि भवन्तमाद्यं
न हि प्रजानामि तव प्रवृत्तिम्।। ३१

Arjuna said

15. O God, I see in Your body all the gods as well as groups of differ-entiated beings, Brahma, the Lord sitting on the lotus seat, all the seers, as well as celestial serpents.

16. I see You having many arms, bellies, faces, eyes, with unending forms in all directions. O Sovereign of the universe, bearing uni-versal forms, I see not Your end nor the middle nor again Your beginning.

17. *I see You bearing a crown, a mace, a discus; You are a heap of light effulgent in all directions, very difficult to look at, immeasurable, and all around brilliant like a blazing fire and the sun.*

18. *You are the indestructible syllable, the supreme object of knowledge; You are the transcendental repository of this universe; You are the immutable One, the guardian of eternal law (dharma). I believe You to be the eternal Spirit.*

19. *I see You without beginning, middle, or end; of unending virility, with endless arms, with the moon and the sun for Your eyes; Your face like a blazing fire that receives oblation offerings, scorching this universe with your effulgence.*

20. *This interval between heaven and earth is indeed pervaded by You alone, and so are all the points of the compass. Seeing this fearsome, wondrous form, all the three worlds are disquieted, O Great-souled One.*

21. *Those groups of gods are entering You, some of them affeared, singing praises to You with hands clasped. The groups of great sages and adepts saying "may it fare well" praise you with ample hymns.*

22. *Rudras, Adityas, Vasus, Sadhyas, Vishve-devas, Ashvins, Maruts, Ushmapas, Gandharvas, Yakshas, Asuras, and Siddhas, in many groups, look at you and are all amazed.*

23. *Your great form with many faces and eyes, O Mighty-armed One, with many arms, thighs, and feet, with many bellies, terrible with many jaws—seeing it, all the worlds are troubled with fear, and so am I.*

24. *Touching the sky, blazing with many hues, with mouth wide open, with huge, burning eyes—-seeing You, with my inner self trembling in fear, I do not find consolation or peace, O Vishnu.*

25. *Seeing Your mouths terrible with jaws that appear like the fire of time, I lose the sense of direction and find no solace. Be pleased, O Lord of gods, the dwelling place of the universe.*

26. *Those sons of Dhritarashtra together with all the groups of kings, Bhishma, Drona, and Suta's son Kama together with our own chief warriors—*

27. *They hasten and enter Your mouths, which are fearsome and awful with jaws; some, stuck in the interstices of Your teeth, are seen with their heads crushed to powder.*

28. *As the many flows of the waters of rivers run only toward the ocean, so the brave warriors of the human world burning on all sides are entering Your mouths.*

29. *As moths with increasing speed enter the blazing fire for their destruction, similarly the worlds with increased speed also enter Your mouths toward their destruction.*

30. *With flaming tongues You are swallowing from all sides all the worlds with burning mouths. Filling the entire world with efful- gences. Your terrible lights are scorching it, O Vishnu.*

31. *Do tell me who are You of fearsome form? Salutations to You, Best of gods. Do be pleased. I wish to know You, the first One; do not know Your movement at all*

Arjuna, having seen the cosmic form of the divine Lord, is aston- ished and terrified. That vision overwhelms him, and he says, "O Lord, I see in Your cosmic body all the divine powers, the king of Gods, Brahma, seated on the lotus, sages, and serpents." He sees that the Lord of lords is not only merciful but also the cruel fire of annihilation. To accept life and the universe with all its diversities is wisdom.

That which is pleasant is not necessarily good, and that which is good is not necessarily pleasant. Pain and pleasure are inseparably mingled. They have separate realities only on the gross level of consciousness. That which is visualized by the ordinary man is limited because of his limited sense perception. When consciousness travels upward toward the higher realms of life, the vision is completely different. That which is pleasant or painful on the gross level of consciousness is not then pleasant or painful but is something different and extraordinary in its nature.

When the mind becomes inward, it encounters the reality of inner dimensions of life, and one is astonished to see how the sense percep- tions are distorted on the gross level of consciousness. Here one can examine, analyze, and understand the limitations of sense perception.

When the whole mind becomes an eye, it captures the vision of the subtle realms within, with all their profundities. It is able to grasp unfathomable levels by itself, without the help of the sense organs. It is able to analyze and judge as a witness, as a seer of the unknown and unfathomable levels of life.

When the mind floats in the divine consciousness of infinite knowledge, it is able to see the causes of all the gross manifestations seen by the sense organs. That diversity which is seen on the gross level of consciousness does not exist in the inner world because in the causal world everything remains inseparably mingled. That which is lawful and unlawful, good and bad, pleasant and unpleasant in the external world is not experienced in the same way. That which is seen as a tree, a mountain, or an ocean in the external world is seen in the causal realm as a seed in its subtle potential form. In that realm apprehension and comprehension are totally different.

The sage sees things as they are in their totality, in an unbroken undivided form, whereas the ordinary mind is unable to have the vision of the whole for lack of a divine eye. Prolonged association with the objects of the world creates attachment for the human mind and obscures the vision of the whole. But when the divine eye is opened, one's previous values regarding the objects of the world change, and a new level of life is fathomed. Then the reality is experienced in an entirely different light.

The aspirant who has not raised the primal force, kundalini, experiences the lowest and grossest level of life, the projections of his lower mind, and sees only evil, devils, and demons because he is under the influence of his lower nature. But when the primal force is awakened and when this ascending force of consciousness fathoms higher and more subtle levels of life, the aspirant has the vision of the finer forces of life related to the aesthetic sense of mind. He then sees all things as beautiful. If one sees something from one angle it looks ugly, but if he sees the same thing from a different angle it looks exceedingly beautiful. It depends upon one's vantage point. When one attains a higher level of consciousness with the force of the ascending divinity within, he sees things entirely differently: he experiences joy, happiness, and peace. One experiences no confusion or conflict, for there one neither sees divisions, nor does he see things in a partial way. Then he is aware of one unbroken entity.

If we view all these things—the gross, subtle, and subtlest levels–at one glance and put them together and see them as a whole rather than separately, that vision will be overwhelming. When one goes to the innermost level of consciousness from which spring all the diverse forms of the universe, he comes to know that the manifestation of diversity has only one source, which we call unity. Unity in diversity is the law of life. When one is able to visualize both, he becomes astonished at the difference between the apparent reality and the underlying Reality.

With his divine eye, Arjuna is able to have the profound vision of the whole universe being born and dying, going to the depths of the unmanifested One, and then all forms arising anew. That vision makes him realize that his grief and despondency are self-created because of his attachment to objects and relationships of the mundane world. With the grace of God, a sage, or a competent teacher, the yogi is able to have divine vision. When the ascending force of human endeavor has attained its height, then dawns Shakti, the grace of the higher Self. Those who are fortunate to have that grace receive knowledge through vision and not through the mind.

The question arises: Why didn't Sri Krishna give Arjuna the divine eye in the very beginning? The answer is that Arjuna was not then prepared to have that vision. His mind was confused and plunged into sorrow. In the modern world, too, the aspirant goes to his teacher confused, and the teacher prepares him for experiencing the higher levels of consciousness. But until the student is fully prepared, the teacher does not impart the subtle knowledge and techniques. After Arjuna has accepted Sri Krishna as Lord incarnate and received the knowledge of life and the universe, he becomes eager to have a vision of the whole of the universe. After examining the objects of the world in a divided way, Arjuna now wants to see the whole form of the Lord, which contains all the innumerable forms of the universe. Yet that vision terrifies and astonishes Arjuna. When the student awakens the kundalini, he has similar experiences and sometimes becomes so terrified that he wants to abandon his practices. During that period the competent teacher helps him to continue his practices and to attain the highest level of consciousness.

श्री भगवानुवाच

कालोऽस्मि लोकक्षयकृत्प्रवृद्धो

लोकान् समाहर्तुमिह प्रवृत्तः।

ऋतेऽपि त्वां न भविष्यन्ति सर्वे

येऽवस्थिताः प्रत्यनीकेषु योधाः।। ३२

तस्मात्त्वमुत्तिष्ठ यशो लभस्व

जित्वा शत्रून् भुङ्क्ष्व राज्यं समृद्धम्।

मयैवैते निहताः पूर्वमेव

निमित्तमात्रं भव सव्यसाचिन्।। ३३

द्रोणं च भीष्मं च जयद्रथं च

कर्णं तथान्यानपि योधवीरान्।

मया हतांस्त्वं जहि मा व्यथिष्ठा

युध्यस्व जेतासि रणे सपत्नान्।। ३४

The Blessed Lord said

32. *I am time waxing, destroyer of the worlds, moving here to gather back the worlds. Even with you all these will cease to be, the warriors who are standing in each of the armies.*

33. *Therefore rise and gain reputation; conquering the enemy, enjoy the prosperous kingdom. They are already killed by you; you become merely an instrument, O Expert at Shooting with the Left Hand.*

34. *Drona, Bhishma, Jayadratha, Karna as well as all the brave warriors—they are already killed by Me. Destroy them; do not suffer hesitation. Fight! You are going to be a winner of enemies in the battle.*

Arjuna is convinced yet bewildered by the vision, and he wants Sri Krishna to remove his confusion concerning the destructive aspect of the Lord. Sri Krishna says to Arjuna that the highest Lord has the capacity to annihilate and assimilate all the manifestations and beings in the same way that he has the capacity to create them. His power of annihilation should not be misunderstood as cruelty, for the Lord is compassionate and loves His children in exactly the same way that a loving mother loves her children. But if there is an abscess anywhere in the body, the mother takes her child to the surgeon to have it removed. It is a painful experience for the child, and he cries in the pain and agony that is experienced, but the mother knows that if the abscess is not removed it will infect the whole body. Similarly, Arjuna is aware of the fact that the army standing before him is unjust and unrighteous and that if it is not destroyed the unjust and unrighteous rulers will rule in unlawful ways and thus destroy the whole nation. Sri Krishna says to Arjuna, "Consider them already dead. Have you not seen them being annihilated by My force of destruction? Have you not seen them being swallowed by kala (time)? All things in this mortal world are subject to time; everything is annihilated by time. Therefore, Arjuna, you are only an instrument. Fight the battle, for it is the battle of the upward march to final liberation. You should accomplish the mission of your life by establishing the kingdom of dharma. You are only an instrument."

सञ्जय उवाच

एतच्छ्रुत्वा वचनं केशवस्य
 कृतांजलिर्वेपमानः किरीटी।
नमस्कृत्वा भूय एवाह कृष्णं
 सगद्गदं भीतभीतः प्रणम्य।। ३५

अर्जुन उवाच

स्थाने हृषीकेश तव प्रकीर्त्या
 जगत्प्रहृष्यत्यनुरज्यते च।
रक्षांसि भीतानि दिशो द्रवन्ति
 सर्वे नमस्यन्ति च सिद्धसंघाः।। ३६

कस्माच्च ते न नमेरन्महात्मन्।
 गरीयसे ब्रह्मणोऽप्यादिकर्त्रे।
अनन्त देवेश जगन्निवास

त्वमक्षरं सदसत्तत्परं यत्।। ३७

त्वमादिदेवः पुरुषः पुराण-

स्त्वमस्य विश्वस्य परं निधानम्।

वेत्तासि वेद्यं च परं च धाम

त्वया ततं विश्वमनन्तरूप।। ३८

वायुर्यमोऽग्निर्वरुणः शशांकः

प्रजापतिस्त्वं प्रपितामहश्च।

नमो नमस्तेऽस्तु सहस्रकृत्वः

पुनश्च भूयोऽपि नमो नमस्ते।। ३९

नमः पुरस्तादथ पृष्ठतस्ते

नमोऽस्तु ते सर्वत एव सर्व।

अनन्तवीर्यामितविक्रमस्त्वं

सर्वं समाप्नोषि ततोऽसि सर्वः।। ४०

सखेति मत्वा प्रसभं यदुक्तं

हे कृष्ण हे यादव हे सखेति।

अजानता महिमानं तवेदं

मया प्रमादात् प्रणयेन वापि।। ४१

यच्चावहासार्थमसत्कृतोऽसि

विहारशय्यासनभोजनेषु।

एकोऽथवाप्यच्युत तत्समक्षं

तत्क्षामये त्वामहमप्रमेयम्।। ४२

पितासि लोकस्य चराचरस्य

त्वमस्य पूज्यश्च गुरुर्गरीयान्।

न त्वत्समोऽस्त्यभ्यधिकः कुतोऽन्यो

लोकत्रयेऽप्यप्रतिमप्रभाव।। ४३

तस्मात्प्रणम्य प्रणिधाय कायं

प्रसादये त्वामहमीशमीड्यम्।

पितेव पुत्रस्य सखेव सख्युः

प्रियः प्रियायार्हसि देव सोढुम्।। ४४

अदृष्टपूर्वं हृषितोऽस्मि दृष्ट्वा

भयेन च प्रव्यथितं मनो मे।

तदेव मे दर्शय देव रूपं

प्रसीद देवेश जगन्निवास।। ४५

किरीटिनं गदिनं चक्रहस्त-

मिच्छामि त्वां द्रष्टुमहं तथैव।

तेनैव रूपेण चतुर्भुजेन

सहस्रबाहो भव विश्वमूर्ते।। ४६

Sanjaya said

35. *Hearing these words of Keshava, his hands clasped, trembling, wearing a crown, bowing again and again, Arjuna addressed Krishna with a trembling voice, exceedingly afraid, prostrating.*

Arjuna said

36. *Aptly, O Lord of Senses, by glorifying You the world rejoices and is attracted with love toward You; the demonic ones are running in all directions, afraid; the multitudes of adepts are all bowing to you.*

37. *Wherefore should they not bow to You, O Great-souled One, the greatest, the creator even of Brahma in the beginning, endless. Lord of the gods, the dwelling place of the world. You the indestructible syllable, existent, nonexistent, and whatever is beyond these.*

38. *You are the first god, the ancient Spirit; You are the transcendental repository of this universe; You are the knower, the object of knowledge, and the transcendent abode. O, You of endless forms, this universe is spanned and permeated by You.*

39. *You are Vayu, Yama, Agni, Varuna, the moon, the progenitor, and great grandfather! Salutations, salutations be to You a thousand times, and again and even more again salutations, salutations to You.*

40. *Salutations in front of You and behind You; salutations be to You from all sides, O All. You of endless power and immeasurable*

stride fill and pervade everything totally. Therefore You are All.

41. *Thinking You my friend, whatever I said impetuously—O Krishna! O Yadova! O friend!—not knowing this glory of Yours, inadvertently as well as out of affection,*

42. *As I have been disrespectful out of jest in occasions of sport, sleep, or dining, alone or in the presence of others, O Infallible One, I beg You, who are immeasurable, to forgive me.*

43. *You are the father of the moving and unmoving world; You are the honorable, greatest guru. There is no one equal to You. How can anyone excel even in the three worlds, O You of unequalled power?*

44. *Therefore, bowing, with lowered body I seek your indulgence, You, who are the sovereign object of praises; like father to son, like friend to friend, like a dear one to the beloved O God You must forgive me.*

45. *Happy at seeing what was never seen before, yet my mind is trembling with fear. Show me, God, the same previous form; be pleased, O Sovereign of gods, dwelling place of the worlds.*

46. *I want to see You the same way as before, wearing crown, bearing mace, with discus in hand. Be of the same four-armed form, O Thousand-armed One whose form is the universe.*

Listening to Sri Krishna tell him that his enemies are already dead and that he should simply become an instrument to secure victory, the thought arises in Arjuna's mind that the Lord has done so much for him. He realizes that he is not accepting the victory that is so kindly being granted to him. Trembling with fear and humility, he salutes the Lord and praises Him. "Trembling with fear" here means that when one encounters his own weaknesses and inadequacies he first tries to deny them. But when he faces them he becomes overwhelmed with emotion. He realizes his inadequacies, becomes humble, and wants to remove them. Sanjaya narrates this whole situation to the blind King Dhritarashtra.

The true yogi and aspirant always finds delight in exclaiming the qualities and powers of the Lord. He is devoted and thinks of the Lord all the time. He does not know how to think otherwise. He remains overwhelmingly inspired by his experiences and thoughts of the divine. The wicked, however, do not make efforts to understand and know the glory of the Lord. They do not like to hear about the Lord, for in their egoism they consider themselves lords unto themselves. They keep themselves away from *satsanga* (company of the sages). But the day comes when even the wicked become disappointed with the fleeting enjoyments of the world. Then they realize the existence of God and pray to Him for His forgiveness.

Only the humble and awakened enjoy listening to the talks of the great sages. Those who are awakened know that the Lord is the first cause of the whole universe, the fountainhead of all knowledge, the One who is the final abode of all. He manifests this universe and pervades it. His is the only power that appears in many ways such as agni (fire) and *vayu* (the vital breath). The fire of life and the vital breath are thus the Lord's own aspects. He is infinite, having infinite forms. It is the Lord alone who protects; He is the teacher of teachers, and His glory cannot be equaled.

Those who are aware of the greatness of God remain in delight and sing the praises of the Lord. There are only a fortunate few who are in love with the Lord. The wicked remain away. The Lord of life and the universe is the first cause, complete in Itself. Therefore He is worthy of salutations. The sages follow the path of divinity, for there is only one truth without a second.

When one realizes that unity in diversity and knows that there is only one truth and that all forms are but the forms of only One, then service to all becomes service to oneself. Hating others is hating oneself; loving all is loving oneself. On this code is founded the dharma of mankind. The duty of mankind is to love all and exclude none.

Many enjoy singing the song of the Lord when they see the excellence of the Lord in the universe. Whether they know the Lord or not and whether they are conscious of it or not, admiring the beauty of any aspect of the Lord is in fact admiring the highest Lord. Both the wicked and the sage are manifestations of the Lord. Anything that exists in the universe is His manifestation. Whenever a person is attracted to anything, he is in fact drawn to the glory possessed by the Lord. The sages and yogis experience and realize that truth, whereas others spontaneously appreciate God's creation but are not aware of the omnipresence of the Lord. The ignorant person acts under the influence of his ignorance. If he first acquires right knowledge and then learns to admire God's creation, he will be liberated. The mind of an ignorant person is delighted by the charms and temptations of the world and in fact the delight, too, is part of the Lord's nature. Whatever man describes, acts, and feels is actually the description of the Lord only. The Lord is the first cause of all. He is complete in Himself. The wicked are afraid of Him, but the accomplished yogi delightfully salutes Him.

All the things existing and nonexistant, animate and inanimate, and beyond these are but the Lord's own form. Whatever is beyond *sat* (that which exists) and *asat* (that which does not exist) is also the Lord's form. His external gross form is called asat, for it goes through change and destruction, but His subtlest form is not subject to change. The Lord is most ancient, ever existent, and the refuge of the whole universe. He is the object, the knowledge, and the knower. In any direction one moves, he cannot go anywhere but to the Lord, who has countless forms: Vayu (the vital breath), Yama (the Lord of Death), Agni (fire), Varuna (the Lord of Water), Chandra (the moon), Prajapati, Vishnu, Shankara and so on. All there is is the Lord Himself. All these aspects of the divinity have different functions, but they function because of the power of the Lord. As one human being plays many roles and is called by various names according to the actions and roles he performs, so is the case with the Lord, whose aspects of manifestation differ in quality, action, and form yet have arisen from one absolute truth: Brahman.

Arjuna formerly related to Sri Krishna merely as a friend, for he did not know his greatness. Now that Arjuna has seen the cosmic form of the Lord, he asks to be pardoned for having treated Sri Krishna lightly. He prays to Sri Krishna to forgive him for any disrespect. Most people jokingly lie or say things that are not true because they are not aware of the truth. They do not know that the Lord is both within and without and that all the strength for whatever one does is received from one and the same source: the Lord. Arjuna, whose heart is purified by Sri Krishna, realizes that, but those whose hearts are not pure do not realize the truth. The Lord is the father of all that moves and moves not. He is the highest of ail preceptors. There is none equivalent to Him. In all three realms of consciousness—gross, subtle, and subtlest—there is only One present all the time, and that is the Lord.

One who devotes his life to the Lord alone is forgiven by the Lord as good parents forgive their child. The Lord is very kind and forgives all those who pray to Him. The aspirant should pray to the Lord for forgiveness of his blunders. Prayer strengthens constant awareness. Without constant awareness one slips from the path and wastes his time and energy doing things that are harmful to himself and others. Prayer gives strength, and repentance prevents the aspirant from doing that which is harmful.

Astonished by what he has been shown and still fearful, Arjuna says, "O Lord, be pleased and show me Thy gentle form." Arjuna prays to Sri Krishna, who shows him *chaturbhuja* (his four-armed form). Having heard this request Sri Krishna, with full affection for his dear devotee, looks at Arjuna and responds.

श्री भगवानुवाच
मया प्रसन्नेन तवार्जुनेदं
रूपं परं दर्शितमात्मयोगात्।
तेजोमयं विश्वमनन्तमाद्यं
यन्मे त्वदन्येन न दृष्टपूर्वम्।। ४७
न वेदयज्ञाध्ययनैर्न दानै-
र्न च क्रियाभिर्न तपोभिरुग्रैः।
एवंरूपः शक्य अहं नृलोके
द्रष्टुं त्वदन्येन कुरुप्रवीर।। ४८
मा ते व्यथा मा च विमूढभावो
दृष्टा रूपं घोरमीदृङ् ममेदम्।
व्यपेतभीः प्रीतमनाः पुनस्त्वं
तदेव मे रूपमिदं प्रपश्य।। ४९

सञ्जय उवाच
इत्यर्जुनं वासुदेवस्तथोक्त्वा
स्वकं रूपं दर्शयामास भूयः।
आश्वासयामास च भीतमेनं
भूत्वा पुनः सौम्यवपुर्महात्मा।। ५०

The Blessed Lord said

47. *Pleased with you, O Arjuna, I have shown you through the yoga of Self, this transcendent form of Mine-—consisting of light, being universal, being endless, being the first one—which was never seen by anyone other than you before.*

48. *Neither through the Vedas, sacrifices, or studies, nor by charities, nor by actions, nor by fierce ascetic observances, can I be seen in this form in the human world by anyone other than you, O the Bravest among Kurus.*

49. *Be not afeared, nor be confused seeing this, such a fearsome form of Mine. Dismissing your fear, with a happy mind, see again this same previous form of Mine.*

Sanjaya said

50. *The indwelling One having addressed Arjuna thus, showed him again his own previous form and consoled him, as he was afraid, the great-souled One again assuming a pleasant-looking body.*

These verses indicate that the universal form of the Lord can indeed be visualized. The aspirant can attain this profound vision of the form of the Lord by practicing *atma yoga,* by making full efforts, utilizing all human resources, and by the grace of the Lord. Anyone who dedicates himself to the Lord can have such a vision. True dedication requires that one attain non-attachment and tranquility, surrender the fruits of his action to the Lord only, and remember the Lord in every breath of his life. The Lord of life has a threefold mission: protection of the good, annihilation of evil, and establishment of the good conduct of life. Arjuna, having seen the cosmic vision of the Lord, dedicates himself to the Lord's mission.

Any aspirant who dedicates himself to the Lord will be able to see the universal form of the Lord as Arjuna did. But if the aspirant thinks that he can attain that profound vision through scriptural knowledge, by giving gifts, by doing good actions, or by performing rituals he is wrong, for that is not possible. There are two conditions that enable one to have such a vision of the Lord. First one should know atma yoga, and second he must receive the grace of the mighty Lord.

Sri Krishna says that the universal form of the Lord was never seen by anyone before. That means that only a fortunate few can have such a vision; it does not mean that no aspirant can ever have that vision. It should be remembered here that Sanjaya is also gifted with a divine eye, and he is equally astonished to see the vision of the cosmic Lord. Sri Krishna says, "O Arjuna, do not be frightened or dismayed by the cosmic form that you have seen. Maintain your balance and keep your mind tranquil, and now be aware of My human form once again."

The aspirant who practices kundalini yoga under the competent guidance of a yogi also attains profound visions while traversing from one level of consciousness to another. But only dedicated yogis who practice atma yoga and who deserve the grace of the Lord are able to see the vision described here in all its glory.

अर्जुन उवाच

दृष्ट्वेदं मानुषं रूपं तव सौम्यं जनार्दन।
इदानीमस्मि संवृत्तः सचेताः प्रकृतिं गतः।। ५१

Arjuna said

51. Seeing this pleasant, human form of Yours, O Krishna, I have recovered my senses and returned to my natural feelings.

Arjuna says, "Lord, having seen Thy human form, I have recovered my normal consciousness and have come back to my usual nature." This verse indicates that Arjuna's consciousness during the period in which he had the cosmic vision of the Lord was quite different from the experience one usually has during the waking state. Surely he was not dreaming either. It is a state of expanded consciousness and not of unconsciousness, for in a state of unconsciousness one does not remember what he sees or visualizes. It is a consciousness similar to that of samadhi, in which the mind remains tranquil yet the aspirant remains fully conscious. In fact it is a state between the sleeping state and samadhi. During *yoga nidra* (yogic sleep) the student learns to expand his consciousness yet remains in deep sleep. This can be called sleepless sleep. That which cannot be known during the waking, dreaming, and sleeping states can be known during yogic sleep. Opening the divine eye is similar to yogic sleep but not exactly the same. It is possible only when a perfect yogi does shakti pata, bestows grace to that student who has been faithfully practicing yoga and who has already attained a deep state of concentration and meditation yet still finds himself incapable of attaining the highest state of samadhi. One cannot attain samadhi by the application of human efforts alone: grace helps him to remove the last stumbling block.

Seeing a vision or opening the divine eye is a case of shakti pata in which the yogi opens the aspirant's third eye with his touch or gaze. But this is done only in rare cases and not in the way modern teachers claim to do it with anyone and everyone. Sri Krishna says that by practicing atma yoga and with the grace of God, the aspirant can also have a similar vision.

श्री भगवानुवाच
सुदुर्दर्शमिदं रूपं दृष्टवानसि यन्मम।
देवा अप्यस्य रूपस्य नित्यं दर्शनकांक्षिणः।। ५२
नाहं वेदैर्न तपसा न दानेन न चेज्यया।
शक्य एवंविधो द्रष्टुं दृष्टवानसि मां यथा।। ५३
भक्त्या त्वनन्यया शक्य अहमेवंविधोऽर्जुन।
ज्ञातुं द्रष्टुं च तत्त्वेन प्रवेष्टुं च परंतप।। ५४

मत्कर्मकृन्मत्परमो मद्भक्तः सङ्गवर्जितः।
निर्वैरः सर्वभूतेषु यः स मामेति पाण्डव।। ५५

The Blessed Lord said

52. *This form of Mine, very difficult to see, that you have seen— even gods are ever desirous of seeing this form.*

53. *Not through the Vedas, nor by ascetic observances, nor by charity, nor through sacrifices can I be seen in this nature as you have seen Me.*

54. *O Arjuna, only through devotion directed toward none other can I be seen, and known in reality, and be entered, O Scorcher of Enemies.*

55. *Performing My act, holding Me as supreme, My devotee, devoid of attachments, whoever is free of animosity toward all beings, he comes to Me.*

Sri Krishna says that the profound vision of the cosmic Lord that was seen by Arjuna is extremely difficult to attain. Those who tread the path of divinity aspire to have the same vision, but that vision cannot be received by studying the Vedas, by practicing austerities or self-mortification, by giving gifts, or by performing sacrificial rites. It can be experienced only when one has one-pointed devotion, *ananya bhava*, which means "I am not different." Only when the aspirant completely gives up all attachment to the people and objects of the world, dedicates his whole life to the service of mankind, and performs all his actions for the Lord alone can he visualize the universal form of the Lord and realize the pure Self. When the aspirant constantly practices the method of ananya bhava, he establishes a oneness with his real Self: he does not think of himself as different from the real Self. It is only possible to attain that state when one stops identifying with the objects of the world and establishes himself in his true nature.

Here ends the eleventh chapter, in which profound knowledge and vision of the cosmic Lord is imparted

Chapter Twelve
The Yoga of Devotion

अर्जुन उवाच
एवं सततयुक्ता ये भक्तास्त्वां पर्युपासते।
ये चाप्यक्षरमव्यक्तं तेषां के योगवित्तमाः।। १

Arjuna said

1. *Those devotees ever joined in yoga who worship You thus and those who worship the unmanifest indestructible syllable—among them which are the highest masters of yoga?*

Arjuna's vision of the Lord is only momentary, for he has to come down to the world of ordinary reality to perform his duty. But something unique occurs in Arjuna's life at that moment, and he develops great faith in the teachings of Sri Krishna. All miracles and visions experienced by the aspirant are actually the signs and symptoms that are experienced on the path, but they are not signs of attainment or fulfillment. The attainment is Self-realization.

The first verse of the 12th chapter puts forth a question that is raised in Arjuna's mind after he sees the vision of the Lord. Overwhelmed by that vision, Arjuna wants to know whether he should meditate on the form of the Lord or on the formless. The absolute truth is beyond the senses, mind, and intellect, and unless one attains that, final liberation is not possible. But if the final realization is attained, there is still another question to be answered: How should one conduct himself in the world? How should he function? After all, he still lives in the world of apparent reality. Sri Krishna is teaching Arjuna how to live in the external world.

श्री भगवानुवाच
मय्यावेश्य मनो ये मां नित्ययुक्ता उपासते।
श्रद्धया परयोपेतास्ते मे युक्ततमा मताः।। २

The Blessed Lord said

2. *Those who, ever joined in yoga, entering their mind into Me, worship Me, endowed with highest faith, I believe them to be the most united in yoga.*

Most people cannot fathom the idea of meditation on the Absolute, which is formless and attributeless. Only a fortunate few are able to attain that highest state of realization. The path of bhakti (devotion) is considered to be superior for those who are unable to realize the pure Self. It is difficult to conceive of meditating without a form or object on which to focus the mind. Sri Krishna, therefore, advises Arjuna to have a concrete form for the concentration of mind, and he teaches Arjuna to worship the manifest form of the Lord with firm faith. The aspirant cannot concentrate his mind if he has no faith in his heart and if he mechanically practices the technique of concentration. Whether one follows the path of bhakti or the path of jnana (Self-realization), a one-pointed mind is important, and that cannot be achieved without concentration. Concentration of mind and faith are essentials for treading either path. The ordinary sadhaka or aspirant should have a concrete form for concentration and meditation before his mind is prepared for the higher realms.

Sri Krishna says that those who are devoted solely to Him, who worship Him alone, are superior devotees. Such devotees have three positive qualities: full dedication of mind, complete dedication of their whole lives, and worship with full faith. It is only then that the fruit of devotion is secured. Then alone can one be considered to be a great devotee. Sri Krishna advises Arjuna to concentrate on an object that has qualities that will lead him toward reverence and devotion. If an object is chosen for concentration but the meditator does not appreciate its qualities, the mind cannot concentrate on that object. The object chosen for meditation should have qualities that enable the meditator to respond to it. Any manifest form of the Lord possessed of excellence that suits the aspirant can be used as the object of concentration. Any aspect of manifestation that can be concentrated upon with firm faith is helpful to the devotee. One who fully devotes his life to worshiping and concentrating on any aspect of manifestation with unshaken faith can attain perfection.

ये त्वक्षरमनिर्देश्यमव्यक्तं पर्युपासते।
सर्वत्रगमचिन्त्यं च कूटस्थमचलं ध्रुवम्।। ३
सन्नियम्येन्द्रियग्रामं सर्वत्र समबुद्धयः।
ते प्राप्नुवन्ति मामेव सर्वभूतहिते रताः।। ४
क्लेशोऽधिकतरस्तेषामव्यक्तासक्तचेतसाम्।
अव्यक्ता हि गतिर्दुःखं देहवद्भिरवाप्यते।। ५

3. *Those, however, who worship the indestructible syllable, the unmanifest that cannot be specified, the all-pervading, beyond thought, absolute, immovable, permanent One—*
4. *Who control the group of senses well, hold all to be alike everywhere, delight in benefiting all beings, they find only Me.*
5. *They have greater difficulty whose minds are drawn to the unmanifest; the unmanifest way is found with difficulty by those who are dwelling in bodies.*

Those who contemplate on the non-manifest Self beyond all forms think that saguna worship (the worship of form) is inferior to nirguna contemplation. Nirguna contemplation is focused on the absolute truth, which has no form, no name, and therefore no attributes. Although one cannot worship the formless, it can be a subject of contemplation.

Those who find delight in the contemplation of the formless, nameless, and attributeless Brahman think that the worship of God with form and name, with attributes, is inferior. The path of nirguna is difficult, and there are chances for the aspirant to slip. Ordinarily the mind needs a concrete object upon which to focus and rest, for the mind is in the habit of depending on concrete objects. It requires great preparation for the finest faculty of mind, buddhi, to be able to understand the difference between the Self and the non-self, the real and unreal. But when buddhi is sharpened, one has the capacity to go beyond the realm of forms. Only a fortunate few tread the path of pure reason.

ये तु सर्वाणि कर्माणि मयि संन्यस्य मत्पराः।
अनन्येनैव योगेन मां ध्यायन्त उपासते।। ६
तेषामहं समुद्धर्ता मृत्युसंसारसागरात्।
भवामि नचिरात्पार्थ मय्यावेशितचेतसाम्।। ७
मय्येव मन आधत्स्व मयि बुद्धिं निवेशय।
निवसिष्यसि मय्येव अत ऊर्ध्वं न संशयः।। ८

6. *However, they who renounce all actions unto Me, are intent upon Me, they worship Me, meditating with yoga directed to no other.*
7. *Their minds absorbed in Me, I soon become their deliverer from the ocean of death and worldly cycle, O Son of Pritha.*
8. *Settle your mind only in Me, enter your intellect into Me. Henceforth you will live only in Me. There is no doubt.*

Sri Krishna integrates the paths of devotion and knowledge. Seeing Arjuna's conflict in regard to saguna and nirguna practices, Sri Krishna states: (1) The Lord is the one single and highest goal of life; (2) Contemplate and meditate only upon the one truth without a second; (3) Concentration of the mind should not be on any object other than the Lord; (4) The entire sadhana of the aspirant is to be directed to the Lord alone; (5) All the faculties of mind, including buddhi, should be directed toward the Lord alone; (6) Dedicate all your actions and the fruits therein to the Lord alone; (7) Be a yogi; identify yourself with your essential nature instead of with the world. When the aspirant realizes his essential nature and performs his duties skillfully and with non-attachment, he remains victorious and free, liberated. He is free from the snare of death, from the mire of delusion, from the rounds of births and deaths.

The concepts of identification and identity are central to modern psychology. At first the child identifies with his parents. Later he identifies with other aspects of the apparent reality, so much so that he thinks of himself only as the apparent reality. He forms an identity or sense of who he is as a distinct individual, but that identity is actually based on complete confusion, for he has come to think of himself solely in terms of the world of forms and names. He takes certain qualities onto himself and attributes others to the world outside of him. According to yogic science such identifications are completely erroneous and mislead one so that he creates apparent separation, distress, and conflict for himself and others.

Sri Krishna exhorts the sadhaka to give up such false identification and instead of being absorbed in the world to allow himself to become completely absorbed in and identified with the supreme Lord. He tells Arjuna to enter into Him, to become one with Him so that there is no distinction. Then the sadhaka becomes an embodiment of the Lord. All of his actions are no longer his alone but are the actions of the Lord.

Many aspirants misapply this teaching. They think that they can become devoted to their teacher in the same way. And many teachers develop inflated egos and encourage their students to worship them and identify with them. Such identification merely produces carbon copies of the teacher: the aspirants walk like the teacher, dress like the teacher, and talk like the teacher. There are many such foolish students who have merely surrendered to the ego of another and have become dependent. Rather than giving up their illusions, they are ever more identified with and hypnotized by the illusory world of names and forms. Sri Krishna is not like other teachers. He asks the student to become free from the forms and names of the world and to identify instead with that which lies beyond, which is his true essential nature.

अथ चित्तं समाधातुं न शक्नोषि मयि स्थिरम्।
अभ्यासयोगेन ततो मामिच्छाप्तुं धनञ्जय।। ९
अभ्यासेऽप्यसमर्थोऽसि मत्कर्मपरमो भव।
मदर्थमपि कर्माणि कुर्वन्सिद्धिमवाप्स्यसि।। १०
अथैतदप्यशक्तोऽसि कर्तुं मद्योगमाश्रितः।
सर्वकर्मफलत्यागं ततः कुरु यतात्मवान्।। ११

9. *Now, if you cannot harmonize a stilled mind in Me, then desire to find Me through the yoga of practice, O Arjuna.*
10. *If you are not even capable of practicing, then become intent on My acts. Even performing actions for My sake, you will gain fulfillment.*
11. *Now, if you are unable to do even this, then resorting to My yoga, do renounce the fruits of all actions, with your mind and self under control.*

It should be understood that Arjuna is not only speaking for himself but represents all seekers and that Sri Krishna answers Arjuna's questions for all aspirants. Sri Krishna says to Arjuna, "If you cannot concentrate your mind on the form or on the formless Brahman, if you are not able to practice the worship of saguna or the path of nirguna, if you are not able to concentrate on Me, you can practice *abhyasa*, the path of performing actions for the Lord only. Even for the aspirant who cannot concentrate, meditate, or contemplate, there is a way to attain spirituality. Abhyasa means practicing, repeating the same method again and again until the goal is attained. In the path of spirituality the student may find himself incapable of attending to his sadhana regularly and punctually. For lack of discipline and orderliness, the aspirant may slip back to his old habit patterns. In such cases he should not abandon the path of spirituality but should again make sincere efforts and practice his sadhana and make it a regular routine.

Abhyasa should be done in an unbroken way; steady practice is needed. If the aspirant thinks that practicing sadhana for some time and then abandoning it for awhile will help him, he is wrong. One must make sincere and constant effort, regularly and punctually, toward the goal. If for some reason, such as ill health, an accident, or any other obstacle that arises, one cannot do his meditation, he should learn to dedicate the prime actions he performs—eating, drinking, sleeping, and so on—so that he can maintain constant awareness of the supreme Lord. He should say to himself, "I will do all actions for Brahman and dedicate all the fruits of my actions to Brahman." With that determination the mind starts flowing in only one direction. This form of practice is equally beneficial.

Many beginning students are stirred emotionally and overdo meditation. Then after a few days or months, they abandon their practices. It is not helpful to do that. One should be aware of his own capacity and improve himself gradually and steadily instead of being emotional, overdoing things, and sometimes going beyond his capacity. The motivation for doing sadhana should be strengthened gradually. A moderate way of life in eating, sleeping, and performing other duties should be developed.

In the beginning the student should learn to dedicate his prime actions, and gradually to dedicate all his actions. That brings about unbroken consciousness and awareness of Brahman. If the student is unable to dedicate all his actions, there is yet another way for him to become free from the bondage created by his actions: he should learn to dedicate or give up the fruits of his actions. If one lacks self-control, concentration of mind, and zeal to dedicate all his actions, then giving up the fruits of his actions is a way toward perfection. When the aspirant practices surrendering the fruits of his actions, in due course this way of being becomes part of his life. It is a profound and concrete worship.

Dedicating the fruits of one's actions is the easiest way for most people. But those who cannot even do that should learn to practice self-control according to their capacities and abilities and should cultivate the desire to have union with the Lord and to surrender whatever they can. Whatever act, great or small, that one can perform, surrendering its fruits will be helpful for his growth. If the aspirant follows a particular code of conduct according to which the fruits of his actions are not to be kept for his enjoyment, and if he gradually practices dedicating those fruits, slowly his desire for enjoyment will be reduced. Finally it will be reduced to the point of zero, and such desirelessness is a state of perfection.

श्रेयो हि ज्ञानमभ्यासात् ज्ञानाद्ध्यानं विशिष्यते।
ध्यानात्कर्मफलत्यागस्त्यागाच्छान्तिरनन्तरम्।। १२

12. Knowledge is better than practice; meditation is distinguished as greater than knowledge. Higher than meditation is renouncing the fruits of actions. Immediately after renunciation comes peace.

Continuing his comparison of various paths, Sri Krishna says that superior to sadhana is the path of knowledge, and higher than knowledge is the path of dhyana (meditation). The path of knowledge was discussed in the second chapter, and the method of dhyana was briefly described in the sixth chapter. In the eighth verse of this chapter the method Sri Krishna imparts is to focus the mind, intellect, and heart on the highest Self alone. But the aspirants who are not able to practice these paths should dedicate the fruits of their actions to the Lord. If the fruits of one's actions are not dedicated, no path of sadhana is helpful. Only by dedicating the fruits of his actions does one attain peace.

अद्वेष्टा सर्वभूतानां मैत्र: करुण एव च।
निर्ममो निरहंकार: समदु:खसुख: क्षमी।। १३
संतुष्ट: सततं योगी यतात्मा दृढनिश्चय:।
मय्यर्पितमनोबुद्धियों मद्भक्त: स मे प्रिय:।। १४
यस्मान्नोद्विजते लोको लोकान्नोद्विजते च य:।
हर्षामर्षभयोद्वेगैर्मुक्तो य: स च मे प्रिय:।। १५
अनपेक्ष: शुचिर्दक्ष उदासीनो गतव्यथ:।

सर्वारम्भपरित्यागी यो मद्भक्तः स मे प्रियः।। १६
यो न हृष्यति न द्वेष्टि न शोचति न कांक्षति।
शुभाशुभपरित्यागी भक्तिमान्यः स मे प्रियः।। १७
समः शत्रौ च मित्रे च तथा मानापमानयोः।
शीतोष्णसुखदुःखेषु समः संगविवर्जितः।। १८
तुल्यनिन्दास्तुतिर्मौनी संतुष्टो येन केनचित्।
अनिकेतः स्थिरमतिर्भक्तिमान्मे प्रियो नरः।। १९
ये तु धर्म्यामृतमिदं यथोक्तं पर्युपासते।
श्रद्दधाना मत्परमा भक्तास्तेऽतीव मे प्रियाः।। २०

13. *Bearing no animosity toward any being, amiable as well as compassionate, free of I, free of 'mine' holding pain and pleasure as equal, forgiving,*

14. *Always satisfied, with a controlled nature, of firm resolve, a yogi who has surrendered his mind and intelligence unto Me, who is My devotee, he is My beloved.*

15. *He from whom the world does not become excited, and he who does not become excited from the world, liberated from the agitations or exhilaration, intolerance, and fear, he is My beloved.*

16. *Free of expectation, pure, dextrous, neutral, free of insecurities, he who renounces expectations of fruits from all acts that he initiates, who is My devotee, he is My beloved.*

17. *He who neither rejoices nor hates, neither grieves nor desires, he who renounces all that is attractive or unattractive, whosoever is endowed with devotion, he is My beloved.*

18. *A like toward foe or friend, similarly toward honor or dishonor, alike toward cold and heat as well as pain and pleasure, devoid of attachment,*

19. *Equal to praise and censure, maintaining silence, satisfied with whatever; homeless, with stable intelligence, whosoever is endowed with devotion, that man is My beloved.*

20. *Those who follow this virtuous nectar of immortality that I have taught, maintaining faith, holding Me supreme, those devotees are My deeply beloved.*

These verses explain the characteristics of the best of devotees. Such a one hates none and loves all, is kind to all and treats everyone alike. For him there is no attachment to any particular person. He has no pride, regards misery and pleasure alike, forgives all, and practices spiritual sadhana regularly. Through his spiritual discipline he is able to control his senses. It is important to control the senses, for they distract and dissipate the mind. Without control over the mind and senses, sadhana is not possible. One who is not motivated by desire for sense enjoyment, who performs his duty with full determination, and who dedicates his skills to the Lord's work is dear to the Lord. He who does not despise anyone and whom no one despises is not affected by success or failure, anger or fear. He who is single-mindedly devoted to his duty and remains equally non-attached to gain and loss is dear to the Lord. One who is able to attain the state of tranquility, not caring for honor or dishonor, who is free from the pairs of opposites, who maintains silence, does not have any home for himself, whose mind is always one-pointed, and whose heart is full of faith regards the Lord as his own Self. Such a one who has secured the highest of knowledge is a blessed one.

To be perfect is to remove all the imperfections in mind, action, and speech. Verses 13 through 20 describe the following virtues, which an aspirant should acquire on the path of perfection: (1) Hatred is the root cause of all misery, for by hating others one isolates himself from the whole; therefore learn to love and give. (2) One should be a friend to all; he should not feel animosity toward anyone. (3) Kindness teaches one to be merciful and is a practical way of expressing one's love; therefore be kind and give. (4) "Mine and thine" are traps of maya that bind one with strong chains of attachment; do not become attached. (5) Do not possess anything, even a house of your own; preoccupation with accumulating wealth is hoarding and is a reflection of greed. (6) Egoism and pride reduce one to nothingness, for the ego makes one petty and separates him from the whole; full effort should be made to purify the ego. (7) When reaping the fruits of his actions, one should learn to be content; contentment is the highest of all wealth, and without it one remains unsatisfied and frustrated. (8) Expectation is a longing for enjoyment, and whether it is fulfilled or not, it creates dependency and robs the human dignity; expectation should be abandoned. (9) One should practice self-control, without which the mind cannot be made one-pointed and the energies cannot be concentrated. (10) A tranquil mind is undisturbed in all situations, favorable or unfavorable; one who has developed tranquility never grieves and is never deluded. (11) Determination builds courage and will power and leads to success in all spheres of life. (12) Firmness is a virtue that leads to fearlessness and self-reliance. (13) Non-attachment helps one to attain spiritual heights; it is the total absence of the desire for enjoyment. (14) Negative emotions lead one to extremes; positive emotions can be substituted, for example love in place of hate. (15) Giving up the fruits of one's actions brings great joy, freedom, and peace; one who gives up everything is the greatest lover of mankind. (16) One should remain a witness, a seer, not identifying himself with the seen. (17) With mind, action, and speech, one should be pure, free from stains and faults. (18) One should be vigilant, for carelessness becomes a stumbling block. (19) The desire for fruits is a hindrance in the path of skillful actions; give up that desire. (20) One who loves all receives love from all; the expression of love should be practiced in daily behavior by giving the best one has. (21) One who has totally dedicated his mind, heart, and intellect is a true yogi. (22) One who is courageous can face any calamity of life; he remains even in all conditions. (23) Faith is the greatest of all virtues provided it is based on pure reason and not mere belief. All of these virtues are the signs and symptoms of the great devotees of the Lord. Blessed are they who work hard to acquire these virtues and attain perfection.

This chapter is devoted to the path of bhakti yoga, the path of love and devotion. Many students think that this is the easiest path, and many consider it to be a path of emotionalism, but that is not the case. To love and to be in love is not easy. The path of devotion and love is as difficult as the paths of jnana and karma yoga. In fact it is more difficult because it requires single-pointed devotion toward the Lord alone, with purity of mind and heart. It is a conscious dissolution of one's individuality in the love of God. The path of love is full of giving without any expectation of reward whatsoever. It is not mere emotionalism but the height of ecstasy where the lover and beloved become one and inseparable. In this path there is no duality; there is no place for two. As the river meets the ocean, they become inseparably one. So it is in the path of devotion. Fortunate are those who are in love with the mighty Lord and remember His name in every breath. They remain free from the pangs of death. They are free from the rounds of births and deaths, for they remain wedded with the Eternal.

Here ends the twelfth chapter, in which the virtues that lead one to perfection are explained.

Chapter Thirteen

Knowledge of the Field and the Knower

अर्जुन उवाच

प्रकृतिं पुरुषं चैव क्षेत्रं क्षेत्रज्ञमेव च।

एतद्वेदितुमिच्छामि ज्ञानं ज्ञेयं च केशव।। १

श्री भगवानुवाच

इदं शरीरं कौन्तेय क्षेत्रमित्यभिधीयते।

एतद्यो वेत्ति तं प्राहुः क्षेत्रज्ञ इति तद्विदः।। २

Arjuna said

1. *I wish to know your primordial nature (Prakriti) and your conscious principle (Purusha)—the field and the field-knower, knowledge and the knowable—O Krishna.*

The Blessed Lord said

2. *O Son of Kunti, this body is called a field. He who knows this, him the experts in this matter call the field-knower.*

After imparting the knowledge of bhakti yoga, the yoga of divine love, Sri Krishna explains to Arjuna that the body is like a field that yields the ambrosial fruit. When the aspirant knows the importance of this field and knows the difference between the field and its knower, he finally realizes the Self. It is essential to have profound knowledge of the body and to look after it with utmost care. One who knows the importance of this body and knows that it is in the possession of Atman is wise indeed. Such an aspirant uses his body as an instrument to attain the purpose of life. In this chapter the word *kshetra* (field) is used to signify the body and *kshetrajna* (field knower) the individual soul. It is the duty of every human being to fully know the field in the form of the body. The field is both an individual's body and the body of the Lord. When one is realized, he is aware that the whole universe is his body.

The Lord alone is the proprietor of all the bodies in the universe, for He alone pervades all the bodies and has profound knowledge of them. The infinite bodies of this universe are like the fields of one farmer, the Lord. There is nothing that is not known by the Lord. The inner dweller in the human body is Atman, which is eternal and infinite in its essential nature. When the aspirant realizes his true Self, such a Purusha (individual soul) becomes *a purushottama* (the best of souls), for he attains Godhood. When the aspirant knows that there is no difference between himself and the universal form of the Lord, he realizes that he is Atman and that the whole universe is his field. The same Atman that dwells within him dwells in all of the universe. The relationship between Atman and the body, the knower and the field, and that between Atman and the universe is the same. Every aspirant should acquire knowledge of this relationship. If that knowledge is not gained, one's knowledge is false knowledge or illusion. Ordinary human beings suffer because of such false knowledge. Sri Krishna explains to Arjuna that the body is like a field, and the individual soul is the knower. Only the knowledge of both is considered to be true knowledge. Atman is the Lord of the body. As the beads of a necklace have a thread that passes through them, so the multifaceted universe has the universal Self running through and sustaining it.

Body and individual soul are related to one another in the same way that Prakriti is related to Purusha. The universe is the outcome of two fundamental principles of one Absolute without a second: Purusha (consciousness) and Prakriti (primordial matter). From Prakriti and Purusha all the animate and inanimate forms of the world are born, maintained, and destroyed. Nothing can exist without the Lord's Prakriti. All the manifestations in the universe are diverse forms of Prakriti.

क्षेत्रज्ञं चापि मां विद्धि सर्वक्षेत्रेषु भारत।
क्षेत्रक्षेत्रज्ञयोर्ज्ञानं यत्तज्ज्ञानं मतं मम।। ३
यत्क्षेत्रं यच्च यादृक्च यद्विकारि यतश्च यत्।
स च यो यत्प्रभावश्च तत्समासेन मे शृणु।। ४

3. *Know Me, O Descendant of Bharata, as the field-knower in all fields; that which is the knowledge of the field and of the field-knower, I hold that to be the true knowledge.*

4. *What that field is, of what kind, causing what products, and produced from what, and of what power and effect it is, hear that from Me briefly—*

When the aspirant attains profound knowledge of both Atman and the body, jnana and vijnana, he is fulfilled. In Upanishadic philosophy that knowledge is called the knowledge of discrimination through which one knows the difference between the real Self, Atman, and the temporal, mundane, or apparent reality of the phenomenal world. That knowledge should be imparted early in life so that one can know life as it is. During ancient times the serious student, called a brahmachari, lived in an ashram and practiced celibacy until the age of twenty-five. He devoted himself to learning that knowledge with a one-pointed mind. Different words have been used to designate that knowledge, but the knowledge of the Self and non-Self, of Atman and the phenomenal reality, of Purusha and Prakriti, of knower and the field is one and the same. In the *Brahma Sutra* the same knowledge that is imparted here is described in a well preserved and conclusive manner. Many sages of the past have also expounded that knowledge in various ways.

ऋषिभिर्बहुधा गीतं छन्दोभिर्विविधैः पृथक्।
ब्रह्मसूत्रपदैश्चैव हेतुमद्भिर्विनिश्चितैः।। ५
महाभूतान्यहंकारो बुद्धिरव्यक्तमेव च।
इन्द्रियाणि दशैकं च पञ्च चेन्द्रियगोचराः।। ६
इच्छा द्वेषः सुखं दुःखं संघातश्चेतना धृतिः।
एतत्क्षेत्रं समासेन सविकारमुदाहृतम्।। ७

5. *As sung of by the sages variously and by manifold Vedic mantras in different ways, as well as by the words of the sutras that teach about Brahman and that are definitive and logical.*
6. *The five great elements, ego, intelligence, and the unmanifest, the ten and one senses, as well as the five pastures of the senses;*
7. *Desire, aversion, pleasure, pain, the whole organism, awareness, sustenance—this is illustrated briefly as the field together with its products.*

In these verses Sri Krishna lists all of the components of Prakriti, the field. They are the constituents of the human body and the universe: earth, water, fire, wind, and space; ego sense; intelligence; non-manifest Prakriti; the senses of smell, taste, sight, touch, and hearing; the mouth, hands, feet, and the organs of procreation and excretion; mind; the five objects of the senses (smell, taste, form, touch, and sound); desire; hatred, pleasure and pain; the organism— aggregate of all; sentience; and sustenance. With these last seven entities Prakriti becomes thirty-onefold, and that thirty-onefold Prakriti is called the field. All of its constituents go through modification and change by intermixing and are thus able to create different forms. These modifications are constantly changing into various forms. They are the components from which the universe is built.

अमानित्वमदम्भित्वमहिंसा क्षान्तिरार्जवम् ।
आचार्योपासनं शौचं स्थैर्यमात्मविनिग्रहः ।। ८
इन्द्रियार्थेषु वैराग्यमनहंकार एव च ।
जन्ममृत्युजराव्याधिदुःखदोषानुदर्शनम् ।। ९
असक्तिरनभिष्वङ्गः पुत्रदारगृहादिषु ।
नित्यं च समचित्तत्वमिष्टानिष्टोपपत्तिषु ।। १०
मयि चानन्ययोगेन भक्तिरव्यभिचारिणी ।
विविक्तदेशसेवित्वमरतिर्जनसंसदि ।। ११
अध्यात्मज्ञाननित्यत्वं तत्त्वज्ञानार्थदर्शनम् ।
एतज्ज्ञानमिति प्रोक्तमज्ञानं यदतोऽन्यथा ।। १२

8. *Absence of self-praise, freedom from hypocrisy, non-violence, forgiveness, simplicity, service to the teacher, purity, stillness, self control;*

9. *A dispassionate attitude toward the objects of the senses, as well as the absence of ego, observing the flow of painfulness in birth, death, old age, and illness;*

10. *Freedom from attraction, freedom from attachment toward progeny, spouse, home, and so forth, and ever remaining even-minded when confronted with desirables or undesirables;*

11. *Undeviating devotion toward Me with single-minded yoga, fondness for solitary places, not delighting in gatherings of people;*

12. *Always dwelling in spiritual knowledge, insight into the meaning of true nature—this is said to be knowledge. Other than this is ignorance.*

These verses focus on putting knowledge into practice. To merely know something intellectually is not to have profound knowledge of it. We all know what to do and what not to do, but we do not know how to actualize that knowledge. Each of us understands certain fundamental truths about how to live, yet we do not know how to put them into practice. It is important to understand those truths from a practical viewpoint. In childhood one is instructed in all the fundamentals: to be good, nice, kind, and gentle. Yet he is not taught how to bring them into practice. Practicing truth is different from learning to know truth. These five verses describe qualities that are systematically developed in the path of yoga.

Pride, conceit, and thoughts of hurting and injuring others are characteristics of the ignorant. Kindness, gentleness, love, forgiveness, straightforwardness, service to one's elders and preceptors, and the steady practice of spirituality are the virtues and characteristics of the wise aspirant. If those qualities are lacking, one remains ignorant. All the virtues and weaknesses should be understood, and the virtues should be cultivated with all sincerity and firmness of will.

The student should practice these principles, which will enable him to expand his consciousness and to fathom the higher levels of consciousness. Then he is clearly treading the path of spirituality. For example, if one wants to practice loving others he should understand and practice ahimsa—non-harming, non-injuring, and non-hurting. f he is still running after sense enjoyments, craving the pleasures of the world, attached and haunted by worldly desire, then he is ignorant. That is not the path of spirituality. The first step of knowledge makes one aware of his shortcomings, and in the second step he learns to remove them. In the third step he acquires virtues like ahimsa, which is the singular expression of love. In the fourth step one completely abstains from those actions that are injurious to his growth.

Those who have firm faith in the inner dweller and who devotedly love the inner dweller, Atman, as the Lord of life are not attached to spouse, children, or home. When one attains evenness he loses all attachment to externals and strengthens his love for the true Self alone. Such an aspirant isolates himself and devotes his time and energy toward spiritual sadhana. He prefers to be in meditation and to remain in the company of the sages. But those who scratch the surface of the mundane world with their hearts filled with desires and who are not aware of the true Self within are ignorant. By studying the behavior of both the sages and the ignorant, one can see that their paths are totally opposite. One is the path of light and the other the path of darkness; one is the path of knowledge and the other is the path of ignorance. A person's behavior reflects certain characteristics that indicate whether he is knowledgeable or not. By studying human behavior—how one talks, thinks, and acts—we can understand who is on the path of knowledge and who is not. Kindness, forgiveness, non-attachment, and self-control are characteristics of the knowledgeable, whereas pride, conceit, hatred, egotism, attachment, and the desire for worldly enjoyments are characteristics of the ignorant.

ज्ञेयं यत्तत्प्रवक्ष्यामि यज्ज्ञात्वाऽमृतमश्नुते।
अनादिमत्परं ब्रह्म न सत्तन्नासदुच्यते।। १३
सर्वतः पाणिपादं तत्सर्वतोऽक्षिशिरोमुखम्।
सर्वतः श्रुतिमल्लोके सर्वमावृत्य तिष्ठति।। १४
सर्वेन्द्रियगुणाभासं सर्वेन्द्रियविवर्जितम्।
असक्तं सर्वभृच्चैव निर्गुणं गुणभोक्तृ च।। १५
बहिरन्तश्च भूतानामचरं चरमेव च।
सूक्ष्मत्वात्तदविज्ञेयं दूरस्थं चान्तिके च तत्।। १६
अविभक्तं च भूतेषु विभक्तमिव च स्थितम्।
भूतभर्तृ च तज्ज्ञेयं ग्रसिष्णु प्रभविष्णु च।। १७

13. *That which is the worthy object of knowledge I shall teach you, knowing which, one attains immortality. It is beginningless, supreme Brahman, which is said to be neither existent nor non-existent.*

14. *With hands and feet in all directions, with eyes, heads, and faces in all directions, having ears everywhere, He dwells covering everything in the world.*

15. *Appearing as though having attributes of all the senses yet devoid of all senses, unattached yet bearer of all, free of gunas yet receiver of gunas—*

16. *Immobile yet moving inside and outside beings, unknowable because of Its subtlety, It dwells far and is near.*

17. Undivided in the beings yet remaining as though divided, bearer of all the beings is that object of knowledge, the consumer and also the creator.

There is an Upanishadic prayer that states: "Lead me from the unreal to the real, from darkness to light, from mortality to immortality." Since ancient times man has been seeking immortality, something permanent, not darkness but light. The human being is striving to attain immortality, but he does not find anything immortal in the external world. The interior researcher knows that immortality resides in the depths of every human being. To attain that, the aspirant should first dive into the deepest level of his being. The highest of truths is beyond all comprehension by the human senses and mind. One should not waste his time and energy searching outside for that which is deeply buried within the tomb of the human body. That which is imperishable, unchangeable, without beginning and end, completely unattached, and shining with all its splendor resides in Its glory, all-pervading power, and majesty both within and without. It is very near and yet very far, undivided yet appearing to be divided. It is the only One to be known, for It is the highest Self, remaining ever present in the inner chamber of every being.

The student should practice to attain the profound knowledge of the highest Lord. From mortality to immortality, from the temporal to eternity is the only way of realizing the Truth. In this inward path, the student first learns to be non-attached, to have a one-pointed mind, and to remain content. This inward journey finally leads the aspirant to the abode of immortality.

ज्योतिषामपि तज्ज्योतिस्तमसः परमुच्यते।
ज्ञानं ज्ञेयं ज्ञानगम्यं हृदि सर्वस्य विष्ठितम्।। १८
इति क्षेत्रं तथा ज्ञानं ज्ञेयं चोक्तं समासतः।
मद्भक्त एतद्विज्ञाय मद्भावायोपपद्यते।। १९

प्रकृतिं पुरुषं चैव विद्ध्यनादी उभावपि।
विकारांश्च गुणांश्चैव विद्धि प्रकृतिसंभवान्।। २०
कार्यकारणकर्तृत्वे हेतु: प्रकृतिरुच्यते।
पुरुष: सुखदु:खानां भोक्तृत्वे हेतुरुच्यते।। २१

18. *That light of lights is said to be beyond darkness. The knowledge yet the object of knowledge, the goal of knowledge. It is established in the heart of all.*
19. *Thus briefly I have stated the field as well as knowledge and the objects of knowledge. Knowing this My devotee becomes ready for becoming Me.*
20. *Know the primordial nature Prakriti as well as the conscious principle Purusha both to be beginningless. Know the gunas as well as the products (vikaras) to be born of Prakriti.*
21. *Prakriti is said to be the cause in the matter of effect, instrument, and agency. Purusha is said to be the cause in apperception of pleasures and pains.*

When the aspirant understands the temporal and the Absolute, the field and the knower, he attains the highest state of truth. Compared to the knower (the Self), the field (the body) does not last for a long time. But that does not mean that the aspirant should not understand the body or that he should ignore it and not look after it, for the kshetra is the field of action through which creativity, arts, and the sciences find their expression. It is important to understand both units of life: the temporal (body, breath, senses, and mind) and the Self.

The yogi should learn to keep his body healthy so that he can attain the goal of life. Knowledge and the field of its expression should be understood clearly. The body can become a means but if not looked after, it can create a stumbling block and barrier. Loving the Self does not mean ignoring the body any more than loving someone means hating others. Our master used to say that the real Self should be loved, but at the same time hatred should not be created for the body. When the student goes to the deeper levels of his being, there is a tendency to ignore the body. But he should not forget that a healthy body is always a means, whereas a sickly body demands the attention of the sadhaka and interferes with his practice. Both a healthy body and a sound mind are essential for the sadhaka.

Sri Krishna reminds Arjuna that Purusha and Prakriti, the Lord and His power of manifestation, are ancient and without beginning. The student should know the modifications arising out of Prakriti and should know that effect and cause reside together in the causal form in Prakriti. When the individual soul becomes attached to the desire to experience pleasure, it also experiences misery, for in the absence of one the other exists. These two pairs of opposites arise from a single cause; that which is the cause of pleasure is also the cause of misery.

पुरुष: प्रकृतिस्थो हि भुङ्क्ते प्रकृतिजान्गुणान् ।
कारणं गुणसङ्गोऽस्य सदसद्योनिजन्मसु ।। २२
उपद्रष्टानुमन्ता च भर्ता भोक्ता महेश्वर: ।
परमात्मेति चाप्युक्तो देहेऽस्मिन्पुरुष: पर: ।। २३

22. *The conscious spirit Purusha, only dwelling within Prakriti, per-ceives the Prakriti-bound gunas. The cause of His birth in the good and bad bodies is His connection with the gunas.*
23. *Close observer, consenter, bearer and experiencer is the great Sovereign. The supreme Spirit in this body is also called the supreme Self, Parama-atman.*

In these two verses the student is asked to be a witness exactly as one's real Self is a witness. When the student practices meditation and withdraws the senses from the external world, his mind is not dis-tracted and disturbed by the dissipation of the senses. But even at that stage he has to encounter the flow rushing from the unconscious, which is the reservoir of all memories, impressions, samskaras, and merits and demerits of one's current and previous lives. How can one deal with such thoughts when they present themselves during meditation? If the meditator learns to observe his thoughts and all that comes from the unconscious—symbols, ideas, fancies, and fantasies—and does not become involved or identify himself with them, he can remain a witness. Without attaining that state, meditation is incomplete. The One who dwells in the heart of the cosmos is the same One who dwells in the body. In the individual body He is the master, and He is the same master and knower of the universe. Just as one and the same space is in the cup, in the room, and outside, the all-pervading Self is everywhere.

When the student is firmly established in the knowledge that the inner dweller, Atman, the supreme Self, resides in the body and also knows the external, mundane, and temporal world well, then whatever actions he performs do not create bondage for him. The aspirant who knows the pure Self, its manifestation, and its qualities and then learns to live in the world is free from the necessity of rebirth.

य एवं वेत्ति पुरुषं प्रकृतिं च गुणैः सह।
सर्वथा वर्तमानोऽपि न स भूयोऽभिजायते।। २४
ध्यानेनात्मनि पश्यन्ति केचिदात्मानमात्मना।
अन्ये सांख्येन योगेन कर्मयोगेन चापरे।। २५
अन्ये त्वेवमजानन्तः श्रुत्वान्येभ्य उपासते।
तेऽपि चातितरन्त्येव मृत्युं श्रुतिपरायणाः।। २६

24. *He knows the conscious spirit Purusha as well as the primordial nature Prakriti together with the attributes (gunas), even though operating in every way, he is not bound again.*
25. *Some see the Self by the Self within the Self through meditation; others by Samkhya or by yoga and yet others by the yoga of action.*
26. *Others not knowing thus, worship upon hearing from others. They too, intent upon learning from others, yet certainly conquer death.*

Sri Krishna distinguishes between four paths and says that Self-realization can be attained by each of those paths. On one path the aspirants practice the yoga of meditation to attain samadhi. In that path the journey from the gross self to the subtlemost Self is trodden systematically by the raja yogis and dhyana yogis. Those yogis practice *ashtanga yoga,* the eight limbs of yoga: *yama, niyama, asana, pranayama, pratyahara, dharana, dhyana,* and *samadhi.* Yama consists of five practices that help one relate to others with a sense of oneness, and niyama is comprised of five practices that lead to self-purification. Asana helps one to prepare the body for meditation through physical postures. Through pranayama one regulates the lungs, breath, and vital energy. Thus one prepares himself through his actions, postures, and breath to enable him to sit for meditation without being distracted by such things as the remembrance of deeds improperly performed, discomfort of the body, or irregular breathing. The aspirant next learns how to withdraw his senses (pratyahara) and then to concentrate his mind (dharana). Prolonged one-pointed concentration leads to meditation (dhyana), and prolonged steady meditation leads to samadhi.

Other aspirants tread the path of knowledge. They study the scriptures attentively and contemplate on the teachings of the Upanishads, the Brahma Sutra, and the Bhagavad Gita. When their contemplation is strengthened by pure reason, their buddhi becomes discriminative, and they understand the difference between the pure Self and the mere self. That is the path of knowledge, which finally leads the aspirant to Self-realization.

There is another group of aspirants who attain spiritual heights by performing their duties and dedicating all the fruits of their actions. They understand the nature of Prakriti and its gunas: sattva, rajas, and tamas. They perform their actions without any attachment and thus reach the highest level of consciousness. The fourth group of aspirants is not learned. They depend on the teachings imparted to them by the sages, and they strictly follow that knowledge with full faith and devotion. Their path is the path of devotion and faith, and it is faith that leads them across the mire of delusion. Having a pure heart and unflinching faith, they reach the shore of life. Various are the paths followed by the many aspirants for attaining spiritual knowledge. All those who make sincere efforts reach the summit.

यावत्संजायते किंचित्सत्त्वं स्थावरजङ्गमम्।
क्षेत्रक्षेत्रज्ञसंयोगात्तद्विद्धि भरतर्षभ।। २७
समं सर्वेषु भूतेषु तिष्ठन्तं परमेश्वरम्।
विनश्यत्स्वविनश्यन्तं यः पश्यति स पश्यति।। २८

27. *So long as any entities, moving or unmoving, are born, know that to be through the union of the field and the field-knower, O Bull among Bharatas.*
28. *Dwelling alike in all beings, the supreme Sovereign, not perishing among the perishing things—-he who sees Him, he truly sees.*

Teaching the yoga of equanimity, Sri Krishna says to Arjuna that whatever we find in the world, animate and inanimate, is the creation of the Self, Purusha, and its power of manifestation, Prakriti. The Self is the knower, the supreme reality, and Prakriti is its field, the manifestation that we see in various names and forms all over the universe. All that comes into existence, whether sentient or insentient, arises from the union of Purusha and Prakriti. These two fundamental principles are the principles of the one Absolute without a second. Purusha controls Prakriti as the body is controlled by its knower. This very Purusha is called Atman. Atman dwells equally everywhere in all things and beings of the universe. The aspirant who has the profound knowledge of the unchanging, everlasting, and eternal knows the Truth. He sees Truth everywhere and in everything. He remains undisturbed, for he has attained the state of equanimity.

समं पश्यन्हि सर्वत्र समवस्थितमीश्वरम्।
न हिनस्त्यात्मनात्मानं ततो याति परां गतिम्।। २९

29. *Seeing the Lord dwelling in everyone equally, one does not violate the Self by the self. Thereby he reaches the supreme state.*

All living beings and objects of the world appear to be distinct from one another, but in reality they are the modifications of one and the same Truth. Distinctions in name, form, and size are only apparent and not permanent. There are countless ripples, waves, and bubbles in the ocean, but they are one and the same water. As there are innumerable rays of sunlight coming from a single source, the aspirant knows that the different modes of the objects of the universe arise from one and the same Brahman.

प्रकृत्यैव च कर्माणि क्रियमाणानि सर्वशः।
यः पश्यति तथात्मानमकर्तारं स पश्यति।। ३०

30. *He alone sees who sees the Self as not a doer, and who sees that all acts are performed by Prakriti alone in every way,*

The wise person knows that Atman is not the doer, that all actions are carried out by Prakriti. It is the material nature that is responsible for all the actions and happenings going on in the universe and in the individual. Atman remains the witness. One who has attained this knowledge has realized the Self.

यदा भूतपृथग्भावमेकस्थमनुपश्यति।
तत एव च विस्तारं ब्रह्म संपद्यते तदा।। ३१
अनादित्वान्निर्गुणत्वात्परमात्मायमव्ययः।
शरीरस्थोऽपि कौन्तेय न करोति न लिप्यते।। ३२
यथा सर्वगतं सौक्ष्म्यादाकाशं नोपलिप्यते।
सर्वत्रावस्थितो देहे तथात्मा नोपलिप्यते।। ३३
यथा प्रकाशयत्येकः कृत्स्नं लोकमिमं रविः।
क्षेत्रं क्षेत्री तथा कृत्स्नं प्रकाशयति भारत।। ३४

31. *When he observes the separate being of all beings united in one, and all expansion from the very same, then he becomes Brahman.*
32. *Being devoid of attributes, this supreme Self (Parama-atman)— though dwelling in the body, O Son of Kunti—neither acts nor is tainted by action.*
33. *Just as the all-pervading sky is not tainted in its subtleness, similarly, this Atman dwelling everywhere in the body is not smeared.*
34. *Just as the single sun illuminates this entire world, so the field-owner illuminates the entire field O Descendant of Bharata.*

The highest Self is the Self of all without any beginning or end, unborn, and timeless. Therefore it is eternal. A well-known prayer of the Upanishads says that the absolute truth is full and if the full is taken from the full, that fullness is not diminished. If something is added to It, It still remains the same. Subtraction and addition do not create any change, for It is always full. The three qualities of sattva, rajas, and tamas are not in the Self, for the Self is beyond qualities and attributes. It is untainted by the manifestation of illusory forms that appear to be incomplete, in conflict, and in many cases to suffer. It is not tainted by the defects or blemishes of the apparent reality. All actions are performed by the body. The Self remains aloof and unaffected, free from all stains and impurities.

क्षेत्रक्षेत्रज्ञयोरेवमन्तरं ज्ञानचक्षुषा ।
भूतप्रकृतिमोक्षं च ये विदुर्यान्ति ते परम् ।। ३५

35. *Those who thus know with the eye of knowledge the difference between the field and the field-knower, as well as the release from the primordial nature Prakriti, which is the origin of elements, they reach the transcendent.*

Human eyes can only see so far; they have limited capacity and are bound by a limited horizon. But those who have attained intuitive knowledge have divine insight and can fathom all the levels of consciousness within and without. Such wise ones do not suffer from pride, egotism, or self-conceit, for their vision is not hindered by the limitations of the senses and the mind. The knowledge that flows through the ordinary mind is not pure and profound, but the knowledge that is received through divine or yogic insight is perfect. One should remember that such knowledge is not received bit by bit but is received with all its profundity and fullness. That knowledge flows from its timeless and infinite source. It is called intuitive knowledge. Pure, unalloyed knowledge of the infinite alone liberates the aspirant from the cruel clutches of Prakriti. Such an aspirant is detached and performs his duties selflessly. He remains in boundless joy, always full of delight. We human beings are the children of eternity, infinite happiness, and joy, and each of us can experience this true nature of ours.

Here ends the thirteenth chapter, in which the knowledge of the Self and the body, the universe and its Knower, the supreme Self is described.

Chapter Fourteen
The Profound Knowledge of the Three Gunas

श्री भगवानुवाच
परं भूयः प्रवक्ष्यामि ज्ञानानां ज्ञानमुत्तमम् ।
यज्ज्ञात्वा मुनयः सर्वे परां सिद्धिमितो गताः । । १
इदं ज्ञानमुपाश्रित्य मम साधर्म्यमागताः ।
सर्गेऽपि नोपजायन्ते प्रलये न व्यथन्ति च । । २

The Blessed Lord said

1. *Again I shall teach you the transcendent knowledge, the highest of sciences, knowing which, all meditators have gone from here to supreme adepthood.*
2. *Resorting to this knowledge, reaching homogeneity with Me, they are not born even at the new cycle of creation, nor do they suffer at dissolution.*

Having described the field of action and the knower of the field, Sri Krishna now leads Arjuna beyond the spheres of the field so that he can attain supreme knowledge. The knowledge that fulfills the purpose of life and leads one to completeness is considered to be the highest knowledge. There are many steps to that supreme knowledge, the final stage of attainment being complete liberation. When the Self is realized, the aspirant no longer fears birth or death. Here Sri Krishna describes that state that is beyond life here and hereafter. He says that when the universe returns to its primordial state after its dissolution, there is manifestation again. But the realized being remains unaffected by both annihilation and manifestation. He is one with Atman and is not subject to change, death, and rebirth. He has reached a state of immortality that gives him freedom from all bondage.

मम योनिर्महद्ब्रह्म तस्मिन्गर्भं दधाम्यहम्।
संभव: सर्वभूतानां ततो भवति भारत।। ३
सर्वयोनिषु कौन्तेय मूर्तय: संभवन्ति या:।
तासां ब्रह्म महद्योनिरहं बीजप्रद: पिता।। ४

3. *My maya is the womb (yoni), identical with Me, who am the great Brahman; I impregnate that; from there the birth of all beings occurs, O Descendant of Bharata.*
4. *All the forms that arise in all the species, O Son of Kunti, I, Brahman, am their seedgiving father, the great origin (yoni).*

The supreme Self is self-existent and is the father of all, and Prakriti is the mother of the entire universe. The supreme Lord sows Its seed in Prakriti from which are born and arise all beings. Thus the whole universe manifests. Every aspirant should know and remember that his vessel of life contains the seed of the supreme Lord. He is the child of the Lord, and just as a child, he only needs to allow the seed to grow so that he becomes the father. When the student becomes aware of this truth that the supreme imperishable seed of eternal life is already within him, he makes sincere efforts to allow it to grow. Then he attains Godhood: the human being eventually becomes divine.

सत्त्वं रजस्तम इति गुणाः प्रकृतिसंभवाः।
निबध्नन्ति महाबाहो देहे देहिनमव्ययम्।। ५
तत्र सत्त्वं निर्मलत्वात्प्रकाशकमनामयम्।
सुखसङ्गेन बध्नाति ज्ञानसङ्गेन चानघ।। ६
रजो रागात्मकं विद्धि तृष्णासङ्गसमुद्भवम्।
तन्निबध्नाति कौन्तेय कर्मसङ्गेन देहिनम्।। ७
तमस्त्वज्ञानजं विद्धि मोहनं सर्वदेहिनाम्।
प्रमादालस्यनिद्राभिस्तन्निबध्नाति भारत।। ८
सत्त्वं सुखे संजयति रजः कर्मणि भारत।
ज्ञानमावृत्य तु तमः प्रमादे संजयत्युत।। ९

5. *Sattva, rajas, tamas—these attributes born of Prakriti bind the immutable body-bearer in the body, O Mighty-armed One.*
6. *Of these, sattva, illuminator and healthy because of its immaculateness, binds through the attraction of pleasure as well as the attraction of knowledge, O Sinless One.*
7. *Know rajas to have the nature of attraction and color, producing craving and attachment. O Son of Kunti, it binds the body-bearer through attachment to action.*
8. *Know tamas to be born of ignorance, the stupefier of all body-owners. O Descendant of Bharata, it binds through negligence, sloth, and sleep.*
9. *Sattva causes attachment to happiness, rajas to action, O Descendant of Bharata. Tamas, however, veiling knowledge, causes attachment to inattention.*

All that we see here, there, and everywhere, all the objects of this universe, have been manifested by the three gunas of Prakriti. With the help of these three gunas, Prakriti manifests the universe. Sattva, rajas, and tamas are distinct, yet they function in coordination with one another. The sattva guna is peaceful, calm, and serene; rajas is active, sensual, and full of desires, attachments, and enjoyments; tamas produces sloth, inertia, confusion, delusion, and ignorance. The aspirant should always be vigilant, watching that tamas and rajas remain tamed with the help of sattva so that he can continue on the path undisturbed and undistracted. In order to accomplish this, earnest effort should be made, and one should meditate regularly.

When sattva is predominant the aspirant remains serene and happy. Elevating thoughts dawn during that time. The sattva quality is full of delight, enlightening, and very helpful for maintaining mental and emotional equilibrium. Without it, psychosomatic imbalances that lead to various kinds of disorders occur. When the sattva quality is not predominant, one experiences a lack of calmness, happiness, and joy. The mind then remains in a state of turmoil, full of conflict and confusion. But when the sattva quality is cultivated by the aspirant, he remains in a state of perpetual joy.

Rajas creates *raga* (attraction or attachment) and *dvesha* (aversion or hatred) toward the objects of the world. One whose life is controlled by rajas remains continually active, for he constantly pursues the objects of pleasure. He is never satisfied and is always seeking new sources of pleasure. That way of being can lead to hypertension and many other diseases and does not allow the student to discipline and control himself. Often the student functions under the sway of unconscious habits of a rajasic nature and acts without knowing and understanding why he is doing so.

Criminals when interrogated confess that they knew they should not have acted in the way that they did but that they committed their offenses out of habit. It is rajas that led them to act and to create a division within and without. So even when they know what to do, they cannot act on that knowledge. The conflict that is created within by rajas leads to serious crimes, and crime is a disease that needs to be treated. Because of mistakes in the social order, either at home or in school, many people do not get proper attention and education. As a result, they form habits that are injurious to themselves and others. Rajas can also be directed positively and can lead one to be creative and constructive. It is an active force, and if properly utilized, it can do tremendous good for both the individual and mankind.

Tamas is sloth and inertia; it produces ignorance and destroys the sense of discrimination. It creates delusion, and then one cannot decide things on time. Thus it leads one to inaction. A lazy aspirant remains in a state of sleepiness and lethargy, and in such a state of mind the aspirant goes through negative withdrawal. For him life is full of gloom; he does not experience joy or delight. Such people become fat and flabby and are prone to disease. Tamas leads one to many illnesses; tamasic people become passive and suffer from all the diseases related to passivity. They do not want to move; they remain in a semi-conscious state. They are controlled by negative emotions; they are depressed, dependent, and helpless. Life becomes burdensome for them.

The entire universe is a drama enacted by the gunas. The three gunas exist in everything, including all human beings. They are the motivating force in the drama of life. Almost everywhere, one guna is predominant and the other two are relatively dormant. They are hardly ever in a state of equilibrium. Equilibrium is experienced only by those sadhakas who practice physical, mental, and spiritual discipline.

रजस्तमश्चाभिभूय सत्त्वं भवति भारत।
रजः सत्त्वं तमश्चैव तमः सत्त्वं रजस्तथा।। १०
सर्वद्वारेषु देहेऽस्मिन्प्रकाश उपजायते।
ज्ञानं यदा तदा विद्याद्विवृद्धं सत्त्वमित्युत।। ११
लोभः प्रवृत्तिरारम्भः कर्मणामशमः स्पृहा।
रजस्येतानि जायन्ते विवृद्धे भरतर्षभ।। १२
अप्रकाशोऽप्रवृत्तिश्च प्रमादो मोह एव च।
तमस्येतानि जायन्ते विवृद्धे कुरुनन्दन।। १३

10. *Overcoming rajas and tamas, sattva prevails, O Descendant of Bharata; rajas prevails overcoming sattva and tamas; similarly tamas prevails overcoming sattva and rajas.*
11. *When the light of knowledge waxes in all the doors of this body, then one should know sattva to have increased.*

12. Greed, activity, the initiation of actions, absence of peace, compet-
itiveness—these are born when rajas has increased, O Bull among
Bharatas.

13. Absence of light, lack of initiative, inattention as well as stupefac-
tion—these are produced when tamas has increased, O Prince of
the Kurus.

The qualities of sattva, rajas, and tamas dwell in every human mind. According to the circumstances, one is predominant and the other two are relatively inactive. When rajas and tamas remain latent, sattva predominates, and when sattva and rajas remain dormant, tamas comes to the fore. These strands of Prakriti constantly intervene in human life. When sattva guna enables the light of knowledge to dawn, one becomes a sage. When rajas predominates, the desire for enjoyment victimizes the human mind. One then loses all sense of discrimination, and he gears his life toward the attainment of enjoyment. When both sattva and rajas remain latent, one goes to a state of pitifulness; he does nothing creative and thinks nothing useful.

Some commentators and scholars say that one should constantly cultivate the sattva guna in order to attain a state of perfection, and others say one should have equilibrium and balance in the three qualities. There is yet another view that one should go beyond all three gunas. Actually these are progressive steps in the inward journey toward perfection. In the beginning the aspirant should not allow the tamasic quality to raise its head. He should prevent his mind from going to the grooves of negativity and passivity. Lack of confidence and lack of success in life lead one to such a negative state.

In the next step the student should learn not to waste his energy trying to attain the objects of pleasure. Such activity robs one of his inner strength, which is the very basis of human advancement and unfoldment. The student should abstain from actions and activities that lead him to a preoccupation with sense enjoyment. When he is able to tame and keep tamas and rajas under control, he starts to cultivate the sattva quality—a delightful and joyous state of mind that leads one in the path of meditation and contemplation. Without going through the process and establishing sattva guna as the predominant current in one's life, meditation and contemplation remain mere techniques and have little value.

When one breathes primarily from the left nostril, tamas holds sway; when he breathes through the right nostril, a rajasic state is evident; and when the breath flows equally through both nostrils, he is in a sattvic state. To establish sattva guna the aspirant learns to apply sushumna with the help of pranayama techniques and meditation, in which mind and breath are well-coordinated. Then both breaths begin flowing freely rather than one predominating over the other. In such a state the mind experiences joy and likes to meditate instead of wanting to go out to the objects of the world. The mind then prefers to go to the inner recesses where it finds more delight and attains a state of equilibrium.

After cultivating sattva guna, the student progresses to the final state. Then none of the gunas has any hold over him. When the student has realized the Self, he has gone beyond all the gunas and nothing affects him. His vision remains unalloyed, untainted, and pure. Each commentator has his own viewpoint. Here Sri Krishna teaches Arjuna to cultivate sattva and then to perform his actions selflessly.

यदा सत्त्वे प्रवृद्धे तु प्रलयं याति देहभृत्।
तदोत्तमविदां लोकानमलान्प्रतिपद्यते।। १४
रजसि प्रलयं गत्वा कर्मसङ्गिषु जायते।
तथा प्रलीनस्तमसि मूढयोनिषु जायते।। १५

14. *When a body-bearer comes to death during an increase of sattva, then he attains the immaculate worlds of those of high knowledge.*
15. *Upon dying in rajas, one is born among those who are drawn to action. Similarly, dying in tamas, one is born among stupefied species.*

Those who have realized the Self, who are in the Self, and who have become one with the Self are never reborn. Those rare sages become inseparably one with the supreme Self and are beyond the influence of the gunas. They have crossed the mire of delusion and maya. They are liberated forever.

If the sages who have cultivated sattva guna prefer to stay in the highest of heavenly states when they depart from this mortal world, they can do so. And if they wish to be reborn, they take birth in the homes of wise parents. But those people who cast off their bodies under the predominance of rajas are reborn in the homes of those who are active in attaining worldly pleasures and the objects of the world. If tamas is predominant when one drops off the body, he is reborn in a dull, dumb, and desolate family, a family in which sloth and inertia rule.

कर्मणः सुकृतस्याहुः सात्त्विकं निर्मलं फलम्।
रजसस्तु फलं दुःखमज्ञानं तमसः फलम्।। १६
सत्त्वात्संजायते ज्ञानं रजसो लोभ एव च।
प्रमादमोहौ तमसो भवतोऽज्ञानमेव च।। १७
ऊर्ध्वं गच्छन्ति सत्त्वस्था मध्ये तिष्ठन्ति राजसाः।
जघन्यगुणवृत्तिस्था अधो गच्छन्ति तामसाः।। १८

16. *The fruit of a meritorious act is sattvic and stainless, but the fruit of rajas is pain, and the fruit of tamas is ignorance.*
17. *Knowledge is born from sattva and greed from rajas; inattention and stupefaction as well as ignorance arise from tamas.*
18. *The sattva-dwellers rise upward; the rajasic remain in the middle; tamasic ones, remaining under the influence of base qualities, move downward.*

How can one have a pleasant death and prepare himself for the life hereafter? Life is but a brief sentence, ending with a comma and no period. By analyzing life between the two commas of birth and death, the profound knowledge of the whole sentence is not grasped. The whole of life thus remains unknown. Death is a preparation for another birth, and death and birth are two transition points that mark the next step in the path of light. Life should be a preparation for the never ending journey to the infinite.

Those who perform good actions without attachment to the fruits of their actions are *sattvikas*. Their actions and fruits are totally dedicated to the whole of mankind, and they are liberated from the bonds and ties of karma. Even after dropping their mortal bodies, they are born again to perform more actions, for actions are like worship for them. They rejoice in being born again and again to breathe an eternal prayer and to perform their actions skillfully and selflessly. Actions performed in such a way are sattvic and liberating. But those who perform actions with selfish motivation are rajasic, and their actions lead to pain. Such people presume that death is painful and remain tormented by the fear of death. And those who are tamasic remain in the darkness of ignorance, completely dependent on fate. Fate leads them to lowly rebirth.

From sattva arises knowledge, from rajas desire is born, and from tamas comes ignorance. Those who have profound knowledge of sattva march upward toward the summit; those who are rajasic can only go up so far and remain in the middle; those who are tamasic are not aware of their path, their potentials, or the creative aspect of life.

नान्यं गुणेभ्यः कर्तारं यदा द्रष्टानुपश्यति।
गुणेभ्यश्च परं वेत्ति मद्भावं सोऽधिगच्छति।। १९
गुणानेतानतीत्य त्रीन्देही देहसमुद्भवान्।
जन्ममृत्युजराद्ःखैर्विमुक्तोऽमृतमश्नुते।। २०

19. *When the seer observes no agents of action other than the gunas and knows the transcendent beyond the gunas, he attains the state of being Me.*
20. *The body-bearer, transcending these three body-creating gunas, freed from the sorrows called birth, old age, and death, enjoys immortality.*

The perfect seer, well established in the supreme Self, knows that all the gunas create the play of the universe and that Atman is not the doer. Therefore he does not become involved and entangled in the play of the gunas. He knows that the real Self remains above the gunas, unaffected and untouched. The body functions because of the three gunas, but the sage is free from identification with body consciousness. Therefore he is free from death, birth, old age, and misery. He has already attained immortality.

अर्जुन उवाच
कैर्लिङ्गैस्त्रीन्गुणानेतानतीतो भवति प्रभो।
किमाचारः कथं चैतांस्त्रीन्गुणानतिवर्तते।। २१

श्री भगवानुवाच
प्रकाशं च प्रवृत्तिं च मोहमेव च पाण्डव।
न द्वेष्टि संप्रवृत्तानि न निवृत्तानि कांक्षति।। २२

उदासीनवदासीनो गुणैर्यो न विचाल्यते।
गुणा वर्तन्त इत्येव योऽवतिष्ठति नेङ्गते।। २३

समदुःखसुखः स्वस्थः समलोष्ठाश्मकाञ्चनः।
तुल्यप्रियाप्रियो धीरस्तुल्यनिन्दात्मसंस्तुतिः।। २४

मानापमानयोस्तुल्यस्तुल्यो मित्रारिपक्षयोः।
सर्वारम्भपरित्यागी गुणातीतः स उच्यते।। २५

Arjuna asked

21. **With what characteristics is that one endowed who has transcended the three gunas, O Lord? What is his conduct? Having transcended the gunas, in what manner does he conduct himself?**

The Blessed Lord said

22. **Illumination, activity, as well as delusion, O Pandava—he is not adverse to these when they are operant nor does he desire them when they have ceased.**

23. **He who sits in neutrality is not moved by the gunas; he observes**

merely that 'they operate with one another' and does not respond.
24. *Alike to pain and pleasure. Self-dwelling, beholding a lump of clay, stone, and nugget of gold as the same, holding the pleasant and unpleasant as equal, endowed with wisdom, alike to praise or censure,*
25. *Alike in honor and dishonor, equal to the friendly or hostile sides, renouncing all endeavor, he is said to have transcended the gunas.*

Arjuna wants to know how to recognize one who has gone beyond the gunas, and he asks how such a person behaves. Sri Krishna says that sattva emanates light, rajas activity, and tamas delusion. In all conditions, whether he is a success or a failure, the person who is sattvic remains content. Finally he goes beyond all the gunas. He remains aloof and unaffected in all situations. In the midst of the play of the gunas, he is neither inspired by sattva nor angered by the play of tamas. No matter what happens, he remains undisturbed, knowing that all the plays and melodramas are arranged by the gunas. He is not imbalanced in either gain or loss. Sattva does not imbalance him, and he is not affected by the grief and sorrow created by rajas and tamas. He maintains his evenness equally in honor and dishonor. Observing such signs and symptoms, the aspirant can identify one who has risen above the play of the gunas.

मां च योऽव्यभिचारेण भक्तियोगेन सेवते।
स गुणान्समतीत्यैतान्ब्रह्मभूयाय कल्पते।। २६
ब्रह्मणो हि प्रतिष्ठाहममृतस्याव्ययस्य च।
शाश्वतस्य च धर्मस्य सुखस्यैकान्तिकस्य च।। २७

26. *And he who serves Me with an undeviated yoga of devotion, fully transcending the gunas, he is fit to become Brahman.*
27. *I am the fundament of the immortal and immutable Brahman, of eternal law (dharma) and of ultimate happiness.*

To cross the mire of delusion created by the three gunas, the aspirant needs to have one-pointed devotion and complete dedication to the supreme Lord alone. Without purification of mind, single- minded devotion is not possible. And without single-minded devotion, one is not able to attain the highest Brahman. The supreme Lord is the final abode. He is immortal and imperishable. He plans the eternal laws of dharma. He is full of peace and bliss.

Here ends the fourteenth chapter, in which the three gunas and the state beyond are explained.

Chapter Fifteen
The Eternal Tree of Life

श्री भगवानुवाच
ऊर्ध्वमूलमधःशाखं अश्वत्थं प्राहुरव्ययम्।
छन्दांसि यस्य पर्णानि यस्तं वेद स वेदवित्।। १
अधश्चोर्ध्वं प्रसृतास्तस्य शाखा गुणप्रवृद्धा विषयप्रवालाः।
अधश्च मूलान्यनुसंततानि कर्मानुबन्धीनि मनुष्यलोके।। २

The Blessed Lord said

1. *With roots upward, with branches downward, there is said to be an immutable fig tree (ashvattha) whose leaves are the Vedic verses. He who knows that knows the Vedas.*

2. *Above and below are spread out its branches, grown through the gunas, with objects of the senses as the shoots; and the roots are spread out below, resulting in the bondage of actions in the human world.*

The Bhagavad Gita is a modified version of the Vedas and the Upanishads. The eternal tree of the universe described in these verses is also mentioned in the Katha Upanishad, Mundaka Upanishad, Atharva Veda, and Rig Veda. The phenomenal world is compared to a tree whose roots are in the heavens and whose branches spread upward and downward. One who knows that tree is called learned in Vedic knowledge, for that tree contains all the Vedic verses as its leaves. Its shade gives comfort to tired and weary scholars. The gunas cause the pleasant sense objects to blossom in that tree of the universe. Sound, touch, color, form, taste, and smell form additional roots, which spread extensively all over.

The *ashvattha* (cosmic tree) is described here as an imperishable tree, although it has been previously stated that this universe is transitory. The universe is a manifestation of one supreme imperishable reality, and that absolute reality is all-pervading and exists eternally with all its splendor and glory. It is immutable. Yet this universe is transitory, for all the objects of the external universe constantly change as a result of the three gunas, and the universe itself finally is absorbed into the unmanifest. But after the universe returns to its unmanifested form, it eventually comes back again to manifestation exactly as it was before. In this sense it is imperishable. It is sustained by that which is eternal.

In reality the essential potentiality of anything in the world does not change at all. The existence of anything in the world remains unchanged; it is never destroyed. Only the forms and names that it assumes are subject to change, decay, and destruction. For instance, modern astronomers say that in aeons to come the sun will become "dead," that it will lose all its fuel and no longer emanate light. But that is a limited perspective. For the light that the sun is emanating will even then continue to radiate throughout the universe as long as the universe exists. That energy may change form, but it never disappears. And even when the universe itself seems to be dissolved, it still exists in a potential form. The self-existent reality, the very summum bonum of life, remains unchangeable. In human life the body changes but not Atman. Without Atman the body cannot exist; the body exists only because of the existence of Atman. The tree of life is deeply rooted in the soil of nature and the power of Atman. Because Atman is imperishable, the tree of life is also considered to be imperishable.

न रूपमस्येह तथोपलभ्यते
नान्तो न चादिर्न च संप्रतिष्ठा।
अश्वत्थमेनं सुविरूढमूल
मसङ्गशस्त्रेण दृढेन छित्त्वा।। ३
ततः पदं तत्परिमार्गितव्यं
यस्मिन्गता न निवर्तन्ति भूयः।
तमेव चाद्यं पुरुषं प्रपद्ये
यतः प्रवृत्तिः प्रसृता पुराणी।। ४

3. *Its form is not apprehended as it appears; it has no end, no begin-*
   ning, or foundation. Cutting this tree of very firmly grown roots
   with the strong weapon of non-attachment—
4. *That higher state should be searched throughout, arriving at which*
   one no longer returns, saying I take recourse in that very Purusha
   from whom perennial activity commenced.'

The understanding of the ashvattha tree is beyond the grasp and comprehension of ordinary people, for their minds remain engrossed in the objects of enjoyment. They do not think of the consequences that arise from pursuing sense objects. They think that the transitory and temporal world is all there is and thus make the enjoyment of the mundane world the goal of their lives. But those who have carefully examined the phenomenal world know that they are caught by the snare of deaths and births. When they understand the basis of their bondage, they also realize that they can cut themselves free from their entanglements with the powerful weapon of non-attachment. The tree of mundane existence has also grown its roots deeply in the soil of the mind and heart of man. Only with the help of non-attachment can those roots be cut. When non-attachment is practiced, the aspirant becomes free from the bondage created by charms, temptations, and attractions to the objects of the world. The tree of worldly existence does not cause bondage for the aspirants who have attained a state of non-attachment.

In the Mundaka Upanishad it is said that there are two birds sitting on the branches of the same tree of life. One enjoys the fruits of the tree, but the other remains a witness. The one who enjoys also suffers, but the one who witnesses is free. When the individual soul remains attached to that which is in the vast reservoir of the unconscious, the storehouse of merits and demerits, or impressions and samskaras, he suffers. But the moment he becomes non-attached, he is free. The aspirant can attain a profound state of non-attachment and become free forever and ever.

निर्मानमोहा जितसङ्गदोषा
अध्यात्मनित्या विनिवृत्तकामाः।
द्वन्द्वैर्विमुक्ताः सुखदुःखसंज्ञै
र्गच्छन्त्यमूढाः पदमव्ययं तत्।। ५
न तद्भासयते सूर्यो न शशांको न पावकः।
यद्गत्वा न निवर्तन्ते तद्धाम परमं मम।। ६

5. *Free of pride and delusion, having conquered the stain of attachment, permanently dwelling in spiritual knowledge, turned away from desires, liberated from the pairs of opposites named pleasure and pain, the undeluded ones go to that imperishable state.*

6. *Neither the sun nor the moon nor the fire illuminates that, going to which they do not return. That is My supreme abode.*

When the aspirant attains freedom from egotism, pride, delusion, and attachments, he becomes content within. Free from all desires, he attains wisdom and finally the highest state of knowledge, which is imperishable in its nature. That knowledge is profound in itself. The light of the sun, moon, and fire have limitations, but the light of knowledge is the highest of all lights. No light is able to dispel the darkness of ignorance except the light of knowledge. The source of all light is in the depths of Atman—not in the sun, moon, or fire. The latter are just fragments of the Light of lights. The aspirant whose delusion has been completely dispelled by the light of knowledge attains the supreme Brahman. Sri Krishna tells Arjuna that the imperishable Brahman is the final abode of all aspirants.

ममैवांशो जीवलोके जीवभूतः सनातनः।
मनः षष्ठानीन्द्रियाणि प्रकृतिस्थानि कर्षति।। ७
शरीरं यदवाप्नोति यच्चाप्युत्क्रामतीश्वरः।
गृहीत्वैतानि संयाति वायुर्गन्धानिवाशयात्।। ८
श्रोत्रं चक्षुः स्पर्शनं च रसनं घ्राणमेव च।
अधिष्ठाय मनश्चायं विषयानुपसेवते।। ९
उत्क्रामन्तं स्थितं वापि भुञ्जानं वा गुणान्वितम्।
विमूढा नानुपश्यन्ति पश्यन्ति ज्ञानचक्षुषः।। १०
यतन्तो योगिनश्चैनं पश्यन्त्यात्मन्यवस्थितम्।
यतन्तोऽप्यकृतात्मानो नैनं पश्यन्त्यचेतसः।। ११

7. *In the world of the living ones. My own eternal particle has become the soul (jiva); it pulls the senses, with mind as the sixth, whose basis is Prakriti.*
8. *Whichever body this Lord attains and from whichever one He departs, He goes taking the mind and senses along in their repository, like the wind carrying fragrances.*
9. *Ruling over the senses of hearing and taste and touch and smell, as well as the mind, the soul experiences the objects of the senses.*
10. *The stupefied ones do not observe Him, whether endowed with gunas, He is departing or staying or experiencing. Only those with the eyes of knowledge truly see.*
11. *The yogis, endeavoring, see Him dwelling within the Self; the unwise, who have not cultivated the Self, do not see Him even though they endeavor.*

The individual soul is a part of the supreme Self. The individual soul lives consecutively in various bodies. As the breeze carries the fragrance of the flowers, so the individual soul when casting off the body carries the samskaras with it. Those samskaras motivate the individual soul to dress up in another garment, another body, and thus rebirth occurs. The individual soul is the enjoyer, and the body is like a garment that is changed when it is no longer useful to that soul. The ignorant are not aware of this, but the aspirant who follows the path of discipline with full efforts and a one-pointed mind and who has no desire for external enjoyments realizes the Truth.

The jiva (individual soul) is but a fragment, a tiny part of God. The space inside a cup, the space in a room, and the space outside are essentially one and the same. We can impose our own imaginary boundaries on the space, but the space remains one individual entity. No power ever existed or will ever exist that can cut the space or divide it into small or big parts. In the same way, there is no power that can cut the eternal Atman into pieces and make a small fragment into a jiva. When we see a particular human being, his form and size, he appears to be separated from the whole, and we call him an individual. But that experience of separation occurs because the ego is not in the habit of acknowledging the whole. That makes one think that the individual soul is only a fragment of the whole. In reality it is not. When the yogi fathoms all the boundaries from gross to subtle to subtlemost and crosses all the boundaries of individuality, he realizes that there is nothing but the real Self, which is the Self of all.

यदादित्यगतं तेजो जगद् भासयतेऽखिलम्।
यच्चन्द्रमसि यच्चाग्नौ तत्तेजो विद्धि मामकम्।। १२
गामाविश्य च भूतानि धारयाम्यहमोजसा।
पुष्णामि चौषधीः सर्वाः सोमो भूत्वा रसात्मकः।। १३
अहं वैश्वानरो भूत्वा प्राणिनां देहमाश्रितः।
प्राणापानसमायुक्तः पचाम्यन्नं चतुर्विधम्।। १४
सर्वस्य चाहं हृदि सन्निविष्टो मत्तः स्मृतिज्ञानमपोहनं च।
वेदैश्च सर्वैरहमेव वेद्यो वेदान्तकृद्वेदविदेव चाहम्।। १५

12. *That brilliance, which remaining in the sun illuminates the entire world, that which is in the moon as well as in the fire, know that to be My brilliance.*

13. *Having entered the earth, I uphold the beings with energy; I also nourish all the plants, having become soma whose nature is all juice and flavor.*

14. *I, becoming the universal fire in the belly, dwelling in the body of breathing creatures, joined with prana and apana, digest the four kinds of food.*

15. *I am also situated in the heart of all. From Me proceed memory, knowledge, and negation. I am the subject to be known through all the Vedas, the author of Vedanta as well as the knower of the Vedas am I alone.*

The blazing sun, the gentle light of the moon, and the golden flames of the fire belong to the one supreme Self. The power of the supreme Lord expressed through these manifestations enables the plants to grow, and in turn gives the vegetable kingdom the capacity to nourish animals and human beings. The fire of life (prana) that dwells in every human body is the fire given by the supreme Lord. All intelligence and knowledge have only one ultimate source. The power of knowledge in the human mind that enables it to know and to remember also emanates from the supreme Lord. The same power emanated all the Vedas and Vedanta; all discussions and praises of the Vedas and Vedanta are devoted to the source of that power. The supreme Lord exists everywhere. He lives in all beings, and His power prompts all human beings to function and to do their duties.

It is important for the aspirant to realize that there is only one truth within and without. That awareness will lead him to the source of the light that is found in the sun, moon, and stars as well as the light of knowledge, through which the human being understands and realizes the goal of life: the Self of all.

द्वाविमौ पुरुषौ लोके क्षरश्चाक्षर एव च।

क्षरः सर्वाणि भूतानि कूटस्थोऽक्षर उच्यते।। १६

उत्तमः पुरुषस्त्वन्यः परमात्मेत्युदाहृतः।

यो लोकत्रयमाविश्य बिभर्त्यव्यय ईश्वरः।। १७

यस्मात्क्षरमतीतोऽहमक्षरादपि चोत्तमः।

अतोऽस्मि लोके वेदे च प्रथितः पुरुषोत्तमः।। १८

16. *There are two conscious principles (purushas) in the world: per-ishable and imperishable. The perishable one is all the beings, and the absolute one is said to be imperishable.*

17. *But the highest conscious principle, Purusha, is elucidated as the Supreme Self (Parama-atman), the immutable Sovereign, who has entered and then upholds and nurtures the three worlds.*

18. *Because I am higher than the perishable and also beyond the imperishable one, therefore both in the world and in the Vedas I am glorified as the highest Self.*

These verses use two different terms: *kshara* (perishable) and *akshara* (imperishable). In this universe we experience two realities: one is constantly changing, and the other never changing. One goes through constant birth, change, death, and destruction; and the other is everlasting with no change at all. In human life there are three units: one unit is made up of the body, breath, senses, and conscious mind; the second consists of the unconscious mind and the individual soul; and the third is the ultimate eternal reality, the supreme Self. The first unit is subject to change and destruction, the second is semi-immortal, and the third is completely immortal. The first and second exist only because of the power of the third, the supreme Self, which is the source of life and light and which nourishes and supports the whole universe. It is the supreme Self that is the highest of all. The sages and Vedas call Him the supreme Lord.

The aspirant should understand that the body, senses, breath, and conscious mind are one unit—the gross unit of life. That unit constantly undergoes change, from birth to death. The second unit is the unconscious mind, which possesses and stores all the impressions and memories within itself and remains attached as a vehicle to the individual self, jiva. When the first unit separates from the second unit after death, the unconscious mind and individual soul continue to exist. When the individual soul becomes detached from its vehicle and realizes the supreme Self, one is free from the rounds of births and deaths and is liberated. When the realization of the supreme Self is accomplished, the individual soul becomes one with the supreme Self. The student should understand and firmly know that the supreme Self resides in the subtlemost recesses of the body and that the physical body is only an outer and gross sheath. The journey that one should follow in the course of his life is not a journey in the external world but an internal journey leading from gross to subtle and finally to the subtlemost supreme Self.

यो मामेवमसंमूढो जानाति पुरुषोत्तमम्।
स सर्वविद्भजति मां सर्वभावेन भारत।। १९
इति गुह्यतमं शास्त्रमिदमुक्तं मयाऽनघ।
एतद्बुद्ध्वा बुद्धिमान्स्यात्कृतकृत्यश्च भारत।। २०

19. *The undeluded one who knows Me this way as the supreme Spirit, he, all-knowing, devotes himself to Me with his entire being, O Descendant of Bharata.*
20. *I have taught you this secret most science, O Sinless One. Awakening to this, one becomes endowed with wisdom, fulfilled as to all actions, O Descendant of Bharata.*

As long as one is deluded by external allurements and dissipated by their various enjoyments, temptations, and attractions, he remains unaware of the beauty, grandeur, glory, and majesty of the supreme Self. But when the aspirant possesses the knowledge of both the external and internal worlds and knows the highest of all, he serves the supreme Self with his full devotion and dedication. The secret knowledge of the path of Self-realization has been imparted to Arjuna and to other aspirants. The key is to search, look, and see within. One who sees the supreme Lord in His wholeness and then does his duty attains and accomplishes the purpose of life.

Here ends the fifteenth chapter, in which the secret knowledge imparted to those who are on the path of Self-realization is explained.

Chapter Sixteen

The Destiny of the Sages and of the Ignorant

श्री भगवानुवाच
अभयं सत्त्वसंशुद्धिर्ज्ञानयोगव्यवस्थिति: ।
दानं दमश्च यज्ञश्च स्वाध्यायस्तप आर्जवम् ।। १
अहिंसा सत्यमक्रोधस्त्याग: शान्तिरपैशुनम् ।
दया भूतेष्वलोलुप्त्वं मार्दवं ह्रीरचापलम् ।। २
तेज: क्षमा धृति: शौचमद्रोहो नातिमानिता ।
भवन्ति संपदं दैवीमभिजातस्य भारत ।। ३

The Blessed Lord said

1. *Fearlessness, purity of mind, stability in the yoga of knowledge, charity, control, sacrificial observance, self-study, asceticism, and simplicity—*

2. *Non-violence, truth, non-anger, selflessness, peace, and non-gossiping, kindness toward all beings, non-greediness, mildness, modesty, non-fickleness—*

3. *Brilliance of confidence, forgiveness, sustenance, purity, nonanimosity, not seeking of honor—these appear in one who is highborn in divine wealth, O Descendant of Bharata.*

It is important to cultivate the qualities that make one's path easy and smooth. Without certain qualities the stumbling blocks, obstacles, and barriers cannot be removed. For some the path is clear, but for others it is full of obstructions. Those who are endowed with good qualities find their path to be easy, whereas those who do not cultivate good qualities constantly create difficulties for themselves. All follow one and the same path, to the Light of lights, but each person creates his own problems, confrontations, and obstacles along the path. Preparation is important before one begins to tread the path of light. To light the fire one must first gather the scattered twigs of those thoughts, desires, and emotions that dissipate his energy and rob him of dignity, courage, will-power, strength, and love. These qualities are virtues and their opposites vices. We all have the capacity to cultivate virtue, to replace vices with qualities that are genuinely needed to tread the path.

Every human being is endowed with strength that needs to be understood and applied before he prepares himself for the voyage to the unknown. Among all qualities fearlessness is the first and foremost. Purity of heart is another quality. Consistency in pursuing the knowledge that helps the aspirant in the inward journey is another virtue that needs to be cultivated. These qualities lead the aspirant to generosity and the attainment of self-control. They help him learn to give and to study his spiritual progress and the teachings of the sages. The practice of austerity and straightforwardness is also essential in preparing to tread the path.

The aspirant should cultivate and develop these qualities and learn to express them in his daily life. Whatever good is practiced or attained should be applied in one's daily life through both speech and action. The practice of ahimsa (non-injury) helps one to express his love to his fellow beings and fellow creatures. And the practice of non-lying with mind, action, and speech leads one to realization of the Truth. When the aspirant gives up all selfish desires, he finds that agitation and anger also disappear. Gladly and joyfully offering the fruits of actions to others leads one to evenness. Those who are not slanderous and have compassion for all beings, who do not usurp other's wealth and property, who are gentle and abstain from harmful deeds, and who are always steady are indeed on the path. Courageous, they always forgive others, hate none, and are without pride and arrogance. These are the qualities necessary to tread the path of spirituality. The students should remember that on the path of spirituality these essentials are means to make his journey easy and smooth.

दम्भो दर्पोऽभिमानश्च क्रोध: पारुष्यमेव च।
अज्ञानं चाभिजातस्य पार्थ संपदमासुरीम्।। ४

4. *Hypocrisy, pride, seeking of honor, anger, harshness, as well as ignorance—these occur in one born to demonic wealth.*

You are the architect of your own destiny. You are the composer of the songs that you sing. You are the surveyor of all that you survey. You are the redeemer of your life. Your destiny is created by you. A man who suffers as a result of hypocrisy, pride, vanity, anger, and arrogance, and who shows off, is an ignorant man. He constantly creates misery through his self-conceit. The qualities he possesses are of a demonic nature and lead him to darkness.

Yoga therapy and training teach a definite and profound way to replace demonic qualities with the spiritual qualities that are the necessary means to pursue the path of knowledge. There is no such training program offered by modern therapists and psychologists. Modern psychology does not focus on the whole being or on helping one to set up a training program for self-transformation. Modern psychology is still learning to understand the cause of suffering, whereas yoga psychology has discovered the means and methods for self-transformation.

दैवी संपद्विमोक्षाय निबन्धायासुरी मता।
मा शुच: संपदं दैवीमभिजातोऽसि पाण्डव।। ५

5. *The divine wealth leads to freedom; the demonic way is known to lead to bondage. Grieve not; you are born to divine wealth, O Pandava.*

Cultivating good qualities gives one the essential means to follow the path of knowledge, light, and spirituality. It is the means to attain freedom. But those who are not awakened and are not aware of spirituality do not cultivate the necessary means and qualities. They remain in bondage. Here are two important points: The first is that good thoughts, good deeds, and good actions are never lost. The aspirant who has trodden the path of spirituality before is endowed with good qualities by birth. Such a student finds the path easy. The second point is that the teacher should make his students aware of their creative aspect and of the qualities that are healthy and helpful in the path of self-unfoldment. Arjuna is made aware that he is endowed with good qualities by birth.

द्वौ भूतसर्गौ लोकेऽस्मिन् दैव आसुर एव च।
दैवो विस्तरशः प्रोक्त आसुरं पार्थ मे शृणु।। ६

प्रवृत्तिं च निवृत्तिं च जना न विदुरासुराः।
न शौचं नापि चाचारो न सत्यं तेषु विद्यते।। ७

असत्यमप्रतिष्ठं ते जगदाहुरनीश्वरम्।
अपरस्परसंभूतं किमन्यत्कामहैतुकम्।। ८

एतां दृष्टिमवष्टभ्य नष्टात्मानोऽल्पबुद्धयः।
प्रभवन्त्युग्रकर्माणः क्षयाय जगतोऽहिताः।। ९

काममाश्रित्य दुष्पूरं दम्भमानमदान्विताः।
मोहाद्गृहीत्वासद्ग्राहान्प्रवर्तन्तेऽशुचिव्रताः।। १०

चिन्तामपरिमेयां च प्रलयान्तामुपाश्रिताः।
कामोपभोगपरमा एतावदिति निश्चिताः।। ११

आशापाशशतैर्बद्धाः कामक्रोधपरायणाः।
ईहन्ते कामभोगार्थमन्यायेनार्थसञ्चयान्।। १२

इदमद्य मया लब्धमिदं प्राप्स्ये मनोरथम्।
इदमस्तीदमपि मे भविष्यति पुनर्धनम्।। १३

असौ मया हतः शत्रुर्हनिष्ये चापरानपि।
ईश्वरोऽहमहं भोगी सिद्धोऽहं बलवान्सुखी।। १४

आढ्योऽभिजनवानस्मि कोऽन्योऽस्ति सदृशो मया।
यक्ष्ये दास्यामि मोदिष्य इत्यज्ञानविमोहिताः।। १५

अनेकचित्तविभ्रान्ता मोहजालसमावृताः।
प्रसक्ताः कामभोगेषु पतन्ति नरकेऽशुचौ।। १६

आत्मसंभाविताः स्तब्धा धनमानमदान्विताः।
यजन्ते नामयज्ञैस्ते दम्भेनाविधिपूर्वकम्।। १७

अहंकारं बलं दर्प कामं क्रोधं च संश्रिताः।
मामात्मपरदेहेषु प्रद्विषन्तोऽभ्यसूयकाः।। १८

तानहं द्विषतः क्रूरान्संसारेषु नराधमान्।
क्षिपाम्यजस्रमशुभानासुरीष्वेव योनिषु।। १९

आसुरीं योनिमापन्ना मूढा जन्मनि जन्मनि।
मामप्राप्यैव कौन्तेय ततो यान्त्यधमां गतिम्।। २०

6. There are two kinds of created beings in this world: the divine and the demonic. The divine has been explained in detail. Now hear about the demonic from Me, O Son of Pritha.

7. Demonic people know neither right conduct nor prohibition; in them there is neither purity nor character nor truth.

8. They say that the world is untrue, without foundation, and Godless—that it is produced only through sexual union and that it has no cause other than what comes from passion.

9. Blocked by this vision, their true nature destroyed, those of little intelligence, doing fearsome acts, come into power as malefactors for the world.

10. Resorting to passion and desire, which is difficult to fulfill, possessed of hypocrisy, seeking honor and frenzy, they of impure observances operate, seizing upon false holdings, out of delusion.

11. They have recourse only to immeasurable worry that goes on until dissolution. They are certain that the enjoyment of passions is supreme, that it is everything.

12. *Bound by a hundred snares of expectation, intent upon passion and anger, they undertake the gathering of wealth by injustice for the purpose of enjoying passions.*

13. *'This I have received today, this wish of mine I shall gain later; this I have, and this wealth shall yet be mine;*

14. *That enemy I have killed, others too I shall destroy; I am sovereign, I am enjoyer, I am accomplished, strong, happy;*

15. *I am rich, I have influential relations. Who else is equal to me? I shall perform sacrifices, I shall enjoy myself.' Thus deluded in ignorance,*

16. *Confused by the many divisions in their minds, covered by the net of delusion, stuck in the enjoyment of passions, they fall into the impure and lowly place.*

17. *Holding high opinion of themselves, lacking humility, possessed of honor and frenzy due to wealth, they sacrifice by sacrifices in name alone, in hypocrisy, and without regard to correct injunctions.*

18. *Resorting to ego, power, pride, passion, and anger, full of malice, hating Me in the bodies of others and in their own,*

19. *These hateful, cruel, base humans in the world—the ugly ones— I ever throw into demonic species alone.*

20. *Fallen into demonic species, stupefied in life after life, without ever finding Me, O Son of Kunti, they then go to the lowest state.*

Having explained the virtues that the aspirant should cultivate, Sri Krishna now explains that there are two kinds of people in the world: those who are endowed with good qualities and those who are endowed with bad qualities. The latter are not aware of what is good and therefore do not know how to perform good actions. They have no knowledge of either the path of action or the path of renunciation. They cannot discriminate between right and wrong. By habit they do harmful actions and suffer. They only work for sensual enjoyments. They do not have any sense of purity. They delight in lying and do not discriminate between a lie and the truth. Outwardly they may appear to be holy, good, and kind, but within their hearts and minds they are not.

Such people do not believe in God. They do not regard this world as an orderly creation of the powers of the Lord. They think that there is no primary cause behind this world. They think that the pleasures of the world are everything and that the world has neither been created by nor supported by God. Those ignorant people remain inflated and deluded, considering themselves to be great enjoyers. They live according to a materialistic and hedonistic view of the world: they consider the world to be full of objects of enjoyment and think that they should take as much pleasure as they can. Such people continually seek the objects of enjoyment.

Those deluded ones are always competing with others in their desires to be stronger and to have more than others. They do not have enough intelligence to acknowledge the existence of others and are overrun by animosity and thoughts of destruction. Their minds remain busy in securing arms and armaments to destroy others and to become victorious. They only believe in increasing physical power and trust that physical might alone is right. Engrossed in hypocrisy and arrogance, they are deluded by their evil desires and thoughts. They are mean, selfish, vicious, and malicious. They are always puffed up with pride, with the thought that they are great and that society cannot survive without them. Such people are egotistical and think, "I am the Lord of my life. 1 am great because 1 have immense wealth." They perform sacrifices and give gifts with an egotistical attitude and then boast about it. Their ideals are impure and false. They work hard to attain those goals that lead them to ruin.

Having innumerable worries, they are never happy. Therefore they do not have peace of mind. They believe that human life is a means for sensual enjoyment, and that is the goal of their lives. But even if they have many sensual enjoyments, they are never satisfied. They do not care whether they obtain wealth by deceptive or dishonest means, for they have no sense of justice. They have endless desires, and when they are not fulfilled, they commit crimes in order to fulfill them. Deluded by such desires they remain distracted and dissipated and suffer hellish lives both here and hereafter. Conceited, arrogant, full of lust and anger, they disturb and destroy others. They find pleasure in being violent. Full of desires they are always restless, and they fight and kill one another.

The allurements of the external world are but temporary, transitory, and momentary, so no one is ever satisfied with the pursuit of mundane pleasure. Intrinsically the human being is in search of permanent happiness, peace, and bliss. After examining all the objects of the external world, one finally realizes that they offer only a fragment of happiness but are not able to quench one's thirst. Real happiness lies within. But the majority of people are not awakened to the reality that there are other dimensions of life that are more glorious and enlightening. The aspirant should avoid the company of such people, for their influence could be injurious.

These verses harshly condemn those who are caught up in materialism and the pursuit of sensory pleasure. They provide a strong warning to the student to avoid that way of being, to open his eyes to the dire consequences of living that way. But all is not hopeless for those who are caught in the snare of illusion. Though they must undergo many experiences and many births and deaths to satisfy their cravings, they finally become disillusioned with the mundane pleasures of the world, and they too slowly grow toward the Light.

त्रिविधं नरकस्येदं द्वारं नाशनमात्मनः।
कामः क्रोधस्तथा लोभस्तस्मादेतत्त्रयं त्यजेत्।। २१
एतैर्विमुक्तः कौन्तेय तमोद्वारैस्त्रिभिर्नरः।
आचरत्यात्मनः श्रेयस्ततो याति परां गतिम्।। २२

21. *This is the threefold gate of hell that destroys one's self: passion, anger, and greed. Therefore one should give up these three.*
22. *One freed from these three doors of darkness, O Son of Kunti, conducts himself toward benefaction for himself and thereby reaches the highest state.*

This lifetime is just a small passage in the book of life, and it is an essential preparation for the life that lies ahead. Those who cling to life here, who are greedy and passionately desire the objects of sense enjoyment, become angry when they are unsuccessful in obtaining those objects. *Kama, krodha,* and *lobha* (selfish desire, anger, and greed) are three negative emotions that lead the human being to unhappiness and misery here and to a life hereafter that is of the same quality as his life in the body. Having all sorts of objects of pleasure in this world, selfish and greedy people are still unsatisfied. They do not enjoy the objects of pleasure they accumulate, for they are continually afraid of losing what they already have and not gaining what they want. Selfish desire, anger, and greed are harmful emotions that need to be shunned.

Such ignorant people are invariably afraid of dying. They sometimes do charitable things because they foolishly think that they will get returns after death. That is not possible, for whatever we do here in this lifetime, we carry the samskaras of our deeds with us. If one is miserable here, how can he expect to be happy in the life hereafter? Unaware of the power of the soul and lacking inner strength, one remains weak, feeble, deluded, and afraid of death. Selfish desire, anger, and greed disrupt and destroy inner strength. The aspirant should renounce these great obstacles. Selfish desire creates strong bonds of passion, anger, and greed—the three openings to hell. Sri Krishna says, "O Arjuna, one who is able to renounce these three harmful habits is free from these dark openings." If the aspirant genuinely renounces these human weaknesses, he can attain the highest state.

यः शास्त्रविधिमुत्सृज्य वर्तते कामकारतः।
न स सिद्धिमवाप्नोति न सुखं न परां गतिम्।। २३
तस्माच्छास्त्रं प्रमाणं ते कार्याकार्यव्यवस्थितौ।
ज्ञात्वा शास्त्रविधानोक्तं कर्म कर्तुमिहार्हसि।। २४

23. *One who, abandoning the injunctions of the scriptures, conducts himself through actions based on desire does not attain fulfillment or happiness or the highest state.*

24. *Therefore, for you the scripture is the authority in order to determine*

*what ought to be done and what ought not to be done; knowing
the act as taught in the scriptural injunctions, you should perform
your actions.*

To achieve the goal of life, one should learn to follow in the footsteps of the ancients whose experiences are recorded in the scriptures.
The authentic scriptures serve as authorities and guide the aspirant.
One who does not follow the teachings of the great sages but instead
follows his own whims does not attain happiness or the goal of life. The
scriptures are the testimony to guide the aspirant, enabling him to know
what to do and what not to do. Any experience during sadhana should
be examined carefully; the validity of the aspirant's experiences during
spiritual sadhana should be verified by scriptural knowledge. Many
have trodden the path of spirituality before us and have left accurate
records that help one to know if he is properly progressing on the path.
Many fake teachers perform so-called miracles that are never referred
to in the scriptures. They perform those tricks to acquire a large following just to satisfy their egos. The seeker should be careful and should
not follow a modern teacher without knowing him well and compar-
ing his teachings with those of the authentic scriptures. The scriptures
guide the aspirant if they are properly understood and not interpreted
merely according to one's own convenience.

*Here ends the sixteenth chapter, in which the yoga of discrimi-
nation between spirituality and ignorance is described.*

Chapter Seventeen
Three Modes of Conviction

अर्जुन उवाच
ये शास्त्रविधिमुत्सृज्य यजन्ते श्रद्धयान्विताः।
तेषां निष्ठा तु का कृष्ण सत्त्वमाहो रजस्तमः।। १
श्री भगवानुवाच
त्रिविधा भवति श्रद्धा देहिनां सा स्वभावजा।
सात्त्विकी राजसी चैव तामसी चेति तां शृणु।। २
सत्त्वानुरूपा सर्वस्य श्रद्धा भवति भारत।
श्रद्धामयोऽयं पुरुषो यो यच्छ्रद्धः स एव सः।। ३
यजन्ते सात्त्विका देवान्यक्षरक्षांसि राजसाः।
प्रेतान्भूतगणांश्चान्ये यजन्ते तामसा जनाः।। ४

Arjuna asked

1. *Those who sacrifice, endowed with faith but abandoning scriptural injunctions, what is their status, O Krishna, is it sattva or rajas or tamas?*

The Blessed Lord said

2. *The faith of the body-bearers is of three kinds, born of their nature, which is sattvic, rajasic, and tamasic; do hear thereof.*

3. *Everyone's faith develops according to his mind's essence, O Descendant of Bharata. Thus, the person consists of faith. Whatever one's faith, that indeed is he.*

4. *The sattvic ones sacrifice to deities; the rajasic ones to demi-gods and powerful semi-human beings (yakshas and rakshasas); others, the tamasic ones, sacrifice to ghosts and to multitudes of other beings.*

In this chapter Arjuna asks Sri Krishna to describe the various modes of shraddha. The word shraddha means conviction. The devotee reveres the objects of his devotion with full conviction and faith. Human beings can be divided into three categories according to the predominance of sattva, rajas, or tamas. Arjuna wants to know which quality is dominant in those who have shraddha yet do not accept the teachings of the sages and the authority of the scriptures. Sri Krishna replies that the tendency of one guna or another to be predominant is a result of the samskaras that one carries from the past. In spiritual people the sattva guna is predominant; those who are active are motivated by rajas; and those who are inert, lazy, and dull are under the sway of tamas.

The type of faith a human being has is in accordance with this natural disposition. The aspirant who has the sattva quality predominant in his life performs religious rites according to the teachings of the scriptures. One who performs religious rites under the sway of rajas worships the gods with the desire to fulfill his selfish ends. The tamasic person also has faith, but he engages in superstitious worship. That class of people does not make efforts. Those of a sattvic nature devote their time and energy to doing good, whereas rajasic people remain active in fulfilling their desires, and those who are tamasic do not do anything, for although they have expectations and desires they remain dependent on others.

अशास्त्रविहितं घोरं तप्यन्ते ये तपो जनाः।
दम्भाहंकारसंयुक्ताः कामरागबलान्विताः।। ५
कर्शयन्तः शरीरस्थं भूतग्राममचेतसः।
मां चैवान्तः शरीरस्थं तान्विद्ध्यासुरनिश्चयान्।। ६

5. *Those people who undertake terrible ascetic practices, which are not enjoined by the scriptures, conjoined with hypocrisy and ego, possessed of the power of attachment,*
6. *Those unwise ones, weakening the group of elements in the body, and also Me, who dwells within the body—know them to be of demonic determination.*

Those who are influenced by tamas are full of sloth and inertia and always depend on others whom they expect to fulfill their desires. When they do engage in practices, those practices are distorted and reflect their obstinate natures. They sometimes practice severe penances that are contrary to the injunctions of the scriptures. For example, many such aspirants fast for several days to remove their mental blocks. They think that fasting will purify both their minds and bodies. They are obstinate and capriciously make up their own way of sadhana and suffer as a result. They are neither self-reliant nor do they rely on the teachings of the scriptures. They create suffering for themselves and for others. Such aspirants do not improve and are not fit to follow the path of spirituality.

Physical mortification and extremism, such as too much eating, sleeping for long hours, and lying around engrossed in worries, is caused by tamas. The aspirant should create a balance in his day-to-day life. When one learns to observe his capacities and abilities, he does not go to extremes. But the student who torments his body, mind, and soul is not suitable for the path of spirituality.

आहारस्त्वपि सर्वस्य त्रिविधो भवति प्रिय:।
यज्ञस्तपस्तथा दानं तेषां भेदमिमं शृणु।। ७
आयु: सत्त्वबलारोग्यसुखप्रीतिविवर्धना:।
रस्या: स्निग्धा: स्थिरा हृद्या आहारा: सात्त्विकप्रिया:।। ८
कट्वम्ललवणात्युष्णतीक्ष्णरूक्षविदाहिन:।
आहारा राजसस्येष्टा दु:खशोकामयप्रदा:।। ९
यातयामं गतरसं पूति पर्युषितं च यत्।
उच्छिष्टमपि चामेध्यं भोजनं तामसप्रियम्।। १०

7. *The favorite food of everyone is also of three kinds; so also sacrifice, ascetic endeavor, and charity. Listen to their distinctions.*

8. *Those that increase life-span, mental essence, strength, health, comfort, and pleasantness, that are flavorful, unctuous, stable, and satisfying to the heart are the foods that are favored by the sattvic.*

9. *Bitter, sour, salty, excessively hot, pungent, dry, and burning are the foods favored by the rajasic, causing discomfort, depression, and illness.*

10. *Not fully cooked, flavorless, smelly, stale, leftover by others, not fit as an offering is the food favored by the tamasic.*

When one analyzes the behavior of aspirants, three distinct qualities are noticeable in their actions, even when they offer gifts and charity. Those who are sincerely generous and love others do charity without any expectation, but those who perform actions selfishly and do charity with the expectation of acquiring name and fame are rajasic and tamasic people.

We all know that food plays a great part in human life. The best selling of all books are not bibles or other spiritual books but cookbooks. Our eating habits in the modern world both in the East and in the West create disasters in human life. The human being is obsessed with food, so much so that it seems that one is born only for eating. Modern man eats many times a day without knowing what comprises a nutritious diet. Taste has become predominant instead of nutrition in the formation of our dietary habits. Artificial foods are increasing daily. We have lost the sense of food value, and we eat foods that are unhealthy.

Food that is not fresh or nutritious, that is leftover and full of spices or grease is unhealthy. Overeating and eating unfresh food and food that is full of fat and spices create many diseases. The mind and body are inseparable; if proper food is not supplied to the body, the mind is affected. Such tamasic food makes the mind dull, passive, and inert. On the other hand, rajasic food agitates the mind and creates hypertension; it is also unhealthy for the liver and hard on the kidneys. Rajasic food satisfies the senses, but it is not healthy physically or mentally. It is not healthy for those who want to tread the path of spirituality. Aspirants are advised that well-selected and well-prepared vegetarian food is healthier than a meat diet. That food which does not cause inertia and heaviness and does not make one restless, lazy, or sleepy is called sattvic food. Those who eat sattvic food remain calm, quiet, and serene; those who eat rajasic food become agitated, angry, and worried; those who eat impure food and drink liquor are tamasic. Those who eat heavy food full of fat and who drink alcohol excessively suffer both physically and mentally.

Food plays an important role in thought, speech, and action: it has profound effects on all aspects of human behavior. Diet and environment are two important factors that play a great role in sadhana. A calm, quiet, and serene atmosphere and a simple, fresh, and nutritious diet are essential requisites for the sadhaka.

अफलाकांक्षिभिर्यज्ञो विधिदृष्टो य इज्यते।
यष्टव्यमेवेति मनः समाधाय स सात्त्विकः।। ११
अभिसंधाय तु फलं दम्भार्थमपि चैव यत्।
इज्यते भरतश्रेष्ठ तं यज्ञं विद्धि राजसम्।। १२
विधिहीनमसृष्टान्नं मन्त्रहीनमदक्षिणम्।
श्रद्धाविरहितं यज्ञं तामसं परिचक्षते।। १३

11. *That sacrifice performed according to scriptural injunctions by those not desirous of fruit, harmonizing the mind with the thought, 'one must sacrifice,' that is the sattvic sacrifice.*
12. *With the intention of fruit or even of hypocritical purpose, the sacrifice that is performed thus, know it to be rajasic, O Best of the Bharatas.*
13. *Against scriptural injunction, without distributing food, without mantras, without priestly gifts, devoid of faith, such sacrifice is said to be tamasic.*

Sri Krishna explains that sacrifices performed in a serene way with evenmindedness and without any expectation of reward are sattvic. When one performs an action for the sake of others and dedicates the fruits to others without any desire for rewards, that action is true worship. Sacrifice means offering the best one has for the service of the Lord who dwells in everyone's heart. It is an offering to the Lord through action. Such an act performed selflessly is of a sattvic nature, and the scriptures describe such acts as supreme. By contrast, the sacrifices and actions that are performed with the desire to obtain a reward are rajasic, and those that are performed out of superstition and fear of spiritual injunction, without a sense of giving or any consideration for others, are tamasic.

Many people in modern society have not developed an attitude of giving to and doing for others in a sincere way. Such people are often seen in psychotherapy. They are self-preoccupied and continually focus on their own trials and tribulations, worries, disappointments, and expectations. Rather than attempting to resolve their self-created conflicts one by one, if the therapist instead directs such people to turn away from their self-preoccupations and to develop a genuine concern for others, devoting their thoughts and energy to helping others, many of their problems would quickly dissolve and disappear. Such people have never been taught how to give, and if they offer anything, it is not with a deep and sincere feeling of love but to receive in return. Modern therapists would do well to actively guide the thoughts and feelings of their clients toward giving to others rather than passively listening to and reflecting on the drone of their clients' self-preoccupations week after week, year after year.

देवद्विजगुरुप्राज्ञपूजनं शौचमार्जवम् ।
ब्रह्मचर्यमहिंसा च शारीरं तप उच्यते ।। १४

अनुद्वेगकरं वाक्यं सत्यं प्रियहितं च यत् ।
स्वाध्यायाभ्यसनं चैव वाङ्मयं तप उच्यते ।। १५

मनः प्रसादः सौम्यत्वं मौनमात्मविनिग्रहः ।
भावसंशुद्धिरित्येतत्तपो मानसमुच्यते ।। १६

श्रद्धया परया तप्तं तपस्तत्त्रिविधं नरैः ।

अफलाकांक्षिभिर्भक्तैः सात्त्विकं परिचक्षते।। १७
सत्कारमानपूजार्थं तपो दम्भेन चैव यत्।
क्रियते तदिह प्रोक्तं राजसं चलमध्रुवम्।। १८
मूढग्राहेणात्मनो यत्पीडया क्रियते तपः।
परस्योत्सादनार्थं वा तत्तामसमुदाहृतम्।। १९

14. *Service to the deities, the twice-born, the gurus, and the wise men; purity, simplicity, celibacy, and non-violence are said to be physical asceticism.*

15. *Speech that does not agitate, that is true, pleasant, and beneficial, as well as the practice of self-study and japa is said to be the asceticism of speech.*

16. *Clarity and pleasantness of mind, peacefulness, silence, total control of one's self, purification of sentiments—this is said to be mental asceticism.*

17. *Those three kinds of asceticism undertaken by humans with supreme faith when they are not desiring the fruit and are joined in yoga are said to be the sattvic ones.*

18. *With the purpose of gaining respect, honor, and worship and out of hypocrisy, the asceticism that is thus performed, temporary and unstable, is rajasic.*

19. *The asceticism that is performed with stupefied comprehension and with pain or for the purpose of uprooting others, that is said to be tamasic.*

Sri Krishna describes three kinds of austerities. Austerity means refraining from the sense pleasures and from habits that are harmful to oneself and others. Austerities help the aspirant in preparing for spiritual advancement, performing selfless actions, and worshipping the supreme Lord. Although a preliminary step, austerity is nonetheless important in all spiritual paths. The aspirant who has reverence for the yogis, learned people, sages, and wise men; purity of mind and heart; straightforwardness; control of mind, action, and speech; and who practices ahimsa is considered to be austere.

The power of speech has a profound influence on the human mind and heart. One who controls his speech, who does not talk ill of others but speaks gently and never lies, his words are always beneficial and soothing to all. If the aspirant learns not to lie, he speaks the truth. And that truth which is greased with love is very helpful to others. Teaching and interpersonal communication are carried on mainly through the medium of speech. The way we use words makes a difference: if the aspirant learns to speak truth in a gentle way, his speech will have an immense impact on the human mind and soul. But when the aspirant speaks only to fulfill his selfish desires or speaks that which is contrary to his thinking, he continually creates psychological barriers for himself. The *apta,* the great man, speaks in accord with the way he thinks and acts; there is complete coordination in his inward action and speech. He never intends to hurt, harm, or injure anyone through his speech.

Many people waste their time speaking nonsense, talking too much, and gossiping-for no useful reason. In the first stage of practice one should learn to speak little, speaking only when it is necessary. In the second step he should establish regular hours of complete silence every day, and in the third step he should determine not to lie. Austere speech is a great virtue.

The practice of non-lying is important for many reasons. Those who speak lies are afraid and lie because of fear of not being accepted. But the power of speech is lost when one lies, and there is always a conflict in the mind, for one knows that he is lying, yet he continues to lie. Such people can never be known by others; they never prove to be good friends. They become victims of their habits, and then they lose the power of discrimination.

The student should learn the distinction between external and internal austerities. In physical or external austerities one should learn not to do that which is not to be done and to speak the way he thinks, understands, and knows. Mental austerity is also very important. When one practices mental austerity, he maintains serenity and silence and remains vigilant toward his thinking process. He avoids entertaining those thoughts that are disturbing and dissipating. Both mental and physical austerities purify the aspirant and make him fit to follow the path of spirituality. These are called sattvic austerities. When the student purifies his mind, action, and speech with the help of sattvic strength, he attains the higher realms of life.

There is another category of aspirants—those who are rajasic. They also practice austerities but with the desire to be respected and to obtain honors from others. They want others to revere and follow them; their austerities are engrossed with self-interest. Many athletes, dancers, and musicians practice austerities to gain name and fame. They are also motivated by rajas.

Another group of aspirants is tamasic. Their thoughts, actions, and speech are directed toward hurting and injuring others. They are never concerned for others but only do things to fulfill their selfish ends, regardless of how much harm is done to others in the process. These people lie, connive, and use others for their own convenience. They are very obstinate and egotistical, and they torture themselves and others in order to attain their selfish ends.

Austerities are not introduced in the modern educational system. That is one of the reasons modern man becomes selfish and has no consideration for his fellow human beings. The kind of austerities that are introduced to children in religious schools are worse than none at all, for they create guilt, which haunts the child's inner being until the last breath of life. That system of introducing austerity is based on fear, and the religion that teaches fear can never help one on the path to liberation. Religious schools suffer as a result of that serious error. They create guilt by introducing many "don'ts" without explaining their purpose or helping children appreciate the profound positive effects that self-restraint can have on the mind and body. Those who seriously pursue athletics, music, and other endeavors learn to practice austerities by sacrificing pleasures for their single goal. But such austerities are rajasic in nature. Sattvic austerity is seldom taught in modern life.

दातव्यमिति यद्दानं दीयतेऽनुपकारिणे।
देशे काले च पात्रे च तद्दानं सात्त्विकं स्मृतम्।। २०
यत्तु प्रत्युपकारार्थं फलमुद्दिश्य वा पुनः।
दीयते च परिक्लिष्टं तद्दानं राजसं स्मृतम्।। २१

20. *'One ought to give'—the charity that is given thus to someone incapable of returning the favor, that is given at the right place and time toward someone worthy—that charity is remembered as sattvic.*
21. *That which is given with the purpose of gaining a return or aiming at a fruit or given with distress—that charity is remembered as rajasic.*
22. *That which is given at an inappropriate place or time to those unworthy, without respect and insultingly—that charity is said to be tamasic.*

These three verses explain the purpose of charity and why one should be charitable. When is charity useful and necessary in human life? For one who has attained knowledge, doing charitable work and giving gifts to others becomes habitual. It is a superb taste that one acquires after understanding that giving is one of the most profound ways to attain liberation. No human being can remain without doing actions, and every action produces fruits. If the fruits are not given to others, their binding force compels one to do more actions. Thus, the doer becomes lost in the jungle of action. One should learn to do his actions and give away the fruits to others. The aspirant who is aware that charity or giving gifts to those in need is a part of spirituality is called a sattvika.

Those who give gifts and do charity with the expectation that it will be returned by Providence are selfish people. They give with the idea of getting something in return and of having others praise them. Sometimes they do charity to maintain their social status, but they never give selflessly. Such people are rajasic. The gifts that are given in a tamasic state of mind are the lowest form of gifts. Tamasic people give out of compulsion and without joy in giving. They always want to receive gifts from others. These unfortunate people have never learned and enjoyed the law of giving. Demanding and expecting to receive from others becomes their nature. They have no sense of when, how, and where to give.

ओं तत्सदिति निर्देशो ब्रह्मणस्त्रिविधः स्मृतः।
ब्राह्मणास्तेन वेदाश्च यज्ञश्च विहिताः पुरा।। २३
तस्मादोमित्युदाहृत्य यज्ञदानतपःक्रियाः।
प्रवर्तन्ते विधानोक्ताः सततं ब्रह्मवादिनाम्।। २४
तदित्यनभिसंधाय फलं यज्ञतपः क्रियाः।
दानक्रियाश्च विविधाः क्रियन्ते मोक्षकांक्षिभिः।। २५
सद्भावे साधुभावे च सदित्येतत्प्रयुज्यते।
प्रशस्ते कर्मणि तथा सच्छब्दः पार्थ युज्यते।। २६
यज्ञे तपसि दाने च स्थितिः सदिति चोच्यते।
कर्म चैव तदर्थीयं सदित्येवाभिधीयते।। २७

23. OM Tat Sat, 'OM, that is Reality'—this is the threefold statement concerning Brahman; from this the Brahmanas, the Vedas, and the sacrifices were produced in the ancient past.
24. Therefore all the sacrifices, charities, and ascetic acts of those proficient in the knowledge of Brahman, performed according to the ordinance, are commenced daily after enunciating 'OM' thus.
25. After enunciating Tat, 'that,' without the intention of fruit, the sacrificial and ascetic acts, and the various acts of charity are performed by those desiring liberation.
26. The word Sat, 'Reality,' is used to express Reality as well as goodness. Also the word 'Sat' is used to express a praiseworthy act, O Son of Pritha.
27. Stability in sacrifice, asceticism, and charity is also called Sat; also any act for the purpose of these is called Sat alone.

When the aspirant understands the importance of sattvic austerities practiced with mind, action, and speech, and then learns to dedicate the fruits of his actions in order to attain liberation, he is the highest aspirant on the path of yoga. His mind, action, and speech are directed to the supreme Lord alone. Verses 23 to 27 describe the way in which yogis and sages constantly remain conscious of the supreme Lord. Whenever they perform any duties or actions, worship, or give gifts, they remember three words: *OM Tat Sat.* These three words have deep meaning.

OM is the cosmic sound remembered by yogis during meditation. It is considered to be a living force that represents the supreme Lord. There are four states that can be realized by human beings. The first three—waking, dreaming, and sleeping—are experienced by all human beings and creatures. But the fourth state is attained only by the fortunate few accomplished yogis. It is a silent state, the deepest and most profound state of perfect equilibrium. The sound OM expresses the knowledge of these four states of consciousness. The aspirant learns to utter this sound all the time, before he talks to anyone and before he begins any work.

Good action is also called Tat Sat. It is auspicious for the sadhaka to remember the words Tat Sat, for they remind him of the goal of his life. The word Tat means that which exists in itself without the help of any other, and Sat means the absolute reality other than which nothing exists. The words Tat and Sat remind the aspirant of the self-existent glory of the Lord and of his benevolent kindness and goodness. Thus, OM Tat Sat refers to all that exists by itself without any second. These words are used by devotees, sages, and yogis for the supreme Lord.

अश्रद्धया हुतं दत्तं तपस्तप्तं कृतं च यत्।
असदित्युच्यते पार्थ न च तत्प्रेत्य नो इह।। २८

28. *An offering made, charity given, ascetic observance undertaken, or whatever act performed without faith, is called asat (untrue, unreal, evil); it bears nothing, neither here nor after death, O Son of Pritha.*

Sri Krishna tells Arjuna that the actions performed by yogis are selfless, done with absolute non-attachment and dedication to the Lord. They do these actions with perfect love and devotion as worship. The duties and actions that are performed with divine love and devotion are called Sat. But there are those who perform their actions, do charity, give gifts, practice austerities, and perform religious ceremonies without divine love and devotion. The scriptures refer to these actions as asat. Such acts are neither healthy nor helpful and do not bear good fruits, for they are done selfishly. Selfish people are not happy in this world, and they remain unhappy in the life hereafter. They create misery, unhappiness, confusion, and delusion.

Here ends the seventeenth chapter in which love and devotion for the divine is contrasted with lust for the objects of the world.

Chapter Eighteen
The Wisdom of Renunciation and Liberation

अर्जुन उवाच
संन्यासस्य महाबाहो तत्त्वमिच्छामि वेदितुम्।
त्यागस्य च हृषीकेश पृथक्केशिनिषूदन।। १
श्री भगवानुवाच
काम्यानां कर्मणां न्यासं संन्यासं कवयो विदुः।
सर्वकर्मफलत्यागं प्राहुस्त्यागं विचक्षणाः।। २

Arjuna said
1. *O Mighty-armed One, I wish to know the essence of renunciation and of relinquishing the fruits, O Lord of senses, destroyer of sin.*
   The Blessed Lord said
2. *The wise have known that abandoning the desire-fulfilling observances is renunciation; the insightful ones say that relinquishing the fruits of all actions is relinquishing.*

The actions that are helpful and liberating in the path of spirituality have been described. Now Arjuna wants to better understand the profound teachings of the path of renunciation (sannyasa) and of the path of renouncing the fruits of one's actions (tyaga). Aspirants who renounce the desire for pleasure are called sannyasins, and those who perform their duties skillfully and selflessly, giving up the fruits of their actions are called karma yogis. Sri Krishna tells Arjuna that there are characteristic differences between renunciates and those who perform actions but renounce the fruits.

However, from time immemorial there have been two paths: the path of renunciation and the path of action. The majority of people in the world follow the path of action. Only the rare and fortunate few walk the path of renunciation. Only those who have already burned their desires for self-enjoyment can walk that path. Others should not try. For the ordinary human being, the path of action is the way.

When one studies various commentaries on the Bhagavad Gita, he finds an intellectual tug-of-war between two groups of commentators: one pulling toward renunciation and the other toward action. These two paths are distinct and separate, and there is no need to judge one as being better than the other. Those who do are prejudiced and act under the influence of their egos. When one studies the message of the Bhagavad Gita, he realizes that all knowledge originates from one source and finally leads one to that source. That source is pure Atman, from which springs the entire knowledge and toward which it flows through various avenues until it finally meets its source: the ocean of happiness, bliss, and peace.

The Bhagavad Gita's message ends in this eighteenth chapter, which is conclusive and decisive. When he replies to Arjuna's questions, Sri Krishna answers the questions of all aspirants. Which is the path that leads one to the immutable, unchangeable, everlasting bliss? Which is the path that should be followed? What is renunciation, and what is action? Many commentators have drawn certain conclusions because they themselves lust for the enjoyments of the world and because they think that since the majority of people of the world follow the path of action, it is superior to the path of renunciation. But to know Truth, one does not need the support of an army of people. Truth can and should be attained in all possible ways. To attain the absolute truth, there are various paths that lead to the same summit. It is of no use to create a war of arguments, attempting to prove one path superior or inferior to another.

In the ancient tradition, the organization of one's life was guided by the thought that one would live for at least one hundred years. The first twenty-five years were devoted to school and learning. In the next twenty-five one attempted to understand relationships and interaction with others and the creatures of the world. The third quarter of one's life was dedicated to understanding the values of life with its currents and cross currents. The last twenty-five were devoted to spiritual sadhana alone. One would completely wash off the past; he would renounce and become totally non-attached, dedicating himself to the supreme Self alone. These last twenty-five years were devoted to Self-realization. With that systematic way of living, one finally attained the purpose of life. That was considered to be the normal procedure. But even during ancient times a few enlightened ones joined monasteries from a very early age, renounced the normal course of life, and attained Self-realization.

The path of renunciation is meant for only a few, and those who are not prepared should not tread that path. Those who learn to dedicate the fruits of all actions to the Lord and for the well-being of others are on the path. Those who renounce both actions and their fruits also follow the path to Self-realization. In the path of renunciation all action is renounced. Therefore the desire to receive the fruits of action is renounced as well. But in the path of action, action is not renounced; only the fruits are surrendered.

The question might arise: Is it possible for anyone to renounce all actions? This can be answered with another question: When all the actions, desires, and motivations for self-enjoyment are renounced, what is the action to be done and what is the purpose of doing actions? There remains only one action: doing action for the welfare of others. That action which is not done for one's own pleasure but only for the well-being of others does not have the power of bondage. Therefore, such action is allowed to be done in the path of renunciation.

Those who follow the path of action believe that actions such as yajna, charity, and austerities are liberating actions that should be performed. And in the path of renunciation, actions such as meditation, contemplation, and prayer are done with the motivation of attaining liberation. Although it is important and a must in the path of renunciation, liberation is only a step toward Self-realization. Even after one has liberated himself from the bondage of attachment, he has yet to attain unity with the Self of all. Liberating the individual self from the bondage of attachment is not the same as attaining samadhi or Self-realization. Even if one performs actions that are liberating and that do not create further bondage, he still remains an individual and has yet to reach a higher state. He has to learn to expand consciousness and go on expanding it until he realizes universal consciousness.

The goal of the renunciate is to systematically fathom one after another of the various stages of consciousness that lead to the innermost One. The following principles are the basis of the path of renunciation: (1) The renunciate directs all his energy toward the attainment of the goal of life, Self-realization; (2) He does not waste time and energy pursuing desires based on self-interest; (3) The renunciate's journey is inward; it is neither action nor inaction nor retreat. It consists of performing actions mentally and directing the mind and its modifications inward rather than toward the external world; (4) Non-attachment is attained spontaneously because the renunciate is not involved with objects; they have ail been consciously renounced; (5) With pure reason all the samskaras are burned in the fire of knowledge; (6) There remains only one desire: the desire for Self-realization. That desire does not motivate one to do actions in the external world but becomes a means to build determination, will power, and one-pointedness. Therefore, such desire is an essential means rather than an obstacle in the path of sadhana; (7) In the path of renunciation. Self-realization alone is the goal, and any action that does not become a means is firmly rejected and renounced. There is no half-here and half-there; total dedication and devotion are essential limbs for renunciation. This path of the rare few is the highest of all. It is difficult but not impossible. Those who are fully prepared should walk this path of fire and light. They should not listen to the suggestions of those who are not capable of following the path of renunciation.

Those who are not prepared to become renunciates should not think that they cannot realize the Self. That which is important to understand and attain is the state of non-attachment, without which treading either path—renunciation or action—is meaningless. It is important to do actions and duties for the common good and to release oneself from the helpless and inevitable law of karma. Such actions become a means to Self-realization, provided the goal always remains foremost and one's actions are performed with zeal to offer all the fruits to the Lord. That brings freedom from the law of karma. Dedicating all the fruits of action to the Lord is meditation in action, a central theme of the Bhagavad Gita, inspiring Arjuna and all aspirants. In the path of action. Self-realization is said to be attained by performing actions that are not binding, that are performed for the Lord alone. No path is superior or inferior. That which is important is to attain the wisdom of non-attachment.

त्याज्यं दोषवदित्येके कर्म प्राहुर्मनीषिण:।
यज्ञदानतप: कर्म न त्याज्यमिति चापरे।। ३
निश्चयं शृणु मे तत्र त्यागे भरतसत्तम।
त्यागो हि पुरुषव्याघ्र त्रिविध: संप्रकीर्तित:।। ४
यज्ञदानतप: कर्म न त्याज्यं कार्यमेव तत्।
यज्ञो दानं तपश्चैव पावनानि मनीषिणाम्।। ५
एतान्यपि तु कर्माणि सङ्गं त्यक्त्वा फलानि च।
कर्तव्यानीति मे पार्थ निश्चितं मतमुत्तमम्।। ६

3. *Some contemplative thinkers say that action should be abandoned like a fault; others say that sacrifice, charity, and ascetic actions cannot be relinquished.*

4. *In this regard hear my determination concerning relinquishment, O the Best of Bharatas. O Tiger among Men, relinquishment indeed is said to be of three kinds.*

5. *Sacrifice, charity, and asceticism—these acts should not be abandoned; indeed they must be done. Sacrifice, charity, and asceticism are purifiers of the contemplative and the wise.*

6. *Even these acts, however, should be performed after abandoning fruits. O Son of Pritha, this is my definite view.*

Some learned men say that all actions should be given up because actions lead one to an endless chain of reactions, thus creating a whirlpool for the performer of the actions. Once one is caught in that whirlpool, it is difficult to come out of it. There is another group of learned people who believe that good actions should not be abandoned because they need not create bondage. According to them, there are two kinds of works: one leads to bondage and the other does not. Describing both renunciation and action, Sri Krishna advises Arjuna to perform actions without any attachment in order to establish righteousness. He says that the three practices of yajna, charity, and austerity are righteous actions. Those actions performed with non-attachment and without the desire to enjoy the fruits should be practiced by those who cannot follow the path of renunciation.

नियतस्य तु संन्यासः कर्मणो नोपपद्यते।
मोहात्तस्य परित्यागस्तामसः परिकीर्तितः।। ७
दुःखमित्येव यत्कर्म कायक्लेशभयात्त्यजेत्।
स कृत्वा राजसं त्यागं नैव त्यागफलं लभेत्।। ८
कार्यमित्येव यत्कर्म नियतं क्रियतेऽर्जुन।
सङ्गं त्यक्त्वा फलं चैव स त्यागः सात्त्विको मतः।। ९

7. *It is not appropriate to renounce the eternal act; to abandon that out of delusion is said to be tamasic.*

8. *If one abandons an act because 'it is difficult' and out of a fear of discomfort to the body, upon committing such rajasic abandonment one would not gain the result of abandoning.*

9. *The act that is ever performed because 'it ought to be done,' O Arjuna, giving up attachment as well as the fruit—such relinquishment is considered sattvic.*

Sri Krishna tells Arjuna that one should not renounce his duty under the influence of either rajas or tamas. Those who renounce their

duties under the spell of confusion, delusion, or disappointment cannot tread the path of renunciation but descend to the darkness of ignorance. Giving up one's duty in a fit of emotion is tamasic renunciation,
which inevitably creates misery. Those who renounce based on such
motivation become a burden to themselves, to their nation, and to the
whole of mankind. They remain dependent on others for their livelihood and become poor examples to others. Sattvikas alone are capable
of treading the rare path of renunciation. Rajasic and tamasic people
should first learn to practice sattva. They should do their duties and
should never out of disappointment or in a fit of emotion or excitement
think of treading the path of light.

Those who are under the sway of rajas are afraid of afflictions, and
their thoughts of losing and not gaining cause them serious pain. It is
fear that causes them to give up actions. They search for pleasure by
making efforts only to attain their selfish ends. If one renounces the
world because of fear or pain, he gives a bad name to the path of fire
and knowledge. Tamasic people are known for their inertia and sloth;
their inactivity creates misery for themselves and others. They are not
fit for either the path of renunciation or the path of action. They believe
in "eat, drink, and be merry"and remain unconscious of both the internal and external realities. For escape they use all sorts of intoxicants.
The sattvic aspirants never renounce their essential duties, whether they
follow the path of renunciation or the path of action. They work hard,
perform their duties skillfully, and even learn to suffer to make others
happy. Sattvikas are the rare people who are successful and always have
clarity of mind; rajasikas are confused; and tamasikas are ignorant.

न द्वेष्ट्यकुशलं कर्म कुशले नानुषज्जते।
त्यागी सत्त्वसमाविष्टो मेधावी छिन्नसंशयः।। १०
न हि देहभृता शक्यं त्यक्तुं कर्माण्यशेषतः।
यस्तु कर्मफलत्यागी स त्यागीत्यभिधीयते।। ११
अनिष्टमिष्टं मिश्रं च त्रिविधं कर्मणः फलम्।
भवत्यत्यागिनां प्रेत्य न तु संन्यासिनां क्वचित्।। १२

10. *A relinquisher possessed of mental essence, endowed with intuitive wisdom, with his doubts dispelled, neither hates the unhappy deed nor is drawn to the happy act.*
11. *It is not at all possible for a body-bearer to abandon acts in their entirety; he, however, who relinquishes the fruits of action is said to be the relinquisher.*
12. *The fruit of action is threefold: undesirable, desirable, and mixed; such fruit accrues after death to those who do not relinquish; but to the renunciates, there is none.*

Those aspirants who are endowed with the qualities of sattva, who are free from all doubts, do not withdraw themselves from disagreeable work and do not become attached to pleasant work. For them duty is duty, and they perform their duties with an even mind. It is not possible for the ordinary human being to abstain from his duties, for he carries his samskaras from his previous lives. He has those latent tendencies within himself that create his duties, and sooner or later they have to be performed. There is no choice but to perform one's duty, but one can choose to renounce the fruits of his actions. The aspirants who do not relinquish the fruits of their actions receive those fruits, but they are uncertain as to what they will be. Some fruits are agreeable, some are unpleasant, and some are mixed. Those who perform their actions selflessly and skillfully, dedicating all the fruits of their actions, remain unaffected here and hereafter.

पंचैतानि महाबाहो कारणानि निबोध मे।
सांख्ये कृतान्ते प्रोक्तानि सिद्धये सर्वकर्मणाम्।। १३
अधिष्ठानं तथा कर्ता करणं च पृथग्विधम्।
विविधाश्च पृथक्चेष्टा दैवं चैवात्र पञ्चमम्। १४
शरीरवाङ्मनोभिर्यत्कर्म प्रारभते नरः।
न्याय्यं वा विपरीतं वा पंचैते तस्य हेतवः।। १५

13. *Learn these five causes from Me, O Mighty-armed One, taught in Samkhya whore all actions end, for the fulfillment of all actions.*
14. *The substratum, the agent of action, and instrumentality of different kinds, separate motions of various kinds, and the rulership of the deities as the fifth—*
15. *The actions that a human initiates with the body, speech, and mind, whether just or its opposite, these five are its causes.*

According to Samkhya philosophy and science, when an aspirant performs action from a state of equilibrium, it is accomplished without any obstacle. Samkhya explains that five factors are necessary for accomplishing an action. First the doer of actions needs a field for his actions and a dwelling place, called *adhisthana*. The second important factor is the performer of the actions who dwells within the field. He should be skilled in the performance. The third factor is the means and instruments of various kinds that are used by the performer. To attain the desired fruit, it is necessary to have health and appropriate means. The fourth factor is effort, for if a concentrated effort is not made, the desire to accomplish something is wasted. The undertaking should be well planned, and effort should be applied skillfully. The fifth factor is a favorable circumstance. Good actions performed in past lives give one the opportunity to be reborn in a family, environment, and country that offer favorable circumstances.

Some people think that a favorable circumstance is the result of luck. But luck is not a non-human factor; it is not partiality shown toward any one particular individual by a supreme being. A favorable circumstance is self-created. The Bhagavad Gita gives this as the last factor. Human endeavor, sincerity, and effort are the principle virtues, and favorable circumstances follow accordingly. Luck is the joy obtained after one's task has been performed successfully, with skill and selflessness. Luck is within the domain of the individual and not in the hands of Providence. Those who are not aware of the actions they have done in the past to bring about their present good circumstances call it luck and attribute it to chance or to Providence.

तत्रैवं सति कर्तारमात्मानं केवलं तु यः।
पश्यत्यकृतबुद्धित्वान्न स पश्यति दुर्मतिः।। १६
यस्य नाहंकृतो भावो बुद्धिर्यस्य न लिप्यते।
हत्वाऽपि स इमाँल्लोकान्न हन्ति न निबध्यते।। १७

16. *This being the reality, he who sees only the self as the agent, because he has not cultivated his wisdom, such a dull-wit does not see.*
17. *He who does not have the sentiment produced by the thought 'I,' whose intelligence is not defiled, even upon killing these beings, he neither kills nor is bound.*

Samkhya philosophy and science declares that five factors are important for accomplishing an act: place, agent, means, effort, and circumstance. Those who do not understand this truth are inflated with pride; they think that they are the doers. Such people are ignorant and unwise. False pride feeds the ego, which creates the last obstruction in the path of Self-realization. In fact all the negative emotions feed the ego, creating a serious barrier that separates a person from the whole.

The aspirant who does not have a feeling of egoism, who has completely surrendered himself, his deeds, and the fruits of his actions to his single goal, the supreme Lord, is not considered to be an evil doer even if he kills someone in the battlefield, because he has profound knowledge of life, love, and equality, and his actions are completely dedicated to the Lord. He is free from the I-ness of his ego and is a representative of the Lord. He has no intention to injure, hurt, harm, or kill anyone. While protecting the boundaries of their country, soldiers fight for their national cause and kill intruders, yet they are not considered to be killers and murderers. When one who is selfless kills someone while performing his duty, his mind remains unstained, and he is not bound by the law of karma, for he has gone beyond the bonds of individuality and remains one with the Lord.

Of course this should not promote fanaticism. Those who are narrow-minded sometimes become religious fanatics and think that they can misuse this scriptural injunction for their own selfish convenience. The yogi who practices ahimsa with mind, action, and speech never dreams of killing anyone. The question here is whether Arjuna should retire or fight the battle of life. When Arjuna, a hero and leader of a nation, becomes despondent and shrinks from his duty in the battlefield, Sri Krishna teaches him not to resign but to fight, for it is the battle of life in which all human beings are participants. All aspirants are fighters. To attain the highest goal one needs courage, strength, and zeal to fight. That is the true meaning of these verses.

ज्ञानं ज्ञेयं परिज्ञाता त्रिविधा कर्मचोदना ।
करणं कर्म कर्तेति त्रिविधः कर्मसंग्रहः ।। १८
ज्ञानं कर्म च कर्ता च त्रिधैव गुणभेदतः ।
प्रोच्यते गुणसंख्याने यथावच्छृणु तान्यपि ।। १९

18. *Knowledge, the object of knowledge, and the knower—this is the threefold source of impelling the action. The instrument, the act, and the agent—this is the threefold gathering of action.*
19. *The knowledge, action, and doer are said to be of three types through the distinction of gunas, as it is taught in the way of discriminating gunas correctly. Hear of these also.*

To live in the world these three are needed: the object of knowledge, the knower, and the instrument. Actions cannot be performed without these three essentials; one must have profound knowledge of them for the accomplishment of any work. Each of these is again divided according to the gunas.

सर्वभूतेषु येनैकं भावमव्ययमीक्षते ।
अविभक्तं विभक्तेषु तज्ज्ञानं विद्धि सात्त्विकम् ।। २०
पृथक्त्वेन तु यज्ज्ञानं नानाभावान्पृथग्विधान् ।

वेत्ति सर्वेषु भूतेषु तज्ज्ञानं विद्धि राजसम्।। २१

यत्तु कृत्स्नवदेकस्मिन्कार्ये सक्तमहैतुकम्।

अतत्त्वार्थवदल्पं च तत्तामसमुदाहृतम्।। २२

20. *That whereby one sees a single, immutable aspect in all beings, undivided in the divided, know that to be the sattvic knowledge.*

21. *When one knows the knowledge and all the separate kinds of aspects, each divided separately among all beings, know that to be the rajasic knowledge.*

22. *That which is attached to a single effect as though it were the entire, without proper reasoning, devoid of essential meaning and reality, and narrow in scope is said to be tamasic.*

Knowledge is of a threefold nature. Aspirants who have cultivated sattva know that the Self is not subject to change, death, or decomposition. Such aspirants have gone beyond the limitations of ignorance and have acquired the knowledge of the whole. Because they have profound knowledge of the whole, they do not suffer from limited and divided vision. For them death and birth are not occasions for either sadness or joy, pleasure or pain.

The knowledge that prompts one to see the single whole as many has a rajasic quality. There is another kind of knowledge, tamasic, that does not even- recognize multiplicity. It only sees and reacts to what is immediately beneficial. Those possessed of this form of knowledge do not think of the consequences of their actions. They are engrossed in sensual pleasures and act impulsively. Such people treat a part as the whole. Selfishness blinds their vision, and they remain in the darkness of ignorance.

नियतं सङ्गरहितमरागद्वेषतः कृतम्।

अफलप्रेप्सुना कर्म यत्तत्सात्त्विकमुच्यते।। २३

यत्तु कामेप्सुना कर्म साहंकारेण वा पुनः।

क्रियते बहुलायासं तद्राजसमुदाहृतम्।। २४

अनुबन्धं क्षयं हिंसामनवेक्ष्य च पौरुषम्।
मोहादारभ्यते कर्म यत्तत्तामसमुच्यते।। २५

23. *An act performed devoid of attachment and without attraction and aversion, by one desiring no fruit, is called sattvic.*
24. *That act, however, which is performed by one desirous of fruit and possessed with ego with much exertion of many kinds, that is called rajasic.*
25. *Without foreseeing the result, loss, violence, or capacity, the act that is initiated out of delusion is called tamasic.*

All actions are divided into three classes. Sattvic actions are those that are performed selflessly, the fruits being dedicated and offered to the Lord. All yoga practices, including physical exercise, pranayama, and meditation, are considered to be sattvic actions. Prayers, chanting, and charity done selflessly are sattvic in nature.

Actions that are not performed with non-attachment but with desire for self-gratification are rajasic. Such actions are performed with great strain and are enveloped by selfish and egotistical desires. That way of being leads one to be chronically anxious and tense. The majority of people in modern society suffer under the strain of actions motivated by rajas. If modern therapy were to concentrate on helping one develop a sattvic way of being, many of the physical disorders and much of the psychological stress that we see would be eliminated.

Tamasic actions are those undertaken without regard for the consequences. The tamasic person stumbles along, reacting to the moment without regard to the havoc he creates as a result of his capacities or limitations. He may think that he is capable of much more than he really is and thus injures himself and others. Or he may believe that he is incapable, and thus become inert and fail to act. Although such people are unpredictable, one can accurately predict that the results of their actions will be disastrous.

मुक्तसङ्गोऽनहंवादी धृत्युत्साहसमन्वितः।
सिद्ध्यसिद्ध्योर्निर्विकारः कर्ता सात्त्विक उच्यते।। २६
रागी कर्मफलप्रेप्सुर्लुब्धो हिंसात्मकोऽशुचिः।
हर्षशोकान्वितः कर्ता राजसः परिकीर्तितः।। २७
अयुक्तः प्राकृतः स्तब्धः शठो नैष्कृतिकोऽलसः।
विषादी दीर्घसूत्री च कर्ता तामस उच्यते।। २८

26. *Liberated from attachment, not uttering 'I,' endowed with the power to sustain and enthuse, unaffected in fulfillment or failure, such an actor is said to be sattvic.*
27. *Attached, desirous of the fruit of action, greedy, inclined to violence, impure, possessed by exhilaration and depression, such an actor is said to be rajasic.*
28. *Not joined in yoga, unrefined, unbending, a rogue, harming others, lazy, always depressed, a procrastinator, such an actor is said to be tamasic.*

One who is endowed with the sattvic quality is free from attachment and egoism. He is courageous and enthusiastic. With evenmindedness he functions and does his duty. He maintains equilibrium all the time; he is neither inflated by success nor depressed by failure. A man of equilibrium is an example for society, for society needs something more concrete than the teachings of the scriptures. Such people are great assets. By contrast, people who are endowed with a rajasic nature are active and work selfishly for sense gratification. They are greedy people and are harmful to society, for they believe in possessing and hoarding. They readily experience fluctuations of joy and sorrow in their daily lives; they have no control of the mind and senses. Their desires are selfish; such people do everything for the sake of selfish ends. Those who are tamasic do not have any concern for the existence of others. They are inactive, lazy, and hurt and harm others. To obtain sensual joy, they will commit any heinous crime. They are the worst examples in society.

After describing three kinds of performers of actions, Sri Krishna distinguishes between three types of intelligence (buddhi) and three types of resolution or firmness (*dhriti*). Among the four main instruments of antahkarana, buddhi is the discriminative, judging, and deciding faculty through which the light of knowledge comes forward. It is through buddhi that one discriminates and understands, judges, and makes decisions before he performs actions. There are three kinds of buddhi. The buddhi that helps one to discriminate, judge, and decide; to know right from wrong; and to understand what is to be feared and what is not to be feared is called sattvic buddhi. Sattvic buddhi leads the aspirant inward and helps him to fathom the subtler and higher realms of life. Without any distraction, the pure reason of buddhi becomes penetrative and fathoms those levels of life that normally remain unknown to ordinary human beings.

The higher or sattvic buddhi has the following characteristics. (1) The power of discrimination is developed; (2) The buddhi that has learned to discriminate between the Self and non-Self, between the supreme Self in its unmanifest state and its power of manifestation, possesses the power of non-attachment; (3) Such a buddhi has one-pointedness and inwardness; (4) It has attained calmness, quietness, and steadiness; it remains serene, undisturbed, and undissipated; (5) It is free from the desire for sense gratification; (6) It helps one to decide right from wrong and to act in a timely manner; (7) It makes one selfless and giving, without any expectations; (8) It helps one to remain tranquil and even in all conditions; (9) It helps one to remain a witness; (10) It leads one to spiritual heights.

बुद्धेर्भेदं धृतेश्चैव गुणतस्त्रिविधं शृणु।
प्रोच्यमानमशेषेण पृथक्त्वेन धनंजय।। २९
प्रवृत्तिं च निवृत्तिं च कार्याकार्ये भयाभये।
बन्धं मोक्षं च या वेत्ति बुद्धिः सा पार्थ सात्त्विकी।। ३०
यया धर्ममधर्मं च कार्यं चाकार्यमेव च।
अयथावत्प्रजानाति बुद्धिः सा पार्थ राजसी।। ३१
अधर्मं धर्ममिति या मन्यते तमसावृता।
सर्वार्थान्विपरीतांश्च बुद्धिः सा पार्थ तामसी।। ३२

29. *Now hear the threefold division of intelligence and sustenance by their gunas, being taught in entirety and separately, O Arjuna.*
30. *Ordinance and prohibition, what ought to be done or not to be done, dangerous and nondangerous, bondage and liberation—the intelligence that knows these, O Son of Pritha, is the sattvic one.*
31. *That by which one knows incorrectly virtue and vice, what ought to be done or ought not to be done, O Son of Pritha, is rajasic.*
32. *That intelligence, which, covered by darkness, believes vice to be virtue, and all the matters opposite of their reality, O Son of Pritha, is tamasic.*

The buddhi that is of a rajasic quality is incapable of helping one distinguish that which is the righteous path from that which is not. It is unable to discriminate between the real and the unreal. However, the rajasic buddhi is important for gaining external knowledge. Mechanical and scientific knowledge, knowledge of business, and knowledge relating to any aspect of the external world is a result of rajasic buddhi. It is not possible for anyone to function in the external world without it. People of a tamasic nature are ignorant and remain engrossed in sense enjoyment. They act in a manner opposite and contrary to the sattvic quality. Tamasic knowledge leads one to sullenness, sloth, and inertia.

The aspirant should not forget that the three gunas always function together in human life. The difference between one person and another is in the relative strength of each quality. The most important factor is which quality is predominant. If sattva is predominant, life becomes peaceful, joyful, and delightful. If rajas is predominant, one becomes active and hyper, prone to restlessness, and may suffer from psychosomatic and psychological illnesses. If tamas is predominant, everything in life becomes negative and passive. Then one does not experience any happiness or joy. The predominance of one or another of these three qualities is clearly noticed in human behavior. Those who have gone beyond the three gunas, who have realized the Self, and who remain in a state of samadhi are rarely seen. They do exist in our world, but they are one in a hundred million. Those great ones guide humanity in a subtle and profound way, emanating their love and knowledge through their minds, actions, and speech.

धृत्या यया धारयते मन: प्राणेन्द्रियक्रिया:।
योगेनाव्यभिचारिण्या धृति: सा पार्थ सात्त्विकी।। ३३
यया तु धर्मकामार्थान्धृत्या धारयतेऽर्जुन।
प्रसङ्गेन फलाकांक्षी धृति: सा पार्थ राजसी।। ३४
यया स्वप्नं भयं शोकं विषादं मदमेव च।
न विमुंचति दुर्मेधा धृति: सा पार्थ तामसी।। ३५

33. *That undeviating steadfastness (dhriti) which sustains activities of mind, prana, and senses through yoga, is, O Pritha, a sattvic one.*
34. *That by which one sustains virtue, desire, and worldly success, desiring fruits incidentally in the context, that steadfastness (dhriti) is rajasic.*
35. *That by which someone devoid of intuitive wisdom does not give up sleep, fear, grief, and depression, that steadfastness (dhriti), O Son of Pritha, is tamasic.*

In addition to intelligence and knowledge, dhriti (firmness or steadiness) is necessary in the path to infinity. There are aspirants who have knowledge, who know what to do and what not to do, but who lack the inner strength to be steady and firm in doing their practices. Some aspirants are very steady and firm but do not have profound knowledge of spirituality. In the path to Self-realization, sattvic buddhi and sattvic firmness are equally important. The way it is used here, the word dhriti has a meaning more profound than that which is usually attributed to it. It is that inner strength which does not dawn all of a sudden but which is attained only after long spiritual practice under the guidance of an accomplished yogi. Human effort, sincerity, and honesty lead the aspirant to attain that power. For lack of that power, the yogi cannot reach the highest realm of spiritual knowledge.

Dhriti enables one to have a one-pointed mind, and it helps one maintain coordination between the mind and the vital breath and pranic energy. It is a method of applying sushumna, which is important for attaining spiritual knowledge and a state of tranquility, for all inner and external distractions are controlled by sushumna application. Those who systematically learn the method of meditation know that after attaining physical stillness and steadiness, irregularity of the breath continues to disturb the mind. Mental unrest can also disrupt the breath. Breath and mind are two inseparable friends who work together until the last breath of life. An in-depth study of the breath has not yet been undertaken by modern scientists, but the yogis know the subtle function of the breath and are aware that irregular breathing agitates the mind and vice versa. When the breath is calm and serene, when it has no jerks and no long pauses, it does not distract the mind but creates feelings of intense joy and steadiness.

The state in which both mind and breath function in a balanced way is established by dhriti. Dhriti is that which brings mind and breath to a state of balance; it is the power that helps them to work together in a serene way. If one is not able to regulate his mind and breath in a perfectly coordinated way, his meditation will not bear the desired fruit, samadhi, no matter how many hours he practices meditation.

When one's posture is comfortable, still, and steady and when the mind is focused on the bridge between the nostrils, then sushumna is applied. Prior to the application of sushumna, the practice of even breathing, alternate nostril breathing, and inner and outer retention of the breath should be perfected. These exercises should be practiced only under the guidance of a yogi, not just with instructions from books and manuals.

Firmness or determination is of three kinds: sattvic, rajasic, and tamasic. It is sattvic when it is able to direct the power of mind, senses, and breath to bring about balance, and when the mind and breath mutually help one another in a coordinated way. It is sattvic when used for spiritual attainment and selfless actions. When used for selfish desire and self-enjoyment, it is rajasic. Rajas-endowed dhriti prompts one to perform actions or religious acts with a desire to enjoy the fruits of those actions. Tamasic dhriti produces excessive and long hours of sleep with numerous and disturbing dreams. It also creates fears, makes one timid and sorrowful, and leads one to cry without valid reason. It makes one arrogant and self-conceited. The firmness of tamasic people is expressed in obstinacy and conceit.

Psychotherapists encounter tamasic dhriti in the passive-aggressive personality, in clients who show willful resistance and negativity, and in those who tenaciously hold on to their symptomatic behaviors despite their superficial pleas that their therapists rid them of such behaviors. If the therapist can help such clients to use that firmness in the context of rajas and sattva, that force which is being used in a negative way can serve a positive and useful function. It is not to be eliminated but rather to be redirected so that it becomes an instrument to help one achieve positive goals.

सुखं त्विदानीं त्रिविधं शृणु मे भरतर्षभ।
अभ्यासाद्रमते यत्र दुःखान्तं च निगच्छति।। ३ ६
यत्तदग्रे विषमिव परिणामेऽमृतोपमम्।
तत्सुखं सात्त्विकं प्रोक्तमात्मबुद्धिप्रसादजम्।। ३७
विषयेन्द्रियसंयोगाद्यत्तदग्रेऽमृतोपमम्।
परिणामे विषमिव तत्सुखं राजसं स्मृतम्।। ३८
यदग्रे चानुबन्धे च सुखं मोहनमात्मनः।
निद्रालस्यप्रमादोत्थं तत्तामसमुदाहृतम्।। ३९

36. *Now hear from Me the three kinds of happiness in which one delights through practice and definitely finds the end of sorrow.*
37. *That which initially is like poison but is in effect like elixir, that happiness is called sattvic born of the pleasantness of one's intelligence.*
38. *That which appears initially like elixir through the union of senses and their objects, but in effect is like a poison, that happiness is considered rajasic.*

39. *That happiness which both initially and in the end result deludes one's self, arising from sleep, laziness, and inattention, that is said to be the tamasic.*

These verses describe three kinds of joy. When first encountered the highest joy seems like a poison or at least a bitter medicine to those who are used to the gross worldly pleasure. But when one becomes familiar with its subtle qualities, that joy becomes a nectar, a joy so subtle that it cannot even be imagined by one who has tasted only worldly pleasures. It is said "A bitter pill has a blessed effect," and such is the case with sattvic joy.

What is joy? That which makes one happy, that which is not disturbing or painful is joy. The whole of mankind and all creatures of this universe are searching for perennial joy. They seem to find a bit of it in relating to different objects of the world, but alas those joys soon diminish for two reasons: the object of joy changes, and the enjoyer's concept of joy also changes. Nothing is permanent in the mundane and temporal world. Creatures other than human beings are controlled by nature, but human beings have a will of their own and a power unique in itself that helps them to continue in search of the imperishable, unfettered joy. When one becomes tired of the fleeting joys of the mundane world, he looks and searches within, in his inner world which he has never tried to know and understand. In the inner world there is a fountain that ultimately quenches the thirst of those seekers who genuinely search for it. If the seeker gets the opportunity and learns the way of fathoming all the levels of life, he will find that there is a source and that there are profound ways to go to that source, from which flows perennially the joy divine.

Discontent is seen on the face of everyone. No one seems to be happy and joyous, even if they have all the desired objects of the world. But the day comes when one awakens to the reality that searching in the external world is in vain, that only the search within is rewarding and satisfying. Then one begins following the path of the inward journey. The Bhagavad Gita says that when the individual self finds delight and joy in the Self, that is the highest of all joys. It is called love without an object, meditation without form, love without desire, and meditation without an obstacle. That is sattva-endowed joy. Such joy is born only after the serenity of Self-knowledge is attained. All the pleasure experienced by the senses is but momentary, and it is also the source of pain. But the profound joy that is attained by Self-realization is permanent and everlasting, for the Self knows no pain, no misery, and no worry.

The joy experienced by rajas-endowed people arises from the contact of the senses with the objects of the world. It is relished like nectar in the beginning, but it is like poison in the end. Tamasic pleasure deludes the human mind in both the beginning and the end. It springs from the ignorance of sleep, laziness, and negligence.

न तदस्ति पृथिव्यां वा दिवि देवेषु वा पुनः।
सत्त्वं प्रकृतिजैर्मुक्तं यदेभिः स्यात्त्रिभिर्गुणैः।। ४०

40. There is no essence in the earth, in heaven, or even among gods that may be free of these nature-born gunas.

All that exists on this earth, in the sky, and in the heavens is enveloped by the three gunas. These three qualities stage a drama for mankind, and all kinds of people participate in that drama. Some are called sattvic, some rajasic, and some tamasic. Everyone plays his role according to his nature.

ब्राह्मणक्षत्रियविशां शूद्राणां च परंतप।
कर्माणि प्रविभक्तानि स्वभावप्रभवैर्गुणैः।। ४१
शमो दमस्तपः शौचं क्षान्तिरार्जवमेव च।
ज्ञानं विज्ञानमास्तिक्यं ब्रह्मकर्म स्वभावजम्।। ४२
शौर्यं तेजो धृतिर्दाक्ष्यं युद्धे चाप्यपलायनम्।
दानमीश्वरभावश्च क्षात्रं कर्म स्वभावजम्।। ४३
कृषिगौरक्ष्यवाणिज्यं वैश्यकर्म स्वभावजम्।
परिचर्यात्मकं कर्म शूद्रस्यापि स्वभावजम्।। ४४

41. *The actions of the brahmanas, kshatriyas, vaishyas, and shudras, O Scorcher of Enemies, are properly divided by the gunas born of the primordial nature Prakriti.*
42. *Peace, control, asceticism, purity, forgiveness, simplicity, knowledge, realization, and positive belief are the actions of a brahmana produced by nature.*
43. *Bravery, confidence, steadfastness, dexterity, not escaping a battle, charity, and expressing sovereign power are the actions of a kshatriya, born of nature.*
44. *Farming, husbandry, and trading are the actions of a vaishya, born of nature, and the actions of a shudra, consisting of service, are also born of nature.*

Sri Krishna describes four kinds of people according to their innate qualities and dispositions. Birth does not take place by chance; it is not accidental. Our desires and actions from the past lead us to our circumstances, abilities, and desires in this birth, and that which we desire and do now determines our future. We experience desires, and we also act according to the qualities or samskaras that we carry from our past. We carry our samskaras from here to the hereafter and are reborn according to our own choices. As we have already noted, human beings can be broadly divided into four categories according to their inherent qualities and dispositions. In the Bhagavad Gita they are called brahmana, kshatriya, vaishya, and shudra.

The brahmana quality is found in spiritually inclined people who know that the purpose of life is to attain tranquility. These aspirants practice self-restraint and self-control, and they gain knowledge of both the internal and external worlds. They also have a profound knowledge of life here and hereafter. They are endowed with the sattva quality because they have strengthened that quality in the past. These brahmanas are called brahmanas not because they have inherited wisdom from their ancestors but because they cultivated that disposition with sincere efforts in their past lives. Sattva is not received through inheritance, but it is the result of one's own efforts. Many times we find that a vagabond or ill-mannered and irresponsible person is born into a family of brahmanas, and often a man of brahmanic qualities and disposition is born into a shudra family. It is said that everyone is like a shudra by birth, but one becomes a brahmana only by his own efforts. It is one's samskaras that create his disposition. One who has the qualities of a brahmana is led toward a virtuous and spiritual way of life, and he is able to teach the art and science of life.

Rajasic qualities are seen in the personalities of kshatriyas. They have valor, courage, and the ability to administer and rule. The rajasic quality and disposition leads one toward an active and creative way of life. The vaishyas are another class of people; they are less endowed with sattvic and rajasic qualities than the people in the first two categories. They like to trade and conduct business. Shudra is the category of people who are not fit enough to tread the path of spirituality. They do not have zeal to be active, they lack courage, and they are not fit for trade and business. Their duty is that of service.

In ancient times this division into classes was the basis for the distribution of labor. It was designed for the well-being of society. One's position and work was determined according to the qualities he possessed. Over time, however, this concept of categorizing individuals according to their abilities has become distorted and used to separate people based on their caste, color, race, culture, or religion. That creates both psychological divisiveness and conflicts in the individual, community, and nation, and it devalues human life. Many great cultures have suffered as a result of false standards fostered by the priesthood and so-called religious leaders who have used religion and scripture to feed their own egocentric and selfish philosophies. These people are supposed to be the custodians of culture and religion, but they become caught up in the cult that serves their selfishness instead of propagating the fundamentals of truth. Instead of teaching unity, they teach diversity. Many societal diseases such as disparity, illiteracy, malnutrition, and discrimination between the poor and rich, the knowledgeable and innocent, have degraded the human being so much that we have forgotten the truth that all human beings breathe the same air supplied by one and the same Lord.

No human being has a right to despise and look down on others and make others suffer. And any nation that desires to advance and march forward should first abolish such rules, ideas, customs, and systems that are the main barriers to the integration of the nation. The sense of inferiority and superiority and the resulting complexes are created by human society and not by God. Everyone should have the opportunity to rise, to think freely, and to contribute what he can for the well-being of society. Society generally considers those who performed services to be the lower class, but the Bhagavad Gita teaches that service is the highest of all actions, for it leads to liberation. Those who serve society in a way that others cannot should be adored and respected. There is nothing good or bad as far as work is concerned. Why should one think a leader is higher than a barber or garbage collector? Such erroneous ideas cause suffering to both the individual and to the whole of society.

The Bhagavad Gita integrates different elements of society into one, without which the survival of a society is ultimately at stake. The grouping of people described in the Bhagavad Gita is not meant to create disparity, caste, or rigid categories based on birth in a particular family. That would be opposed to the central theme of this sacred text.

स्वे स्वे कर्मण्यभिरतः संसिद्धिं लभते नरः।
स्वकर्मनिरतः सिद्धिं यथा विन्दति तच्छृणु॥ ४५

यतः प्रवृत्तिर्भूतानां येन सर्वमिदं ततम्।
स्वकर्मणा तमभ्यर्च्य सिद्धिं विन्दति मानवः॥ ४६

45. *A person attains perfection when absorbed and delighting in his own act. Hear how one who is content in his own actions finds perfection:*
46. *Worshipping Him with his act he from Whom begins all activity of beings, by Whom all this is spanned and pervaded, a child of Manu finds perfection.*

Verses 45 and 46 are conclusive as far as the caste system is concerned. These verses say that anyone who is sincerely devoted to his own duty is successful. Not only brahmanas, kshatriyas, vaishyas, and shudras, but anyone who is devoted to his duty can attain perfection. The aspirant attains success when he regards his duty as worship to the supreme Brahman from whom all human beings spring and by whose power they are able to do their work. One who surrenders himself with mind, action, and speech and makes Brahman the goal of his worship reaches Brahman. The student should remember that self-surrender—when one learns to surrender all that he thinks is his own—is the highest of yogas.

Total surrender means total acceptance of the supreme Self in the place of the individual self. This should not be misunderstood and thus lead one to become inert and lazy but should instead lead one to do all that can be done for the Lord. The attitude, "I am Thine and Thou art mine" is the first step in the practice of self-surrender. The second step is "Thou art everything," and the last step is "All that is conceivable and comprehended, all that exists is Thou alone." That state of Self-realization is attained by very few, only by those who have completely surrendered their egos and have realized the beauty and grandeur of the Lord of life. That realization is beyond I-ness and my-ness. It is timeless and infinite.

श्रेयान्स्वधर्मो विगुणः परधर्मात्स्वनुष्ठितात् ।
स्वभावनियतं कर्म कुर्वन्नाप्नोति किल्बिषम् ।। ४७
सहजं कर्म कौन्तेय सदोषमपि न त्यजेत् ।
सर्वारम्भा हि दोषेण धूमेनाग्निरिवावृताः ।। ४८
असक्तबुद्धिः सर्वत्र जितात्मा विगतस्पृहः ।
नैष्कर्म्यसिद्धिं परमां संन्यासेनाधिगच्छति ।। ४९

47. *Better one's own duty (dharma) even devoid of quality, rather than another's duty, even though well performed. By performing the act determined by nature, one does not gather stain.*

48. *One should not give up one's inborn act even though faulty; all endeavors are accompanied by some fault, like fire covered with smoke.*

49. *One whose intellect is not attached, whose inner instrument is conquered in every way, one whose attraction is gone, attains through renunciation the perfection of actionlessness.*

Sri Krishna explains that one should always try to understand his own character, abilities, and capacities and that all duties should be undertaken according to one's own character. One should not abandon his own duty and attempt to do the duty of others. No matter how beneficial it might seem, abandoning one's own duty is unhealthy.

If one abandons his duties and takes up the duty of another, there will be serious disorder in society. Good and bad are two values that we project onto circumstances according to our own viewpoints. Though one's natural duty may appear to be tainted with faults, one should realize that all actions are tainted with defects. As fire, which is lustrous, contains smoke, likewise no action is perfect in itself. One who is completely non-attached and continues to do his duty as best he can, renouncing the fruits of his actions, is a true renunciate. He attains the highest of perfection.

Every action in the phenomenal world is defective. No matter how good one's intentions, no action is perfect. If one gives something to another person with love and kindness, that action will produce pain if the object given is lost or broken or if another person becomes envious. If one wants to practice non-injury and therefore avoids eating meat, he nevertheless must kill plants and other forms of life in order to survive. If Arjuna fights in the battle of Kurukshetra and becomes victorious, he will help his nation overcome evil, but in the process he will create immense suffering. One must be courageous and act to the best of his knowledge and ability in spite of the inevitable imperfections of his actions, and he should remain non-attached to the fruits.

सिद्धिं प्राप्तो यथा ब्रह्म तथाप्नोति निबोध मे।
समासेनैव कौन्तेय निष्ठा ज्ञानस्य या परा।। ५०
बुद्धया विशुद्धया युक्तो धृत्यात्मानं नियम्य च।

शब्दादीन्विषयांस्त्यक्त्वा रागद्वेषौ व्युदस्य च।। ५१
विविक्तसेवी लघ्वाशी यतवाक्कायमानसः।
ध्यानयोगपरो नित्यं वैराग्यं समुपाश्रितः।। ५२
अहंकारं बलं दर्पं कामं क्रोधं परिग्रहम्।
विमुच्य निर्ममः शान्तो ब्रह्मभूयाय कल्पते।। ५३
ब्रह्मभूतः प्रसन्नात्मा न शोचति न कांक्षति।
समः सर्वेषु भूतेषु मद्भक्तिं लभते परम्।। ५४
भक्त्या मामभिजानाति यावान्यश्चास्मि तत्त्वतः।
ततो मां तत्त्वतो ज्ञात्वा विशते तदनन्तरम्।। ५५
सर्वकर्माण्यपि सदा कुर्वाणो मद्व्यपाश्रयः।
मत्प्रसादादवाप्नोति शाश्वतं पदमव्ययम्। ५६

50. *How one, having attained perfection, attains Brahman, learn from Me—as well as the final determination of knowledge.*

51. *Endowed with purified intelligence, controlling himself with sustenance (dhriti), abandoning the objects of senses such as sound, and casting away attraction and aversion;*

52. *Enjoying solitary places, eating lightly, with speech, body, and mind controlled, unceasingly intent on the yoga of meditation, having perfect recourse to dispassion;*

53. *Having abandoned ego, pride, passion, and anger, not receiving sense inputs, free of 'mine,' the pacified one is fit to become Brahman.*

54. *Having become Brahman, with pleasant and clear self, one neither grieves nor desires; alike toward all beings he gains the highest devotion toward Me.*

55. *Through devotion he recognizes Me, how expansive and who I am in reality. Then knowing Me in reality, he enters Me immediately.*

56. *Even performing all the actions at all times depending entirety on Me, through My grace he attains the eternal, imperishable state.*

Sri Krishna briefly explains how the accomplished yogi attains the highest Brahman. The yogi has to attain many realms of wisdom before he can attain the highest Brahman. In the first step he learns to develop control over his senses through self-restraint. In the second step he concentrates the mind, not allowing it to become distracted and dissipated. Next he makes his mind one-pointed by practicing both meditation and non-attachment. In the next step he becomes a witness and does not identify himself with the objects of the world. In a still higher stage he establishes himself in his true nature: peace, happiness, and bliss. At the final state he realizes his Self as the Self of all. Each of the stages of wisdom is valuable and is an accomplishment, but the highest of perfection is attained when the individual soul is united with the absolute Self. The yogi who has attained that does not suffer as a result of the negative emotions that have such a powerful impact on the minds and hearts of ordinary people. The realized yogi is tranquil, for he has already attained Brahman, and for him there is nothing more to be attained. He has no desires; his whole life is devoted to the Lord alone. He has profound knowledge through direct experience of the greatness of the Lord, and he remains one with the Lord. Such a yogi performs his actions with an attitude of worship. His whole life is devoted to the Lord, and the eternal becomes his permanent abode.

चेतसा सर्वकर्माणि मयि संन्यस्य मत्परः।
बुद्धियोगमुपाश्रित्य मच्चित्तः सततं भव।। ५७
मच्चित्तः सर्वदुर्गाणि मत्प्रसादात्तरिष्यसि।
अथ चेत्त्वमहंकारान्न श्रोष्यसि विनंक्ष्यसि।। ५८

57. *Renouncing all acts to Me with the mind intent upon Me, resorting to the yoga of wisdom, always hold your mind in Me.*

58. *Holding your mind in Me, you will go across difficult passages through My grace; if, however, out of ego you will not listen, you will perish completely.*

These two verses give instructions to Arjuna, who follows the path of action, not of renunciation. One who follows the path of action should dedicate his thoughts, actions, and speech to the Lord. If one keeps his mind fixed on the Lord, it enables him to give up and offer the fruits of his actions. The aspirant who attains that crosses the mire of delusion through the grace of God. When human endeavor and efforts have been exhausted, then dawns the grace of the descending force of the compassionate Lord of life. But if the aspirant does not follow this path and instead is caught by his egoism, the purpose of his life is not achieved.

यदहंकारमाश्रित्य न योत्स्य इति मन्यसे।
मिथ्यैव व्यवसायस्ते प्रकृतिस्त्वां नियोक्ष्यति।। ५९
स्वभावजेन कौन्तेय निबद्धः स्वेन कर्मणा।
कर्तुं नेच्छसि यन्मोहात्करिष्यस्यवशोऽपि तत्।। ६०

59. *If, resorting to ego, you think, I shall not fight,' this, your resolve, is a false one; nature will impel you.*
60. *Bound by your nature-born act, O Son of Kunti, what you do not wish to do out of confusion, even that you will do helplessly.*

If one becomes obstinate and thinks that he will not do something that he has to do, he can waste time and he can suffer, but his nature will eventually force him to do it. Although he is a warrior and a leader and a descendant of Bharata, Arjuna withdraws himself from the field of action and wants to retreat. Because he is confused and deluded, he forgets to do his duty and becomes caught up in attachment. But Sri Krishna tells him, "You must perform your duty. You have to do your dharma, and for performing your duty you must be non-attached, free from pride, prejudice, and the bonds of ego." The aspirant should always remember and follow his inborn nature and potential, with the help of which he should learn to unfold, improve, and accomplish the purpose of life. Often occasions come that lead one to deviate from the path, but then he should again make sincere attempts to tread his path. Every human being is endowed and gifted with some great and profound quality that can be called his inborn nature. If the aspirant does something that he is not meant to do, his inborn nature will compel him to do that for which he is meant. Suppose the aspirant follows the path of renunciation sincerely with his mind and heart but becomes distracted along the way. He will invariably come back again to the path because his deep-seated desire to follow the path of renunciation, motivated by his inborn qualities, will again bring him back to his path.

ईश्वरः सर्वभूतानां हृद्देशेऽर्जुन तिष्ठति।
भ्रामयन्सर्वभूतानि यन्त्रारूढानि मायया।। ६१

तमेव शरणं गच्छ सर्वभावेन भारत।
तत्प्रसादात्परां शान्तिं स्थानं प्राप्स्यसि शाश्वतम्।। ६२

इति ते ज्ञानमाख्यातं गुह्याद् गुह्यतरं मया।
विमृश्यैतदशेषेण यथेच्छसि तथा कुरु।। ६३

61. *The sovereign God dwells in the heart space of all beings, O Arjuna, making all beings move with His maya as though they were mounted on a machine.*
62. *Go and take refuge only in Him with your entire being, O Descendant of Bharata. By His grace you will attain the highest peace and eternal station.*
63. *I have taught you this knowledge, more secret than any secret. After contemplating it in entirety, do as you wish.*

In Verse 61 there is a subtle and profound teaching. Sri Krishna says, "O Arjuna, the supreme Lord is the inner dweller in everyone's heart." That the Lord is the inner dweller should be understood by all aspirants, but with that knowledge alone, one cannot directly attain wisdom. He will have to learn to practice to see and realize the Lord himself first; then he can grasp and comprehend that the Lord dwells in every heart. The mere knowing of a principle is not the same as realizing it.

Those who do not realize that the Lord dwells in the hearts of all remain attached to the vehicles of nature. They are compelled as though they are being used as puppets. Therefore Sri Krishna says, "O Arjuna, surrender yourself to the Lord alone, and once you have surrendered, then by grace you can attain the state of tranquility and thus will be liberated." That is the secret of secrets that is imparted to Arjuna. After that secret is imparted, one is left alone to decide for himself what is right for him. When a teacher imparts knowledge, he wants his student to use his free will, to be courageous, and to make experiments to experience and then to realize what is right for him. Spiritual teachings should not be forced on students as commandments. But there is a commitment between the teacher and the student, and once the teacher has completed his commitment, it is up to the student to choose, practice, and do as he likes. Thus, in the path of spiritual knowledge, fifty percent of the responsibility lies with the teacher and fifty percent with the student.

सर्वगुह्यतमं भूयः शृणु मे परमं वचः।
इष्टोऽसि मे दृढमिति ततो वक्ष्यामि ते हितम्।। ६४
मन्मना भव मद्भक्तो मद्याजी मां नमस्कुरु।
मामेवैष्यसि सत्यं ते प्रतिजाने प्रियोऽसि मे।। ६५
सर्वधर्मान्परित्यज्य मामेकं शरणं व्रज।
अहं त्वा सर्वपापेभ्यो मोक्षयिष्यामि मा शुचः।। ६६

64. *Again hear My final words, the most secret of all: you are firmly My favorite; therefore I shall say what is beneficial to you.*
65. *Let your mind be in Me; My devotee, sacrificing to Me, offer salutations to Me; you wilt come only to Me truly; I avow you are My beloved.*
66. *Abandoning all virtue, come and take refuge in Me alone; I shall liberate you from all evil; grieve not.*

The teacher's love for his student is immense and immeasurable. It is always selfless and of the highest quality. Such love cannot be found in any other relationship in the world. With his immortal love for Arjuna, Sri Krishna says, "Listen to my words of wisdom. I am imparting the secret of secrets because you are my beloved disciple. This is for your good."

Students are many, but disciples are rare. A student can join a school and can also leave it. He comes to a spiritual teacher, studies with him for some time, and then leaves forever. But when the spiritual commitment is made by both the teacher and disciple, it is impossible for the teacher not to impart to his disciple all the secrets that he himself has realized. The true disciple always remains eager to learn the subtle secrets that fulfill the purpose of his spiritual commitment.

When the disciple learns to fix his mind on the Lord alone and dedicates his entire life to the Lord, he attains the kingdom of eternity, where the Lord resides unattached in His splendid glory. Knowledge of the path of devotion and of the way in which God is attained is a secret imparted only to the very dear disciple. Sri Krishna says, "O Arjuna, forsake all religious works whatsoever and make the supreme Lord your final and sole refuge. Grieve not, for you will be free and released from all sins." The 66th verse contains the teachings of the Bhagavad Gita in a nutshell: renounce all actions and come to the Lord alone, for your stains will be washed by the Lord. Ordinarily if one abandons his duties, he suffers and plunges into sorrow. But if one renounces a lesser duty in order to perform a greater duty, his sin is forgiven. If the cause is higher and more profound than the duty that is abandoned, that duty should be renounced delightfully. Suppose one renounces his home, he will suffer the consequences of renouncing his duties, but he will be free from that suffering if he takes on a duty greater than the duties he was performing before. If one renounces his country for the service of mankind, he is performing a higher duty. And if one renounces everything and devotes all his time and energy to deep and profound meditation and contemplation, he is the highest of all devotees, and his stains are washed off by his pure devotion.

Serious questions arise here: Since Arjuna was prepared to renounce the world in the beginning, why was he not allowed to do so? And why is the secret of secrets, that one should abandon all duties and that the Lord will wash away all his stains and sins, being imparted here? In the beginning Arjuna wanted to withdraw himself and to abandon his duty in a state of confusion and despondency. He was not renouncing in a state of wisdom but in a deep state of sorrow and out of fear, attachment, and confusion. These verses teach the aspirant that the highest of all is that path in which one devotes and dedicates all that he has and all that he is to the Lord. Such a lost lover of the Lord is the highest of all aspirants. Whether he follows the path of renunciation or the path of action, he is liberated here and now, and he enjoys eternal happiness.

इदं ते नातपस्काय नाभक्ताय कदाचन।
न चाशुश्रूषवे वाच्यं न च मां योऽभ्यसूयति।। ६७
य इदं परमं गुह्यं मद्भक्तेष्वभिधास्यति।
भक्तिं मयि परां कृत्वा मामेवैष्यत्यसंशयः।। ६८
न च तस्मान्मनुष्येषु कश्चिन्मे प्रियकृत्तमः।
भविता न च मे तस्मादन्यः प्रियतरो भुवि।। ६९
अध्येष्यते च य इमं धर्म्यं संवादमावयोः।
ज्ञानयज्ञेन तेनाहमिष्टः स्यामिति मे मतिः।। ७०
श्रद्धावाननसूयश्च शृणुयादपि यो नरः।
सोऽपि मुक्तः शुभाँल्लोकान्प्राप्नुयात्पुण्यकर्मणाम्।। ७१

67. *This should never be taught by you to a non-ascetic or a non-devotee nor to someone inattentive nor to one who defames Me.*

68. *He who narrates this supreme secret to My devotees, completing his highest devotion toward Me, will come to Me alone, without doubt.*

69. *Among human beings, there is no one who causes Me greater pleasure nor shall there be anyone more beloved of Me on earth than*

70. *One who will read this virtuous dialogue that has occurred between us. Let him sacrifice unto Me with the sacrificial observance of knowledge; this is My view.*

71. Endowed with faith and without calumny, whichever human would hear this, even he, liberated, would obtain the beautiful worlds of those with meritorious acts.

The great sages like to impart their knowledge to their loving disciples. Their teachings are called secret knowledge because they cannot be comprehended by the ordinary mind. The teacher imparts such knowledge to his close disciples only. It would be a waste of time and energy to impart such knowledge to those who are not prepared, for it would be like Greek or Latin to them. There is no reason to discuss the spiritual depths with those who are not at all proficient in the path of spirituality. The supreme secrets of spiritual knowledge are imparted only to the dear and true devotees who have already trodden the path and who have still to attain.

One who imparts the knowledge of devotion and dedication to those weary, tired, and old travelers who are on the path but still stumbling is dear to the Lord. Such teachings help both the teacher and the student. The greatest of all professions is the teaching profession, and among all the branches of knowledge, spiritual teaching is the highest. Among the many spiritual paths, the path of complete devotion and dedication is the highest. Thus, the teacher who imparts his spiritual knowledge is the highest of all teachers. Teaching spirituality is the highest of actions and is pleasing to the Lord of life. There is no one higher than the sage who propagates the truth lovingly and selflessly.

One who studies, practices, and propagates the dialogue between Sri Krishna and Arjuna with all his heart and mind is the greatest of all devotees. By studying and practicing the teachings of the Bhagavad Gita, one is in fact worshipping the supreme Lord. One who listens to the discourse of the Bhagavad Gita with unquestioned faith is a holy man. Such a man becomes free from stains and fears. One who contemplates upon the teachings imparted through the dialogue between Sri Krishna and Arjuna is released from bondage and attains a high state of spirituality. Among all the offerings made by human beings, the sacrifice that is made by imparting the knowledge of the Bhagavad Gita is the highest of all. The knowledge imparted by the Bhagavad Gita is beneficial for all people in all times.

कच्चिदेतच्छ्रुतं पार्थ त्वयैकाग्रेण चेतसा।
कच्चिदज्ञानसंमोहः प्रनष्टस्ते धनंजय।। ७२

अर्जुन उवाच

नष्टो मोहः स्मृतिर्लब्धा त्वत्प्रसादान्मयाऽच्युत।
स्थितोऽस्मि गतसन्देहः करिष्ये वचनं तव।। ७

72. *Did you perchance hear this, O Son of Pritha, with a one-pointed mind? Did your delusion of ignorance perchance vanish, O Arjuna?*
   Arjuna said
73. *The delusion has vanished by Your grace; I have received remembrance, O Infallible One. I stand here free of doubts; I shall act according to your word.*

Throughout the dialogue between Sri Krishna and Arjuna, it has been Arjuna who has asked the questions. But here Sri Krishna asks questions of Arjuna: "Is your delusion dispelled? Has your ignorance vanished? As a result of knowledge imparted by me, are all your questions answered, or is there still doubt lingering in your mind?" Arjuna replies, "O Enlightened One, my ignorance has been dispelled, and my doubts have been resolved by the teachings you have imparted to me. 1 have no doubt in my mind and no conflict about doing my duties. 1 will fight with all my might. You have inspired me, and 1 have regained my inner strength. 1 will perform my duties according to my dharma. Now 1 am able to perform them skillfully and selflessly without any attachment."

Those like Arjuna who plunge into sorrow and delusion lose their memories of their true nature and of the source from which they came. But Sri Krishna has led Arjuna to the awareness of that which he had forgotten. Arjuna now realizes his unity with the Self of all.

संजय उवाच
इत्यहं वासुदेवस्य पार्थस्य च महात्मनः।
संवादमिममश्रौषमद्भुतं रोमहर्षणम्।। ७४
व्यासप्रसादाच्छुतवानेतद्गुह्यमहं परम्।
योगं योगेश्वरात्कृष्णात्साक्षात्कथयतः स्वयम्।। ७५
राजन्संस्मृत्य संस्मृत्य संवादमिममद्भुतम्।
केशवार्जुनयोः पुण्यं हृष्यामि च मुहुर्मुहुः।। ७६
तच्च संस्मृत्य संस्मृत्य रूपमत्यद्भुतं हरेः।
विस्मयो मे महान्राजन्हृष्यामि च पुनः पुनः।। ७७
यत्र योगेश्वरः कृष्णो यत्र पार्थो धनुर्धरः।
तत्र श्रीर्विजयो भूतिर्ध्रुवा नीतिर्मतिर्मम।। ७८

Sanjaya said

74. *I heard this wondrous dialogue, making my hair stand on end, between the indwelling One and the great-souled Son of Pritha.*

75. *By the grace of Vyasa I heard this secret most, supreme yoga from Krishna, the Lord of yoga, personally teaching it Himself.*

76. *O King, remembering again and again this wondrous, virtuous dialogue between Krishna and Arjuna, I rejoice again and again.*

77. *And remembering that very wondrous form of the Lord, there is great amazement in me, O Lord, and I rejoice again and again.*

78. *Where there is Krishna, the Lord of Yoga, and where there is the bowbearer, Son of Pritha, there glory, victory, success, and polity are definite. This I believe.*

Sanjaya, the narrator of the dialogue between Sri Krishna and Arjuna, speaks to King Dhritarashtra. The compiler of this dialogue is the sage Vyasa who gave the power of vision to Sanjaya, enabling him to narrate what occurs on the battlefield. Sanjaya says, "O Dhritarashtra, I have heard the supreme and profound wisdom and the knowledge of life and the universe and that which is beyond from the master of yoga.

1 am describing it to you exactly as 1 heard it. When 1 recall these profound teachings my hair still stands on end. With great joy 1 saw the vision of the Lord of the universe, and the joyous and delightful memory of that experience is still with me. I firmly assert that where there is a great hero like Arjuna and a perfect yogi like Sri Krishna helping him, that side is sure to be forever victorious in all ways."

The dialogue between Sri Krishna and Arjuna gives deep insight into the philosophy of life and its practical application. These teachings describe the eternal wisdom of the infinite Lord and the ways in which that wisdom can be attained. When a good student has a perfect preceptor, attainment is sure.

Here ends the profound and unique teachings of the Bhagavad Gita. In this concluding chapter Yogeshvar Krishna imparts the art and science of renunciation.

Glossary of Sanskrit Terms

Words set in SMALL CAPS are defined elsewhere in the Glossary.

ABHYASA. Practice. The Bhagavad Gita suggests two means to attain mastery over the mind and its modifications: abhyasa, which is a systematic spiritual practice or instruction given by a master, and VAIRAGYA. which means detachment.

ACHARYA. A spiritual teacher or instructor. Literally, one whose character and behavior should be followed by others.

ADHIBHUTA. That which is related or belongs to the elements or which resides in the elements.

ADHIDAIVATA. That which is related or belongs to the bright beings (gods) or resides in the gods.

ADHISTHANA. Base, foundation, or seat. In the Bhagavad Gita, the senses, mind, and buddhi are said to be the seat of attachment and anger through which the ever-shining light of ATMAN is covered, just as the fetus is covered with the membrane of the amniotic sac and fire is covered with smoke.

ADHIYAJNA. That which resides in sacrifice. SRI KRISHNA says, "I, the supreme Lord, am the indweller or presiding God of all rituals."

ADHYATMA. That which is related to, belongs to, or resides in ATMAN.

ADVAITA. Non-dual; single reality. In the Vedanta system, the Self or the absolute Reality is said to be the non-dual, single principle.

AGATASU. A living being; one whose life force has not departed or been disconnected from the body. According to the Bhagavad Gita, the soul never dies and is never born; death is a habit of the body. As long as there is breath, a person is called alive, but the moment the breath ceases, one is declared to be dead. *See* GATASU.

AGNI. Fire.

AGRA BHAGE. In the front. In this context it refers to the base of the juncture that separates the two nostrils. *See* NASAGRE.

AHIMSA. Non-injury, non-hurting, and non-killing. It is one of the YAMAS, also known as the "great DHARMA," the highest of all observances leading to spiritual goals.

AJAPA JAPA. Repetition of the MANTRA done spontaneously throughout the day and night without any effort. The state of ajapa japa comes when a student has practiced his or her MANTRA for a long period of time, uninterruptedly and sincerely. Then, as a result, the unconscious mind is filled with the vibration of the MANTRA.

AJNA CHAKRA. That center of consciousness located between the eyebrows; literally, "command center." At this center the command of spiritual guidance from the higher CHAKRAS is received. It is the seat of the mind.

AKSHARA. Indestructible. According to the Bhagavad Gita, absolute Reality, Consciousness, or the pure Self is indestructible. It also means a unit of speech.

AMRITA. Ambrosia, nectar. According to legend, the gods and demons churned the ocean, and as a result found nectar. The gods, however, knew the art of drinking the nectar and thus became immortal, while the demons remained subject to death and rebirth.

ANASAKTI YOGA. The spiritual path that emphasizes performing one's actions without becoming attached to their fruits. It is an alternative path for those who do not choose to follow the path of renunciation.

ANANYA BHAVA. One-pointed devotion; literally, the attitude of "I am not different" from the object of devotion.

ANITYA. Non-eternal. Except ATMAN, the pure Consciousness, all that which seems to exist is non-eternal, illusory, and impermanent. *See* NITYA.

ANTAHKARANA. The inner instrument. The intellect (BUDDHI), ego (ahamkara), sensory-motor mind (MANAS), and storehouse of memories (chitta) are considered to be the inner instruments of cognition.

ANTAHKARANA CHATUSHTAYA. The group of four functions of the inner instrument: intellect, ego, sensory-motor mind, and the storehouse of memories.

ANTAR YAJNA. Inner sacrifice or inner ritual. It signifies the knowledge through which a yogi burns all past SAMSKARAS and VASANAS and attains freedom from them forever.

ANTAR YOGA. Internal yoga characterized by meditation, as opposed to external rituals and physical yoga postures.

APANA. A kind of vital force (PRANA) ordinarily identified with exhalation. *See* PRANA.

APTA. A trustworthy person, a great person, one who speaks in accord with the way he thinks and acts, one whose speech and actions convey truth.

ARDHA PADMASANA. The half-lotus posture, used for meditation.

ARJUNA. The protagonist of the Bhagavad Gita, who chose SRI KRISHNA as his charioteer in the war against the KAURAVAS. Arjuna represents the individual self or the student, and KRISHNA is the universal Self or teacher. Arjuna means "one who makes sincere efforts." Historically, Arjuna belongs to the famous royal clan Bharata, after which the subcontinent India (called BHARATA in Hindi) is named.

ARYA. Fully civilized.

ASANA. Posture. This is the third rung of RAJA YOGA, consisting of HATHA YOGA postures or asanas. This term refers especially to the one seated pose used for meditation.

ASAT. That which is non-existent. *See* SAT.

ASHRAM. A community of spiritual aspirants where discipline, practice, and study are pursued. It also denotes the place where such a community resides.

ASHRAMA. The stages of life. In the Indian tradition the life span is ideally divided into four parts. The first is called BRAHMACHARYA, which covers the first twenty-five years of life and is devoted to study, self-discipline, and self-transformation. The next twenty-five years, GRIHASTHA, the householder's life, is spent in skillfully and selflessly carrying on one's duties toward family and society. The third stage, VANAPRASTHA, retirement, consists of preparation for renouncing the world and cultivating the courage to attain the goal of life. In the fourth and last stage, SANNYASA, one develops a completely detached attitude and establishes himself in the knowledge of the pure Self, leaving the external world behind.

ASHTANGA YOGA. The eight-limbed yoga described by PATANJALI, also called RAJA YOGA.

ASHVATTHA. A tree that, because of its immensity and roots that grow downward from branches above, is compared with the imperishable Reality, and vice versa. (*See Bhagavad Gita* XV. 1-2).

ASU. PRANA, the life force.

ATMA YOGA. The yoga of ATMAN; a spiritual path that leads the aspirant to the realization of ATMAN.

ATMAN. The pure Self. According to Indian philosophy, the Self is eternal, and its essential nature is existence, consciousness, and bliss. It permeates the waking, dreaming, and deep sleep states and remains above all mundane pains and pleasures.

AUM. The phonetic spelling of OM, indicating the three sounds A, U, M, which designate the three states of waking, dreaming, and sleeping.

AVATARA. A divine incarnation. After death, realized beings can choose to incarnate onto the physical plane in order to serve humanity. Ordinary mortals are merely reborn to continue their growth process and do not have the choice of remaining beyond.

AVATI ITI OM. An etymological meaning of OM: "One who protects is called OM."

AVYAKATA. Unmanifest, the unmanifest primordial nature. Under the guidance and direction of the supreme Lord, this unmanifest primordial nature produces the entire universe. *See* VYAKTA.

BANDHAS. Locks. The various locks practiced by yogis, such as the root lock, navel lock, and tongue lock, are engaged in order to hold and channel energy and thereby enhance spiritual practice.

BHAGAVAN. The glorious one. The supreme Lord is called Bhagavan because He is the One whose glory is this entire Universe. He is the almighty creator, preserver, and annihilator.

BHAKTI YOGA. The yoga of love and devotion.

BHARATA. Lover of knowledge. It also refers to the ancient wise King Bharata and his descendants. Since ARJUNA is a lover of knowledge as well as a descendant of King Bharata, this epithet is also given to him. It also refers to the nation of India.

BHAVA. Mood, emotion, positive feeling, mental creation. In order to cultivate bhava, the Bhagavad Gita advises the aspirant to change his mental state from its ordinary course and channel it to awareness of the Self, ATMAN.

BHUTA. The elements, the past tense, departed souls, or individuals who are born. According to the Bhagavad Gita, something cannot come out of nothing, and that which exists cannot be made to be non-existent. It is a misconception to think that a soul comes into existence at birth and then becomes non-existent after death. The soul remains unaffected while the body, breath, and mind go through birth and death.

BHUTI. Victory, happiness, and strength.

BRAHMA. Creator of the universe. In Sanskrit the term "BRAHMA" refers to the immanent aspect, while the term "BRAHMAN" refers to the absolute transcendent Reality. Another similar term, BRAHMANA, refers to those who are knowers of BRAHMAN or sometimes (but never in the Bhagavad Gita) to the BRAHMANA caste, the intellectual class of Hindu society.

BRAHMACHARI. One who walks or lives in BRAHMAN consciousness. In usual usage it also means one who is in the celibate student phase of life and one who does not indulge in sensual pleasures.

BRAHMACHARYA. The first phase of life, from birth to twenty-five years. The focus of this phase is study, self-discipline, and self-transformation. *See* ASHRAMA.

BRAHMAN. The absolute Reality, pure Consciousness. According to ADVAITA VEDANTA philosophy. Brahman is the Absolute non-dual Reality, and Its essential nature is existence, consciousness, and bliss. There is a perfect identity between the Self and Brahman; the difference or duality between Brahman and the Self is mere illusion.

BRAHMANA. The knower of BRAHMAN. Brahmana is a specific title given to one who has attained the profound knowledge of Atman and who experiences the unity between his self and the Self of all. It also refers to members of the priestly class, who are scholarly and sattvic in nature. The anglicized version of the word is "Brahmin."

BRAHMA NIRVANA. Absorption in BRAHMAN.

BRAHMA RANDHRA. The divine hollow. In yogic literature it refers to the gateway leading to the highest of all centers of consciousness.

BRAHMA SUTRA. The first codified philosophical work on VEDANTA, by Badarayana. Many scholars have written commentaries on this work. Among them, that of SANKARA is the foremost and most profound.

BRAHMA VIDYA. The science of Brahman, the absolute Reality, which includes philosophical and practical disciplines that lead one to the spiritual goal.

BRAHMA YAJNA. A sacrifice performed for attaining BRAHMAN. It is purely internal and does not require any external rituals.

BUDDHI. Intellect, the decisive faculty of the inner instrument. This is the first evolute of PRAKRITI. closest to PURUSHA.

BUDDHI YOGA. The yoga of intellect. It is almost the same as JNANA YOGA.

CHAKRA. Wheel or circle. In the yogic tradition, it refers to a center of consciousness. There are said to be seven or more of these located within the human being, ranging from the base of the spine to the top of the head.

CHATURBHUJA. With four hands. In his anthropomorphic form. Lord VISHNU, preserver of the universe, is described as having four arms. Thus the epithet "Four-armed" is given to him.

DEVAS. Bright beings or celestial beings. According to the Bhagavad Gita, any kind of activity, whether physical, verbal, or mental, if endowed with a sattvic quality, belongs to the realm of the devas. Devas are said to be superior to other beings because of the predominance of sattva in them.

DHARMA. The eternal law that holds and maintains the individual as well as social life. In the Eastern tradition, it signifies philosophy, spirituality, and discipline, which if practiced could guide humanity toward its highest destiny. It also refers to one's duty or destiny in life.

DHRITARASHTRA. The blind king, father of DURYODHANA. leader of the KAURAVAS.

DHRITI. The quality of resolution or firmness. It is one of the essentials on the path of spirituality, ensuring the sincere aspirants success in attaining the highest goal.

DHUMA. Smoke. It symbolizes the dark aspect of the human personality or the dark forces that try to hide the light of Truth.

DHYANA YOGA. The systematic practice of meditation; one of the paths described in the Bhagavad Gita.

DIVYACHAKSHU. Divine vision. In the yogic tradition, it is said that a person with a divine eye can see the phenomena of past, present, and future.

DURYODHANA. The unjust king who dishonestly usurped the kingdom of the PANDAVAS, thus creating the situation that caused the great war of the

MAHABHARATA.

DVESHA. Aversion. According to the Bhagavad Gita, in order to attain peace and happiness, one needs to eliminate RAGA (attachment) and DVESHA (aversion). As a result, control and mastery over the senses as well as transparency of mind or real happiness ensue.

EKOHAM BAHU SYAM. A famous statement from the Upanishads meaning, "I am One; let me become many." This indicates that the divine will or divine determination is the cause of the manifestation of the universe.

ESHANAS. Desires. Out of the numberless desires, there are three main ones. First, the desire for a spouse and children; second, the desire for wealth, and third, the desire for name and fame. The SANNYASIN must renounce these.

GANAPATI. The deity of Indian mythology who has the head of an elephant and the body of a human being. The popular name of this god is *Ganesha*. His vehicle is a mouse, who has sharp teeth symbolizing the sharpness of Ganapati's intellect and discrimination, capable of cutting the fetters of bondage and removing the obstacles.

GATASU. One whose prana has departed from the body. According to the Bhagavad Gita, the departure of prana from the body never means the death of the soul. Death and birth are habits of the body and the self. An individual suffers on account of his or her attachment to the body-mind organism.

GUHYA. Secret or hidden. Advanced spiritual instruction is said to be secret or hidden because it can be imparted only by a competent master to a deserving student.

GUNAS. Attributes of nature. According to SAMKHYA philosophy, PRAKRITI, the primordial nature, has three qualities: SATTVA, RAJAS, and TAMAS. SATTVA signifies brightness and lightness; RAJAS indicates movement; while TAMAS indicates heaviness, inertia, and darkness. For spiritual growth, SATTVA is helpful and should be cultivated.

GURU. The popular term used for a spiritual master who reveals the path of divinity to his students. GURUDEVA is the proper appellation for such a teacher.

GURUDEVA. The term used for the spiritual teacher, indicating great reverence and humility. Traditionally the term "guru" is not used by itself without "deva." Literally it means "the bright being who dispels the darkness of ignorance."

GURUKULA. The place where the GURU resides and imparts secular and spiritual wisdom to his students. Literally, it means "the guru's family."

HANUMAN. A great warrior entirely devoted to Lord Rama. He was king of a race that is described as resembling monkeys. His exploits are described in the RAMAYANA.

HATHA YOGA. The yoga comprising the first five rungs of RAJA YOGA: YAMA, NIYAMA, ASANA, PRANAYAMA, and PRATYAHARA.

IDA. The subtle energy channel on the left side of SUSHUMNA, opposite to PINGALA on the right. See NADI.

INDRA. King of the gods. Entymologically, Indra means the master of the senses. Indra is depicted as a student having an enormous amount of patience and a burning desire to realize the Truth.

ISHVARA. The almighty God residing in everyone's heart and directing all human activities. The manifest Lord or personal deity.

JANMA. Birth. According to the Bhagavad Gita, birth simply means coming to an external state of existence. The soul is exactly the same before and after birth.

JAPA. Repetition of the MANTRA, whether verbal or silent.

JIGYASA. The desire to know. In a spiritual context, it means a burning desire to learn and follow the path of BRAHMA VIDYA.

JITATMA. One who has conquered the appetite of the lower self.

JIVA. The individuated soul. Because of its association with MAYA or PRAKRITI, the soul becomes subject to bondage and thus seeks liberation.

JIVA ATMA YAJNA. Internal yajna in which the individual self, or lower self, offers itself to the higher Self, ATMAN.

JNANA. Knowledge of the Absolute. Here it means experiential knowledge leading the individual to union with the Supreme.

JNANA NISHTHA. A firm commitment to follow the path of knowledge.

JNANA YAJNA. Wisdom sacrifice. The Bhagavad Gita offers various interpretations of ritual or sacrifice and suggests the internalization of external ritual by offering various attitudes and tendencies into the fire of higher knowledge. For jnana yajna, the Bhagavad Gita suggests the offering of the sense of duality and multiplicity into the fire of non-dual knowledge. Thereby one attains freedom and immortality.

JNANA YOGA. The yoga of knowledge as expounded by VEDANTA.

JYOTI. Light.

KALA. The time principle. According to the Bhagavad Gita, good and bad, construction and destruction, all occur within the range of time. Everything originates and ultimately dissolves into the mouth of time. Here time is identical with the supreme Reality.

KALPA. A measure of time; a day and night of Brahma. A set of four YUGAS is called a MAHAYUGA. One thousand MAHAYUGAS constitute the period of creation (one day of Brahma), and another thousand comprise the period of dissolution (one night of Brahma). Two thousand such MAHAYUGAS are called a kalpa, which is 8,652,000,000 years. See YUGA.

KAMA. Kama is the prime desire that gives birth to anger, greed, attachment, jealousy, and pride.

KARIKA. A commentary in verse form. In this context it refers to the special commentary written by Gaudapada on the Mandukya Upanishad.

KARMA. Action. According to yoga traditions, the karma that is performed with any selfish motive brings about bondage, while performing the same karma selflessly for the sake of duty alone brings freedom.

KARMA NISHTHA. A firm conviction to follow the path of action.

KARMA YOGA. The yoga of selfless and skillful action.

KAURAVAS. The sons of Kuru, led by DUROYODHANA, who fought against the PANDAVAS, led by ARJUNA.

KHECHARI MUDRA. A yogic practice performed by stretching the tongue behind the palate. This stimulates the ambrosial nectar (AMRITA) to drip from the lambini CHAKRA, located near the pituitary or pineal glands, thus rejuvenating the body.

KRIPA. Grace, favor. Grace is considered to be the direct cause of the highest spiritual achievement.

KRISHNA. Sri Krishna represents the pure Self, the center of consciousness, who instructs Arjuna, the individual self.

KRISHNA. Darkness.

KRIYA. Washes and methods of purification. These include the upper wash, lower wash, complete wash, and various internal kriyas, which are usually combined with advanced techniques of PRANAYAMA.

KRODHA. Anger.

KSHARA. Perishable. One experiences two kinds of reality: the one that is constantly changing (kshara) and the one that never changes, (AKSHARA).

KSHATRIYA. The warrior and governing class. The duties of warriors include protecting and serving all of humanity.

KSHETRA. Field. Here field means the primordial nature (PRAKRTI) and all its evolutes. Since nature is unconscious, it cannot know itself; its knower is the conscious principle, PURUSHA.

KSHETRAJNA. Knower of the field; PURUSHA, the ever-illumined pure Self.

KUNDALINI. The divine energy, which ordinarily remains latent, sleeping at the base of the spine. The goal of yoga is to awaken this force and lead it upward to unite with supreme Consciousness, thus yielding unitary bliss.

KURUKSHETRA. The field on which everyone has to perform his actions. This is also the name of a place with a profound historical, religious, and spiritual significance, situated in modern Hiriyana not far from Delhi, where the battle described in the Bhagavad Gita is said to have taken place.

KUSHA. A kind of grass with very sharp points. Kusha grass is considered to be very holy and is traditionally used for rituals. It is woven into meditation mats because it is a very poor conductor of energy. Thus, the energy accumulated in meditation is not dissipated through contact with the earth or any other object.

LOBHA. Greed.

LOKA SANGRAHA. Actions performed only for the sake of others.

MAHABHARATA. A great Sanskrit epic containing 100,000 verses. Although it describes the story of two great kings, it also contains vast knowledge on subjects such as ethics, morality, social laws, philosophy, metaphysics, and spirituality. This book is considered to be the inexhaustable source of Eastern wisdom.

MAHATMA. A great soul. A spiritually evolved person who through his wisdom has broken the limited boundary of ego and thus sees himself in all beings.

MAHAYUGA. A set of four YUGAS; 4,326,000 years. *See* KALPA.

MANAS. Mind. According to VEDANTA it is one of the four functions of the inner instruments, ANTAHKARANA. Manas is the sensory-motor mind, characterized by indecision and doubtful thinking.

MANTRA. Divine seed syllables which, through constant repetition and remembrance, lead students toward higher spiritual achievements.

MANUS. The law-givers. In the Indian tradition, it is believed that at the beginning of each cycle of creation there is born such a seer of Truth who makes laws for human beings of that period.

MAUNA. Silence.

MAYA. The power of BRAHMAN; the illusory force through which Reality enacts the drama of illusory appearance and disappearance of the external world as well as bondage and liberation. Maya has two functions: the power to veil Reality and the power to project the unreal in place of the Real.

MOKSHA JNANA YAJNA. Internal sacrifice leading to the attainment of final liberation.

MUKTA. A liberated one; one who is not in the bondage of pain because he realizes his essential nature.

MUKTI. Liberation.

MULA PRAKRITI. "Mula" means root, "prakriti" means primordial nature. Combined together this means "the root cause of the entire universe."

MUNI. One who practices silence.

NADI. An energy channel. According to the yogic tradition, there are 72,000 nadis of which 14 are the important ones. Out of these fourteen, IDA, PINGALA, and SHUSHMNA are the most important nadis, especially for spiritual purposes.

NASA. Nose.

NASAGRE. At the front of the nose. Practically, it is the juncture at which the nostrils are separated. *See* AGRA BHAGE.

NIDIDHY ASANA. Pondering over the Truth and applying it in one's daily life.

According to JNANA YOGA, one attains identity with supreme knowledge in three successive stages: studying or listening to the teaching (SRAVANA), thinking about and analyzing them (MANANA), and applying them practically and assimilating them into one's personality (NIDIDHYASANA).

NIRGUNA. Without attributes. In Indian philosophy, reality is said to have two states: reality without attributes and reality with attributes. The former remains uninvolved with worldly phenomena while the latter is the cause of manifestation, preservation, and annihilation of the universe. *See also* SAGUNA.

NISHTHA. Firm conviction or a well-thought-out and firm decision, free from doubt. *See* JNANA NISHTHA *and* KARMA NISHTHA.

NITYA. Eternal; that which is not affected by the laws of time, space, and causation and which remains unchanged and unaffected forever.

NIYAMA. Restraints; disciplinary guidelines for self-transformation and self-improvement. This is the second rung of the eightfold path of RAJA YOGA. It consists of purity, contentment, austerity, self-study, and dedication or surrender to God.

OM TAT SAT. OM, that alone is real.

PANDAVAS. The five sons of Pandu, among whom Yuhdishthira was the eldest. For the sake of righteousness and under the guidance of Lord KRISHNA, they fought and defeated the KAURAVAS. ARJUNA was a Pandava.

PANDIT. A learned man. One who is well versed in the scriptures and who follows the path of spirituality.

PARA. Beyond. Here it is used to indicate the knowledge of the Supreme, which cannot be achieved through books and other methods of conventional study and education.

PATANJALI. The codifier of the Yoga Sutras.

PINGALA. The subtle energy channel on the right side of sushumna, opposite to IDA on the left. *See* NADI.

PRABHU. All-pervading and omnipresent. This is the title given to one who has attained mastery over the senses and mind.

PRAJAPATI. The lord of all subjects; a term for the creator of the universe.

PRAKRITI. Primordial nature. According to the SAMKHYA and YOGA systems of philosophy, there are two eternal realities: PURUSHA and PRAKRITI. PURUSHA is the conscious principle, and PRAKRITI is the unconscious principle, PURUSHA is the pure witness, the subject, consciousness, PRAKRITI is unconscious, the object, the cause of all worldly phenomena. Through association with PURUSHA, PRAKRITI becomes the enjoyer of pain, pleasure, and indifference. The universe comes into existence when PURUSHA and PRAKRITI join each other and apparently share each other's qualities.

PRANA. The life force. In the yogic tradition the life force prana is said to be tenfold, depending on its nature and function. Of the ten, PRANA and APANA are the most important ones. PRANA is ordinarily identified with inhalation and APANA with exhalation. According to the Bhagavad Gita, a yogi should balance and control the movement of prana and APANA in order to have control over the modifications of the mind and thus attain SAMADHI.

PRANAVA. The eternal sound "OM."

PRANAYAMA. Breath control; breathing exercise; the fourth rung of RAJA YOGA.

PRATYAHARA. Withdrawal of the senses; the fifth rung of RAJA YOGA.

PURUSHA. The conscious principle; the pure Self. *See* PRAKRITI.

PURUSHOTTAMA. Best among all the purushas. This is an epithet given to Lord KRISHNA.

RAGA. Attachment.

RAJA VIDYA. Royal knowledge; a well-defined spiritual path leading to the highest goal of life.

RAJA YOGA. The royal path of yoga. The great sage PATANJALI codified the system of raja yoga, which has eight successive stages: YAMA, NIYAMA, ASANA, PRANAYAMA, PRATYAHARA, DHARANA, DHYANA, and SAMADHI. *See* ASTANGA YOGA.

RAJAS. The GUNA of activity or motion. *See* GUNA.

RAMAYANA. The earliest epic in Sanskrit literature, attributed to the poet sage Valmiki. It describes the life story of Lord Rama and all of his great works.

RATRI. Night, symbolizing the lunar energy.

SADHAKA. One who follows the spiritual path.

SADHANA. Spiritual practice.

SAGUNA. With attributes; the lower aspect of the Reality also known as Iswara (God). This state of reality is endowed with MAYA and thus is the cause of manifestation, preservation, and annihilation of the universe. *See* NIRGUNA.

SAHASRARA. The thousand petaled lotus, the crown CHAKRA. In the yoga tradition there are seven main centers of consciousness; among them, sahasrara is the highest. Because of its anatomical location at the top of the head it is called the crown center.

SAKAMA. Actions performed with certain motives.

SAKAMA UPASANA. Worship or meditation with motives.

SAKSHATKARA. Direct realization of Truth from within. In contrast to perceptual, inferential, and any other kind of ordinary knowledge, it signifies the inner, intuitive, spontaneous revelation of the Truth in its totality and purity.

SAMADHI. Spiritual absorption; the eighth rung of RAJA YOGA. As long as a yogi is aware of the process of meditation, the object of meditation, and the meditator, such a state is called samadhi with seed. When the yogi merges into unitary consciousness, such a state is called samadhi without seed.

SAMAHITA. A yogi whose mind is calm and tranquil and who is thus established in the inner Self; the state in which all questions are answered.

SAMATVAM. The sense of equanimity. It is the characteristic of a yogi who is ever established in knowledge. Such a yogi sees no difference between gold and dirt, heat and cold, pain and pleasure, and so on.

SAMA VIDYA. Knowledge of meditation and devotion.

SAMKALPA. Firm resolve. Samkalpa means to decide to do something, and VIKALPA means to remain doubtful about such decision.

SAMKALPA SHAKTI The power of determination. In spiritual practice; this power is the foundation of progress.

SAMKALPA VIKALPA ATMAKA. That which is characterized by indecision and uncertainty. This is the definition of mind in Indian philosophy.

SAMKHYA. The system of Indian philosophy that posits the existence of two realities, PURUSHA and PRAKRITI, the conscious and unconscious principles.

SAMSKARAS. Subtle impressions of past actions.

SAMYAMA. Discipline. In order to shake off laziness, inertia, and lack of motivation, discipline is required. The main characteristic of discipline is the purification and control of thought, speech, and action.

SANJAYA. The narrator of the Bhagavad Gita, who had the extraordinary power to see and hear things happening at a distance. Because of this ability, he was able to explain to King DHRITARASHTRA in his palace the events of the war as well as the knowledge imparted by SRI KRISHNA to ARJUNA.

SANNYASA. Renunciation. See ASHRAMA and ESHANAS.

SANNYASIN. A renunciate, one who is not attached to any worldly things or to the fruits of his actions.

SAT. That which is existent.

SATSANGA. Company of the sages.

SATTVA. The GUNA of light, brightness, and peace. *See* GUNA.

SATTVIKAS. Aspirants whose actions are performed selflessly with a motive to serve others, those who are based in SATTVA GUNA.

SATYAM. Truth. Absolute Reality is supposed to be endowed with three inherent properties: SATYAM, SHIVAM, and SUNDARAM.

SHAKTI. The primal force that resides within.

SHAKTI PATA. Spontaneous spiritual transformation resulting from divine grace through the touch or gaze of a realized master.

SHANKARA. The great sage who founded the monastic order of yogis and wrote commentaries on the principle UPANISHADS, the Bhagavad Gita, and the

Brahma Sutra, expounding the theory of non-dualism, ADVAITA VEDANTA.

SHANTI PARVA. The cantos of the MAHABHARATA in which the grandfather of ARJUNA imparts the knowledge related to all aspects of life and society.

SHIVAM. Auspicious.

SHRADDHA. Faith. Faith is a divine quality and an essential aspect of one's spiritual practice. Such faith does not rely on the knowledge of the scriptures; rather it comes through spontaneous experience from within.

SHUDRA. The working class of society.

SHUKLA. White, symbolizing the bright aspect of the personality; the solar energy.

SIDDHASANA. The accomplished posture, recommended by yogis as a meditation pose for sincere students.

SOMA. A specific species of plant or the juice extracted from it. In ancient times there were sacrifices in which the juice from the soma plant was offered into a ritual fire with the desire to achieve mundane goals or heaven.

SHRAVANA. Listening to teachings and studying the scriptures, the first step in the path of JNANA YOGA, the yoga of knowledge. VEDANTA and JNANA YOGA describe spiritual practice in three successive stages: listening to teachings and studying the scriptures (sravana); pondering and contemplating the truths explained in the scriptures (manana); and practicing those truths in daily life (NIDIDHYASANA).

SRI. A title of respect.

STHITA PRAJNA. Steady insight. One whose wisdom is established in his inner Self. The Bhagavad Gita explains the nature and behavior of such evolved spiritual souls in great detail.

SUKHASANA. The comfortable posture, a pose prescribed for meditation.

SUKTA VIDYA. The knowledge of good utterances and thoughts.

SUNDARAM. Beauty.

SUSHUMNA. The central NADI, the inner channel corresponding to the spinal column. This NADI has profound significance in yogic practices, especially in the practice of KUNDALINI yoga. Only competent masters know how to open SUSHUMNA and direct the dormant divine force KUNDALINI through it, leading it to SAHASRARA, the thousand petal led center. When the breath flows freely and equally through both nostrils, SUSHUMNA is engaged.

SUYATE. To bring forth or bring about prosperity. In the Bhagavad Gita SRI KRISHNA says, "Under My direction PRAKRITI brings forth all animate and inanimate existence."

SVABHAVA PRAKRITI. One's own habitual tendencies that have become inseparable from his personality. These innate tendencies cause certain SAMSKARAS to become conscious and cloud the conscious part of the mind, forcing an individual to desire and become involved in certain actions..

SWAMI. A yogi who is the master of his senses and mind. It is also the title usually given to any of the monks of the Shankaracharya order. It can also refer to God, since He is the Master of all.

TAMAS. The GUNA of inertia, heaviness, and darkness. *See* GUNA.

TAT SAT. "That is real;" Truth; that Reality which is beyond time, space, and causation, and which cannot be grasped by speech and mind.

TRATAKA. Gazing on external objects. It is a complete science in itself. An experienced yogi can prescribe the proper object and specific method of gazing for attaining concentration and one-pointedness of mind or for improving the eyesight.

TURIYA. The state beyond the waking, dreaming, and deep sleep states. This state is the essential nature of the Self, in which the Self is established in its pure existence, consciousness, and bliss.

TYAGA. Giving up possessions. It is one of the two essential requirements of the path of renunciation. Under the law of tyaga one gives up all that he possesses and enjoys the freedom that comes from non-possessiveness. Under the other requirement, non-attachment (VAIRAGYA), the basic necessities that cannot be given up have to be used without attachment.

UPANISHADS. The end of the Vedas. Texts that should be studied while sitting at the feet of the teacher. The Upanishads are the books of wisdom endowed with profound philosophical and practical instruction. Of the more than 200 Upanishads, 10 are of major importance. The Upanishads are the foundation of VEDANTA philosophy.

VAIRAGYA. Dispassion or non-attachment. According to the Bhagavad Gita one does not necessarily need to renounce the world or what one needs, but one should perform his duties lovingly, skillfully, and selflessly, remaining unattached to the fruits of his actions.

VAISHYA. The business class and landowners.

VAK SHAKTI. The power of speech.

VASANA. Subtle traces of one's thoughts and actions.

VAYU. Air or wind. Here it is used in the sense of the life force, represented by breath.

VEDANTA. The system of Indian philosophy that expounds the theory of non-dualism, ADVAITA.

VEDAS. The sourcebook of knowledge. Veda is revealed wisdom, experienced by the great sages in deep meditation. For many centuries the sages imparted the knowledge of the Vedas orally to their close disciples. Finally the great sage Vyasa, on the basis of topic and practical application, organized the Vedas into four classes and commited them to writing. These four sections are now known as Rig Veda, Sama Veda, Yajur Veda, and Atharva Veda. The Upanishads are the last portions of these four books of the Vedas.

VIBHUTI. The glorious manifestation of God, or the extraordinary powers of the Lord.

VIJNANA. Special or higher knowledge. In contrast to ordinary knowledge of mundane awareness, it refers to spiritual wisdom.

VIJNANA YAJNA. Wisdom sacrifice. In contrast to external rituals and offerings, it signifies internal rituals in which knowledge of duality is offered into the fire of nondual unitary knowledge.

VIKALPA. A state of mind that is unsettled, confused, and doubtful.

VIKARMA. Action that is opposed to right action.

VISHADA. Dejection.

VISHNU. The all-pervading One. Vishnu is one of the gods of the Hindu pantheon. His main characteristic is to maintain and preserve the universe. Sri Krishna is one of the incarnations of Vishnu.

VYAKTA. The manifest aspect of nature. See AVYAKTA.

VYASA. A great sage of Indian spiritual lore. The Bhagavad Gita, the whole MAHABHARATA, and many of the other epics are attributed to Vyasa. According to tradition he was a yogi of extraordinary abilities.

YAJNA. Sacrifice or ritualistic ceremony. In the Bhagavad Gita, it refers to the act that helps an individual to maintain harmony within his individual, social, and cosmic life. Depending on the nature and the goal, there are various kinds of yajnas. These can be categorized in two main classes: the external and the internal.

YAJUR VIDYA. Knowledge of sacrificial acts.

YAMA. Observances. This is the first rung of RAJA YOGA, consisting of non-violence, truthfulness, non-stealing, non-indulgence, and non-possessiveness.

YOGA. The system of Indian philosophy systematized and codified by the sage Patanjali. It also refers to the practical aspect of any philosophy, particularly SAMKHYA. Literally it means "yoke," referring to the uniting of the individual self and the universal Self.

YOGA NIDRA. Yogic sleep. Instead of going through the ordinary dreaming and sleeping states, advanced yogis provide complete rest to their bodies and minds by applying the technique of yoga nidra. It is a complete, scientific method described in yogic texts.

YOGA SADHANA. The practice of yoga.

YOGI. One who practices yoga.

YUGA. Aeon. In the Indian calendar, human civilization is hallmarked by four different stages of growth, called yugas. Although astronomers have given definite time spans for each yuga, these calculations differ considerably, but a yuga encompasses at least several thousand years. A set of four yugas is called a MAHAYUGA, which consists of 4,326,000 years. Two thousand MAHAYUGAS constitute a KALPA. Three hundred and sixty KALPAS make one year of BRAHMA, who lives for one hundred such years.

About Swami Rama

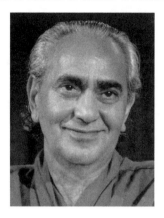

SWAMI RAMA, one of the greatest adepts, teachers, writers, and humanitarians of the 20th century, is the founder of the Himalayan Institute. Born in northern India, he was raised from early childhood by a Himalayan sage, Bengali Baba. Under the guidance of his master, he traveled from monastery to monastery and studied with a variety of Himalayan saints and sages, including his grandmaster who lived in a remote region of Tibet. In addition to this intense spiritual training, Swami Rama received higher education in both India and Europe. From 1949–52, he held the prestigious position of Shankaracharya of Karvirpitham in South India. Thereafter, he returned to his master to receive further training at his cave monastery, and finally, in 1969, came to the United States, where he founded the Himalayan Institute. His best-known work, Living with the Himalayan Masters, reveals the many facets of this singular adept and demonstrates his embodiment of the living tradition of the East.

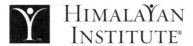

HIMALAYAN
INSTITUTE®

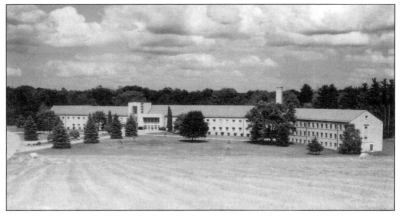

*The main building of the Himalayan Institute headquarters near
Honesdale, Pennsylvania, USA.*

The Himalayan Institute

The Himalayan Institute offers educational programs, services, and tools for yoga, meditation, spiritual development, and holistic health. The Institute's mission is spirituality in action, and includes a range of global humanitarian projects in addition to its educational activities. Founded in 1971 by Swami Rama of the Himalayas, the Institute draws on its roots in the ancient tradition of the Himalayan masters to facilitate personal growth and development and service to humanity.

Our international headquarters is located on a beautiful 400-acre campus in the rolling hills of the Pocono Mountains of northeastern Pennsylvania. Our spiritually vibrant community and peaceful setting provide the perfect atmosphere for seminars and retreats, residential programs, and holistic health services. Students from all over the world join us to attend diverse programs on subjects such as hatha yoga, meditation, stress reduction, ayurveda, yoga, and tantra philosophy.

In addition, the Himalayan Institute offers the following products, services, and programs:

Global Humanitarian Projects

The Himalayan Institute's humanitarian projects bring spirituality into action. Our projects offer education, vocational teaching, healthcare, and environmental regeneration, serving impoverished communities in India, Mexico, and Cameroon, West Africa. Through rural empowerment, our humanitarian projects fight poverty and seek to create lasting social transformation.

Yoga International

Yoga International is the educational division of the organization, connecting practitioners of yoga, meditation, and ayurveda to a timeless and authentic source of wisdom. Steeped in a 5,000-year-old tradition, our expert teachers provide systematic instruction at all levels, both in interactive digital learning environments and through immersive retreats.

Visit YogaInternational.com for full-length online seminars, inspiring articles, and delicious recipes, or to register for a retreat or learn about our yoga certification programs. We offer three membership options, and a basic membership is free. Sign up today!

Publications

The Himalayan Institute publishes over 60 titles on yoga, spirituality, and holistic health, including the best-selling *Living with the Himalayan Masters* by Swami Rama, *The Secret of the Yoga Sutra, Power of Mantra and the Mystery of Initiation, From Death to Birth*, and *Tantra Unveiled* by Pandit Rajmani Tigunait, PhD, and *Yoga: Mastering the Basics* by Sandra Anderson and Rolf Sovik PsyD.

Total Health Center

For over 40 years, the Himalayan Institute Total Health Center has combined Eastern philosophy and Western medicine in an integrated approach to holistic health. It offers individualized programs based on these principles, utilizing holistic medical evaluations, massage, yoga therapy, ayurveda, biofeedback, natural medicines, lifestyle education and counseling for a combined approach that facilitates optimal healing and revitalization in both mind and body.

Total Health Products

The Himalayan Institute Total Health product line includes the original Neti Pot™ and an assortment of natural, homeopathic, holistic, and ayurvedic products. From non-GMO components, petroleum-free biodegrading plastics, and eco-friendly packaging, we create products that have the least impact on the environment. Your patronage is important and appreciated. Part of every purchase supports our Global Humanitarian projects.

For further information about our programs, humanitarian projects, and products,

call: 800-822-4547

e-mail: info@HimalayanInstitute.org

write: The Himalayan Institute
952 Bethany Turnpike
Honesdale, PA 18431

or visit: HimalayanInstitute.org

The Secret is Out!

The *Yoga Sutra* is the living source wisdom of the Yoga tradition. Using it as a guide, we can unlock the hidden power of Yoga and experience the promise of Yoga in our life. The *Yoga Sutra* is as fresh today as it was 2,200 years ago when it was discovered by the sage Patanjali. By applying its living wisdom in our practice, we can achieve the purpose of life—lasting fulfillment and ultimate freedom. *The Secret of the Yoga Sutra: Samadhi Pada* is the first practitioner-oriented commentary that is fully grounded in a living tradition. It shares the essence of Pandit Tigunait's rigorous scholarly understanding of the *Yoga Sutra* through the filter of experiential knowledge gained through decades of advanced yogic practices and enriched by the gift of living wisdom he received from the masters of the Himalayan Tradition.

"From the very first pages of *The Secret of the Yoga Sutra*, the reader can feel the hand of a master—a scholar, a practitioner, a devotee. This commentary is not just about yoga. It *is* yoga."

—Stephen Cope, founder of the Kripalu Institute for Extraordinary Living

"Of the dozens of translations and explications of this text that exist in English alone, few possess the power and reliability of Pandit Rajmani Tigunait's *The Secret of the Yoga Sutra*."

—Robert Svoboda, ayurvedic physician and author

"Pandit Tigunait's commentary on the *Yoga Sutra* offers us a true mystical transmission of the inner teachings of this classic text. Writing from his deep understanding of both the text and the tradition behind it, Panditji also shares the fruit of his own meditative practice. The power of his experience and knowledge radiates through these pages. I especially recommend *The Secret of the Yoga Sutra* to any meditator who wants to understand more deeply the higher stages of meditation."

—Sally Kempton, author of *Meditation for the Love of It* and *Awakening Shakti*

To order: 800-822-4547
Email: mailorder@HimalayanInstitute.org
Visit: HimalayanInstitute.org

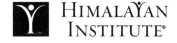

HIMALAYAN
INSTITUTE®

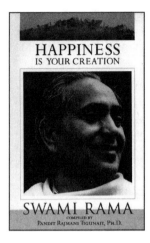

Happiness Is Your Creation
Swami Rama as compiled by Pandit Rajmani Tigunait, PhD

Did you ever pause for a moment and realize that you are the creator of your destiny? In *Happiness Is Your Creation*, Pandit Tigunait gathered the inspirational teachings of his master, the late Swami Rama, on the yogic prescription for happiness. These enriching passages identify the causes of unhappiness and provide direction to remain centered and joyful in everyday life. Learn how to cultivate a positive mind and charge your body and mind through meditation, allowing you to lead a more active and productive life. This motivational book reveals the ancient teachings of self-discipline, self-mastery, and self-realization through yoga and meditation.

Paperback with flaps, 5½" x 8½" , 136 pages
$12.95, ISBN 978-0-89389-246-3

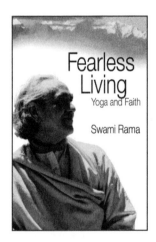

Fearless Living: Yoga and Faith
Swami Rama

Learn to live without fear—to trust a higher power, a divine purpose. In this collection of anecdotes from the astonishing life of Swami Rama, you will understand that there is a way to move beyond mere faith and into the realm of personal revelation. Through his astonishing life experiences we learn about ego and humility, how to overcome fears that inhibit us, discover sacred places and rituals, and learn the importance of a one-pointed, positive mind. Swami Rama teaches us to see with the eyes of faith and move beyond our self imposed limitations.

Paperback with flaps, 5½" x 8½", 160 pages
$12.95, ISBN 978-0-89389-251-7

To order: 800-822-4547
Email: mailorder@HimalayanInstitute.org
Visit: HimalayanInstitute.org

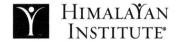
HIMALAYAN INSTITUTE®

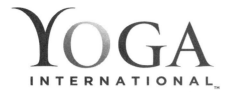
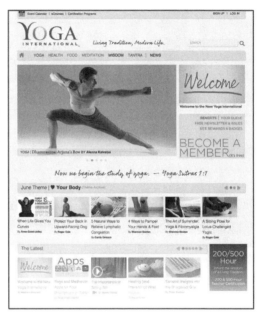

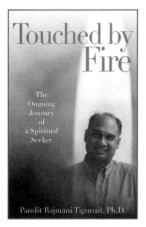

Touched by Fire
Pandit Rajmani Tigunait, PhD

This vivid autobiography of a remarkable spiritual leader—Pandit Rajmani Tigunait, PhD —reveals his experiences and encounters with numerous teachers, sages, and his mentor, the late Swami Rama of the Himalayas. His well-told journey is filled with years of disciplined study and the struggle to master the lessons and skills passed to him. *Touched by Fire* brings Western culture a glimpse of Eastern philosophies in a clear, understandable fashion, and provides numerous photographs showing a part of the world many will never see for themselves.

Paperback with flaps, 5½" x 8½", 296 pages
$16.95, ISBN 0-89389-239-4

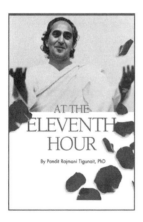

At the Eleventh Hour
Pandit Rajmani Tigunait, PhD

This book is more than the biography of a great sage—it is a revelation of the many astonishing accomplishments Swami Rama achieved in his life. These pages serve as a guide to the more esoteric and advanced practices of yoga and tantra not commonly taught or understood in the West. And they bring you to holy places in India, revealing why these sacred sites are important and how to go about visiting them. The wisdom in these stories penetrates beyond the power of words.

A memorable and impressive picture of a modern-day saint, whose legacy is very much alive in both the East and the West. —Andrew Weil, M.D.

Paperback with flaps, 6" x 9", 448 pages
$18.95, ISBN 0-89389-212-2

To order: 800-822-4547
Email: mailorder@HimalayanInstitute.org
Visit: HimalayanInstitute.org

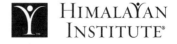

HIMALAYAN INSTITUTE®

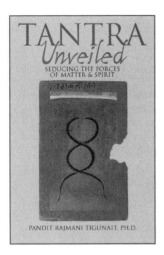

Tantra Unveiled
Pandit Rajmani Tigunait, PhD

This powerful book describes authentic tantra, what distinguishes it from other spiritual paths, and how the tantric way combines hatha yoga, meditation, visualization, ayurveda, and other disciplines. Taking us back to ancient times, Pandit Tigunait shares his experiences with tantric masters and the techniques they taught him. *Tantra Unveiled* is most valuable for those who wish to live the essence of tantra—practicing spirituality while experiencing a rich outer life.

Paperback, 5 ½" x 8 ½", 152 pages
$14.95, ISBN 978-0-89389-158-9

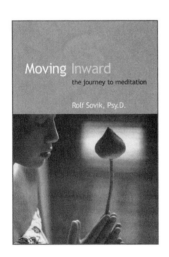

Moving Inward
Rolf Sovik, Psy.D.

Rolf Sovik shows readers of all levels how to transition from asanas to meditation. Combining practical advice on breathing and relaxation with timeless asana postures, he systematically guides us through the process. This book provides a five-stage plan to basic meditation, step-by-step guidelines for perfect postures, and six methods for training the breath. Both the novice and the advanced student will benefit from Sovik's startling insights into the mystery of meditation.

Paperback, 6" x 9", 197 pages
$14.95, ISBN 978-0-89389-247-0

To order: 800-822-4547
Email: mailorder@HimalayanInstitute.org
Visit: www.HimalayanInstitute.org

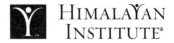

HIMALAYAN
INSTITUTE®

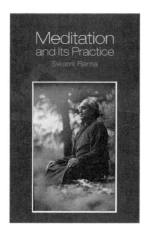

Meditation and Its Practice
Swami Rama

In this practical guide to inner life, Swami Rama teaches us how to slip away from the mental turbulence of our ordinary thought processes into an infinite reservoir of consciousness. This clear, concise meditation manual provides systematic guidance in the techniques of meditation - a powerful tool for transforming our lives and increasing our experience of peace, joy, creativity, and inner tranquility.

Paperback, 128 pages
$12.95 / ₹250

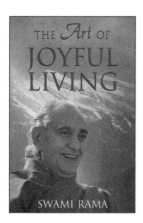

The Art of Joyful Living
Swami Rama

In *The Art of Joyful Living*, Swami Rama imparts a message of inspiration and optimism: that you are responsible for making your life happy and emanating that happiness to others. This book shows you how to maintain a joyful view of life even in difficult times.

It contains sections on transforming habit patterns, working with negative emotions, developing strength and willpower, developing intuition, spirituality in loving relationships, learning to be your own therapist, understanding the process of meditation, and more!

Paperback, 198 pages
$15.95 / ₹295

To order: 800-822-4547
Email: mailorder@HimalayanInstitute.org
Visit: HimalayanInstitute.org

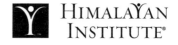

HIMALAYAN
INSTITUTE®